Clinical Manual of Child and Adolescent Psychopharmacology

Clinical Manual of Child and Adolescent Psychopharmacology

Edited by

Robert L. Findling, M.D.

Professor of Psychiatry and Pediatrics and
Director, Division of Child and Adolescent Psychiatry
University Hospitals Case Medical Center
Discovery and Wellness Center for Children
Case Western Reserve University
Cleveland, Ohio

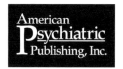

American Psychiatric Publishing, Inc.

Washington, DC
London, England

List of Tables and Figures

Contributors

Boris Birmaher, M.D.
Professor of Psychiatry, University of Pittsburgh Medical Center, Western Psychiatric Institute and Clinic; Co-director, Pittsburgh Bipolar Institute, Pittsburgh, Pennsylvania

John V. Campo, M.D.
Chief of Child and Adolescent Psychiatry, Medical Director of Pediatric Behavioral Health, and Professor of Psychiatry, The Ohio State University and Columbus Children's Hospital, Columbus, Ohio

Craig A. Erickson, M.D.
Child and Adolescent Psychiatry Fellow, Department of Psychiatry, Indiana University School of Medicine; Christian Sarkine Autism Treatment Center at the James Whitcomb Riley Hospital for Children, Indianapolis, Indiana

Robert L. Findling, M.D.
Professor of Psychiatry and Pediatrics and Director, Division of Child and Adolescent Psychiatry, University Hospitals Case Medical Center, Discovery and Wellness Center for Children, Case Western Reserve University, Cleveland, Ohio

Nitin Gogtay, M.D.
Staff Clinician, Child Psychiatry Branch, National Institute of Mental Health, Bethesda, Maryland

Laurence Greenhill, M.D.
Ruane Professor of Clinical Psychiatry, Division of Child and Adolescent Psychiatry, Columbia College of Physicians and Surgeons, Columbia University; Research Psychiatrist II, New York State Psychiatric Institute, New York, New York; Principal Investigator, New York State Research Units on Pediatric Psychopharmacology

Peter S. Jensen, M.D.
Director, The REACH Institute, New York, New York

Kevin W. Kuich, M.D.
Clinical Lecturer; Child and Adolescent Inpatient Faculty; Director, Marketing and Program Development for Inpatient Programs, Section of Child and Adolescent Psychiatry, University of Michigan, Ann Arbor, Michigan

Christopher J. McDougle, M.D.
Albert E. Sterne Professor and Chairman, Department of Psychiatry, Indiana University School of Medicine; Christian Sarkine Autism Treatment Center at the James Whitcomb Riley Hospital for Children, Indianapolis, Indiana

Elizabeth Pappadopulos, Ph.D.
Assistant Director, Center for the Advancement of Children's Mental Health at Columbia University; Assistant Professor, Clinical Psychology (in Psychiatry), Columbia University, New York, New York

Natalya Paykina, M.A.
Project Manager, Columbia College of Physicians and Surgeons, New York State Psychiatric Institute, New York, New York

David J. Posey, M.D.
Associate Professor of Psychiatry, Department of Psychiatry, Indiana University School of Medicine; Christian Sarkine Autism Treatment Center at the James Whitcomb Riley Hospital for Children, Indianapolis, Indiana

Natoshia Raishevich, B.A.
Research Associate, Center for the Advancement of Children's Mental Health at Columbia University, New York, New York

Judith L. Rapoport, M.D.
Chief, Child Psychiatry Branch, National Institute of Mental Health, Bethesda, Maryland

Jennifer Regan, B.A.
Research Assistant, New York State Psychiatric Institute, Columbia University, New York, New York

Moira A. Rynn, M.D.
Associate Professor of Clinical Psychiatry, New York State Psychiatric Institute, Columbia University, New York, New York

Lawrence Scahill, M.S.N., Ph.D.
Professor of Nursing and Child Psychiatry, Yale Child Study Center, New Haven, Connecticut

Phillip Shaw, M.D., Ph.D.
Clinical Fellow, Child Psychiatry Branch, National Institute of Mental Health, Bethesda, Maryland

Kimberly A. Stigler, M.D.
Assistant Professor of Psychiatry, Department of Psychiatry, Indiana University School of Medicine; Christian Sarkine Autism Treatment Center at the James Whitcomb Riley Hospital for Children, Indianapolis, Indiana

Benedetto Vitiello, M.D.
Chief, Child and Adolescent Treatment and Preventive Intervention Research Branch, National Institute of Mental Health, Bethesda, Maryland

Disclosure of Competing Interests

The following authors have competing interests to declare:

Boris Birmaher, M.D.—*Employer:* University of Pittsburgh, University of Pittsburgh Medical Center/Western Psychiatric Institute and Clinic; *Grant support:* National Institute of Mental Health; *Sponsored forum participation:* Solvay, Abcomm. Receives royalties from a book (*New Hope for Children and Teens With Bipolar Disorder*) published by Random House, Inc.

Craig A. Erickson, M.D.—Dr. Erickson received free aripiprazole (Abilify) from Bristol-Myers Squibb in support of a clinical trial.

Robert L. Findling, M.D.—Dr. Findling receives or has received research support, acted as a consultant, and/or served on a speaker's bureau for Abbott, AstraZeneca, Bristol-Myers Squibb, Celltech-Medeva, Forest, GlaxoSmith-Kline, Johnson & Johnson, Eli Lilly, New River, Novartis, Otsuka, Pfizer, Sanofi-Aventis, Shire, Solvay, and Wyeth.

Laurence Greenhill, M.D.—*Consultant:* Pfizer, Janssen, Eli Lilly; *Data and Safety Monitoring Board:* Pfizer (Chair), Janssen, Eli Lilly; *Research contract:* Cephalon, Novartis, Forest; *Scientific Advisory Board:* Eli Lilly.

Peter S. Jensen, M.D.—*Grant support:* McNeil, Pfizer, Eli Lilly; *Speaker's bureau:* CMED, UCB Pharma, PsychCME, CME Outfitters, Neuroscience Education Institute; *Consultant:* Best Practice, Inc., Janssen, Novartis, UCB Pharma.

Christopher J. McDougle, M.D.—*Grant support:* Janssen, Eli Lilly, Bristol-Myers Squibb, Forest Laboratories; *Consultant:* Janssen, Eli Lilly, Bristol-Myers Squibb; *Speaker's bureau:* Pfizer, Bristol-Myers Squibb.

Elizabeth Pappadopulos, Ph.D.—*Honoraria:* Bristol-Myers Squibb.

David J. Posey, M.D.—*Grant support:* Forest, Eli Lilly; *Consultant:* Forest; *Honoraria:* Janssen, Pfizer; *Stock:* Shire.

Moira A. Rynn, M.D.—*Grant support:* Wyeth, Pfizer, Eli Lilly, Astra-Zeneca, Forest; *Speaker's bureau:* Wyeth, Pfizer, Eli Lilly; *Consultant:* Wyeth, Pfizer, Eli Lilly, AstraZeneca.

Lawrence Scahill, M.S.N., Ph.D.—*Consultant:* Janssen, Bristol-Myers Squibb, Supernus. Provided training to Janssen and Bristol-Myers Squibb.

Kimberly A. Stigler, M.D.—*Research support:* Bristol-Myers Squibb, Eli Lilly, Janssen.

The following authors have no competing interests to report:

John V. Campo, M.D.
Nitin Gogtay, M.D.
Kevin W. Kuich, M.D.
Natalya Paykina, M.A.
Natoshia Raishevich, B.A.
Judith L. Rapoport, M.D.
Jennifer Regan, B.A.
Phillip Shaw, M.D., Ph.D.
Benedetto Vitiello, M.D.

Introduction

The topic of pediatric psychopharmacology is compelling and often controversial. In addition, what is known about the psychopharmacological treatment of children and adolescents is rapidly changing. This book, *Clinical Manual of Child and Adolescent Psychopharmacology,* was designed to meet the needs of clinicians who want to provide state-of-the-art care to their patients.

A key focus of this book is to communicate to readers both empirically based and timely, scientifically sound information about pediatric psychopharmacology. However, it is readily appreciated that a substantial gap often exists between what is known about a given topic and the information that is required to meet the needs of an individual patient.

For this reason, leading clinician-scientists were chosen to be authors so they could provide their perspectives on key aspects of the newest research in pediatric psychopharmacology. The authors have also been asked to give commentary regarding the clinical interpretability of the extant scientific literature so that readers might have insights into how to incorporate research results into superb clinical practice.

It has been frequently observed that children and adolescents do not necessarily respond to psychopharmacological treatment the same way as adults. In the first chapter of this book, Benedetto Vitiello reviews potential underpinnings that explain this phenomenon. Topics considered in this chapter include pharmacokinetics and pharmacodynamics, as well as salient issues pertaining to the safety and efficacy of psychopharmacological treatment. In addition, Dr. Vitiello reviews ethical and regulatory considerations pertaining to psychotropic medication research in youths.

Children with attention-deficit/hyperactivity disorder (ADHD) and disruptive behavior disorders often receive psychopharmacological interventions. Stimulants are the psychotropics most commonly prescribed to youths. In Chapter 2, Natalya Paykina and Laurence Greenhill review medication treatments for ADHD. Both stimulant and nonstimulant agents are considered. The authors also review key aspects regarding the implementation and monitoring of patients treated with medications for ADHD.

A substantive amount of research has recently been conducted that pertains to the pharmacotherapy of disruptive behavior disorders in youths. In Chapter 3, Natoshia Raishevich, Elizabeth Pappadopulos, and Peter Jensen review this literature and provide recommendations regarding pharmacological approaches to patients with these disorders based on the extant scientific evidence on this topic.

Anxiety disorders are common in children and adolescents but frequently go undiagnosed and untreated. In Chapter 4, Moira Rynn and Jennifer Regan review the pharmacotherapy of anxiety disorders. The authors focus on both the potential benefits and the potential risks of prescribing medications to these patients. They also consider these drug treatments within the context of psychotherapeutic interventions.

Mood disorders are also relatively common in the young. These conditions are considered in Chapters 5 and 6. First, Boris Birmaher reviews what is known about the pharmacological treatment of juvenile depressive illness. He also thoughtfully considers suicidality, a topic that has recently received a great deal of attention both in the scientific literature and in the lay press. In the next chapter, Kevin Kuich and Robert Findling review the pharmacotherapy of bipolar disorders. Particular attention is paid not only to drug monotherapy trials but also to combination pharmacotherapeutic approaches.

Kimberly Stigler, Craig Erickson, David Posey, and Christopher McDougle, in Chapter 7, review what is known about the pharmacotherapy of the pervasive developmental disorders. The chapter begins with a review of the atypical antipsychotics, followed by a consideration of serotonin selective reuptake inhibitors and other antidepressants. The authors then discuss α_2-adrenergic agonists and psychostimulants. Other agents are then examined in this comprehensive review. The chapter concludes with a section on practical management approaches to these vulnerable patients.

Pharmacological approaches to tic disorders are reviewed in Chapter 8. Lawrence Scahill not only describes agents that might be used to treat tic disorders, but also provides perceptive insights on the pharmacotherapy of tic disorders in patients suffering from comorbid ADHD.

Judith Rapoport, Nitin Gogtay, and Phillip Shaw review the pharmacotherapy of schizophrenia and psychotic illnesses in Chapter 9. Both typical and atypical antipsychotics are considered.

In the last chapter, John Campo reviews the pharmacotherapy of youths who are primarily seen in general medical settings. He examines a variety of conditions, including functional somatic syndromes and somatoform disorders, eating disorders, sleep disorders, elimination disorders, and delirium, to name just a few.

Much thought, energy, and consideration have been given to ensure that *Clinical Manual of Child and Adolescent Psychopharmacology* is a book that is both scientifically sound as well as clinically rich. The ultimate goal of this work is to offer clinicians useful information that will facilitate the care they provide to the children and adolescents they have the privilege of treating. It is hoped that this goal has been successfully achieved.

Robert L. Findling, M.D.

Acknowledgments

This book was truly a collaborative endeavor. As a result, there are many people who deserve to be recognized for their contributions.

All the chapter authors are busy, highly regarded experts who have multiple and frequent demands on their time. It was exceptionally generous of them to dedicate their energy and efforts to this book.

The editorial staff at American Psychiatric Publishing, Inc. (APPI), has also been exceptionally generous with their time, expertise, and patience. Many thanks are owed to Katharine Phillips, M.D., member of the APPI Board of Directors; Robert E. Hales, M.D., Editor-in-Chief; John McDuffie, Editorial Director of the Books Division; and Bessie Jones, Acquisitions Coordinator.

Finally, Corrie Nesselhauf-Zimerla at the Discovery and Wellness Center for Children at University Hospitals Case Medical Center deserves a great deal of thanks. Her meticulous assistance and perseverance have truly helped make the idea of this book become a reality.

1

Developmental Aspects of Pediatric Psychopharmacology

Benedetto Vitiello, M.D.

Pediatric psychopharmacology involves the application of psychotropic agents to the treatment of children and adolescents with mental disorders. The defining elements of this discipline are the developing organism (in particular, the developing brain), psychopathology, chemical compounds that act on the brain, and therapeutic intent. The interplay among these elements determines benefits and toxicity of treatment. In addition, special ethical and regulatory considerations apply when treating children for purposes of either personal care or research.

Disclaimer: The opinions and assertions contained in this chapter are the private views of the author and are not to be construed as official or as reflecting the views of the National Institute of Mental Health, the National Institutes of Health, or the Department of Health and Human Services.

Dr. Vitiello has no financial relationship with pharmaceutical companies.

1

Extrapolation from adult data is insufficient to inform rational pediatric pharmacotherapy. Differences in the way the developing organism treats the drug (pharmacokinetics), how the developing brain reacts to the drug (pharmacodynamics), and how psychopathology is manifested during development all have implications for both efficacy and safety, and call for direct research in children. The considerable expansion of pediatric psychopharmacology research during recent years has started providing the foundation on which evidence-based pharmacotherapy can be built.

The purpose of this chapter is to describe the specific features of pediatric psychopharmacology and how those features make it a distinct discipline at the crossroads of child and adolescent psychiatry, pediatrics, and pharmacology.

Pharmacokinetics

Pharmacokinetics determines the availability of a drug at the site of action and thus directly influences the intensity and duration of the pharmacological activity. The basic pharmacokinetic processes of absorption, distribution, metabolism (biotransformation), and excretion are all influenced by development, as summarized in Tables 1–1 and 1–2. Because knowledge of the pharmacokinetics of a drug is critical to identifying the therapeutic dose range and frequency of administration, pediatric pharmacokinetics studies should precede and inform clinical trials aimed at testing efficacy in children (Findling et al. 2006).

Although children are smaller in body size than adults, they have a greater proportion of liver and kidney parenchyma after adjustment for body weight. Compared with adults, children also have relatively more body water, less fat, and less plasma albumin to which drugs can bind. These structural characteristics result in a smaller volume of distribution for drugs, greater drug extraction during the first pass through the liver after oral administration, lower bioavailability, and faster metabolism and elimination (Table 1–2). Therefore, simply decreasing adult doses on the basis of child weight can result in undertreatment. Adjustment by body surface area would control for both weight and height, but such an approach is usually reserved for administration of drugs with a narrow therapeutic index, such as antineoplastics, and is seldom used in pediatric psychopharmacology.

Table 1–1.   Essential pharmacokinetics terminology

Term	Definition
Absorption	Process by which a drug is absorbed from the site of administration into the systemic circulation
Liver first-pass extraction	Drug metabolism that occurs when a drug goes through the liver soon after intestinal absorption, before reaching the systemic circulation
Bioavailability	Proportion of administered drug that reaches the systemic circulation
Area under the curve (AUC)	Total area under the curve that describes the drug plasma as a function of time
Metabolism (biotransformation)	Phase I: cytochrome P450 (CYP450)–mediated oxidation; hydroxylation Phase II: conjugation reactions (glucuronidation, sulfation, acetylation)
Volume of distribution (V_d)	Apparent volume in which the drug is distributed after absorption (V_d = dose absorbed /C_p)
Concentration in plasma (C_p)	Drug quantity for unit of plasma (C_p = dose absorbed/V_d)
Peak plasma concentration (C_{max})	Highest plasma concentration
Time to C_{max} (T_{max})	Time that it takes from drug administration to reach C_{max}
Clearance (plasma clearance: CL)	Volume of plasma completely cleared of the drug in a unit of time; the cumulative result of drug removal that occurs in the liver, kidney, and other parts of the body (e.g., lungs, skin, bile); CL = dose absorbed/AUC
Elimination half-life ($t_{1/2}$)	Time that it takes, after full drug absorption and distribution in the body, for C_p to be reduced by 50%; a function of CL and V_d ($t_{1/2}$ = 0.693 · V_d/CL)
Steady-state plasma concentration	Stable C_p between doses that is achieved when the rate of elimination equals the rate of absorption; usually achieved after about four half-lives during constant drug administration

Table 1–2. Developmental pharmacokinetics and its implications

Compared with adults, children have	Pharmacokinetics implications	Examples
Smaller body size	Smaller volume of distribution → higher peak plasma concentration	After 20 mg oral fluoxetine, plasma levels are twofold higher in children than in adolescents (Wilens et al. 2002)
More liver parenchyma relative to body size	Relatively greater metabolic capacity → greater first-pass liver drug extraction → reduced bioavailability → faster drug metabolism → greater metabolite/parent drug levels ratio → shorter half-life	Ratio of metabolites to bupropion in plasma is 19%–80% greater in youths than in adults; mean bupropion $t_{1/2}$ is 12 hours in youths vs. 21 hours in adults (Daviss et al. 2005)
Relatively more body water and less adipose tissue	Less accumulation of drug → faster elimination	
More kidney parenchyma relative to body size	Relatively greater clearance capacity → faster drug elimination → shorter time to plasma peak → shorter half-life ($t_{1/2}$)	Lithium $t_{1/2}$: 18±7 hours in children vs. 22±8 hours in adults (Vitiello et al. 1988)

Adolescence is characterized by marked growth in body size and redistribution of body compartments. Differences between sexes become more pronounced. In males, the percentage of total body water increases and that of body fat decreases, while the opposite occurs in females. These changes can produce gender differences in pharmacokinetics.

Drug metabolism consists of biotransformations that turn the drug into derivative products (metabolites) that are more polar and therefore more easily eliminated. Not all drugs undergo metabolism, however. Lithium, for instance, is excreted unchanged through the kidneys. Drug metabolism typically includes two phases: Phase I, during which medications undergo enzymatic oxidative or hydrolytic transformations, and Phase II, during which conjugates between the drug, or its metabolites, and glucuronic acid, sulfate, glutathione, or acetate are formed. Phase I oxidative processes are mediated by cytochrome P450 (CYP450) microsomal enzymes, which are concentrated in the liver, although they are present in small quantities in other tissues too.

The CYP450 system matures rapidly after birth. For instance, liver microsomes have only 1% of the adult 2D6 activity found in the fetus, but this rate increases to about 20% of the adult activity in a 1-month-old infant. The immaturity of the CYP2D6 system at birth is one of the possible explanations for the syndrome of irritability, tachypnea, tremors, and increased muscle that has been observed in newborns whose mothers are taking selective serotonin reuptake inhibitors (SSRIs) (Chambers et al. 1996). An alternative explanation is that the syndrome is a withdrawal reaction from the SSRI (Sanz et al. 2005). In any case, the CYP450 metabolizing capacity is well developed by age 3 years (DeWildt et al. 1999). Because children have proportionally greater liver parenchyma than adults, the weight-adjusted metabolic capacity is greater in childhood.

The two most important CYP450 enzymes in pediatric psychopharmacology are the CYP3A4 and the CYP2D6, which are involved in the metabolism of most psychotropics, as summarized in Table 1–3. Genetic polymorphism has been identified for CYP2D6. About 7%–10% of whites, 1%–8% of Africans, and 1%–3% of East Asians are poor metabolizers. Poor metabolizers have higher drug concentrations in plasma and other body tissues. For example, the mean elimination half-life of atomoxetine is about 5 hours in children or adults who are extensive metabolizers, but 22 hours in poor metabolizers (Sauer et al. 2005). Being a poor metabolizer can have safety implications. One case of death in a 9-year-old child with a CYP2D6 genetic deficiency was associated with unusually high plasma levels of fluoxetine (Sallee et al. 2000). Assaying for genetic polymorphism is currently not considered a routine procedure in pediatric psychopharmacology, but it may be considered on a selective basis for individual patients in the case of long-term treatment with drugs metabolized by CYP450 enzymes with genetic polymorphisms (e.g., 2D6 and 2C19), low therapeutic index of the drug (e.g., tricyclics), polypharmacy, or history of toxicity.

Possible drug–drug and drug–food interactions must also be taken into account, because numerous drugs or food can inhibit, induce, or compete with specific CYP450 enzymes (Table 1–3). Especially important are those genetic polymorphisms and drug interactions that involve drugs with potential toxicities at high plasma concentration. Poor metabolizer status or the concomitant administration of another drug that competes with or inhibits the metabolism of the first drug would result in increased plasma concentrations. For instance, poor CYP2D6 metabolizers could develop toxic levels of tricyclic antidepressant. Concomitant administration of fluvoxamine (inhibitor of CYP3A4) and pimozide (metabolized by 3A4) could lead to high levels of pimozide and prolongation of the QTc (cardiac-corrected) interval. In sexually active female adolescents, use of oral contraceptives can induce CYP enzymes and thus increase drug metabolism and elimination.

The main route of drug elimination is through the kidneys, whereas bile, lungs, and skin account for a much smaller portion. Absolute clearance is usually lower in children than in adults, but weight-adjusted clearance is greater in children than in adults (Table 1–2). Because drug elimination is faster among children, the plasma drug half-life is often shorter in children than in adults (Daviss et al. 2005; Findling et al. 1999, 2000; Vitiello et al. 1988).

A shorter elimination half-life has several clinical implications. Plasma steady state is reached sooner during repeated administration. Elimination is faster and withdrawal symptoms are also more likely. More frequent dosing may be needed to maintain steady state and prevent withdrawal symptoms between doses. Pharmacokinetics can be influenced by the dose of medication and the duration of treatment, as shown by studies of sertraline in adolescents (Axelson et al. 2002). After a single dose of sertraline 50 mg in adolescents, the mean half-life was about 27 hours, but at steady state, after repeated administrations of the drug, it decreased to about 15 hours. In addition, the steady state

Table 1–3. Selected compounds relevant to pediatric pharmacotherapy metabolized by cytochrome P450 (CYP450) enzymes

CYP450 enzyme	Genetic polymorphism	Substrates	Inhibitors	Inducers
3A4	None	sertraline	fluoxetine	carbamazepine
		citalopram	fluvoxamine	phenobarbital
		escitalopram	nefazodone	phenytoin
		bupropion	erythromycin	primidone
		mirtazapine	clarithromycin	topiramate
		aripiprazole	indinavir	oxcarbazepine
		ziprasidone	ritonavir	rifampin
		quetiapine	ketoconazole	dexamethasone
		pimozide	grapefruit juice	St. John's wort[†]
		nefazodone		
		buspirone		
		alprazolam		
		zolpidem		
		ethinyl estradiol		
		erythromycin		
		indinavir		
		saquinavir		
		ritonavir		
2D6	Yes[a]	fluoxetine	fluoxetine	
		venlafaxine	paroxetine	
		paroxetine	haloperidol	
		atomoxetine	amitriptyline	
		risperidone	nortriptyline	
		olanzapine	imipramine	
		aripiprazole	desipramine	
		perphenazine	clomipramine	
		haloperidol	bupropion	
		imipramine		
		desipramine		

Table 1–3.   Selected compounds relevant to pediatric pharmacotherapy metabolized by cytochrome P450 (CYP450) enzymes *(continued)*

CYP450 enzyme	Genetic polymorphism	Substrates	Inhibitors	Inducers
2D6 *(continued)*		amitriptyline nortriptyline fluvoxamine mirtazapine dextromethorphan		
1A2	None	fluvoxamine clozapine olanzapine amitriptyline theophylline caffeine	fluvoxamine erythromycin ciprofloxacin	carbamazepine modafinil tobacco smoke
2C9	Yes[b]	fluoxetine fluvoxamine ibuprofen naproxen	fluoxetine fluvoxamine modafinil sertraline	carbamazepine rifampin
2C19	Yes[c]	citalopram escitalopram clomipramine imipramine amitriptyline diazepam	fluoxetine fluvoxamine modafinil	
2B6	Yes[d]	bupropion		diazepam clonazepam

[†]*Hypericum perforatum.*
[a]Poor metabolizers: 7%–10% of whites, 1%–8% of Africans, and 1%–3% of East Asians. Ultra-fast metabolizers: 1%–3% of whites.
[b]Poor metabolizers: 6%–12% of whites, 4% of Africans, and 3% of East Asians.
[c]Poor metabolizers: 1%–3% of whites, 1%–3% of Africans, and 20% of East Asians.
[d]Reported in white and Japanese populations.

half-life was found to be longer (approximately 20 hours) after administration of higher doses (100–150 mg). The clinical implication is that lower doses (50 mg/day) should be given twice a day to ensure consistent treatment and prevent withdrawal, whereas higher doses can be given once a day.

In the case of medications such as methylphenidate and amphetamines, whose short half-lives result in brief duration of action with consequent need for multiple daily administration, a variety of extended-release formulations have been developed. The first generation of extended-release formulations of methylphenidate consists of tablets with different coatings of immediate- and slower-release medication. Because of considerable intersubject variability in absorption, however, the onset of action may be delayed in the morning and/or the therapeutic effect may attenuate in the afternoon. More recently, a second generation of biphasic extended-release formulations has been introduced. These formulations allow an initial bolus of medication to be absorbed immediately, followed by a second formulation offering a more gradual release. The plasma pharmacokinetics curve thus shows an acute initial peak at about 1.5 hours after dosing, followed by a second peak approximately 3 hours later. The rationale for these biphasic-release formulations rests in the observation that optimal clinical effect occurs at increasing plasma levels of methylphenidate (Swanson et al. 2003). Extended-release preparations can be administered just once a day in the morning, given that they allow adequate control of attention deficit/hyperactivity disorder (ADHD) for 8–10 hours (Stein et al. 2003; Swanson et al. 2004).

Plasma levels are used as an indication (surrogate marker) of drug concentration at the site of action, which, in the case of psychotropics, is not easily accessible. In fact, plasma drug levels are a rather incomplete reflection of the drug concentration in the brain, as is also suggested by the somewhat low correlation between plasma level and clinical effects that is observed for most, though not all, drugs. Proton magnetic resonance spectroscopy has allowed the brain level of several drugs, such as lithium and fluoxetine, to be directly measured. As a result, a direct correlation between serum and brain lithium levels was reported in both children and adults; younger subjects, however, had a lower brain-serum ratio, which suggests they may need higher maintenance serum concentrations of lithium than adults to achieve therapeutic lithium concentrations in the brain (Moore et al. 2002).

Pharmacodynamics

Although the exact mechanism of action responsible for the therapeutic effects of many psychotropics remains unknown, the basic biochemical activity of these medications is generally considered to be similar across all ages. For instance, SSRIs block the reuptake of serotonin in both children and adults, and their antidepressant effect has been found to be associated with the degree of inhibition of the serotonin transporter in platelets (Axelson et al. 2005). However, the possible effects of development on the intensity and specificity of this pharmacological activity have not been systematically evaluated.

Most psychotropics act through neurotransmitters, such as dopamine, serotonin, and norepinephrine, whose receptors undergo major changes during development (Rho and Storey 2001; Wong et al. 1984). Receptor density tends to peak in preschool years and then gradually declines toward adult levels in late adolescence (Chugani et al. 2001). The impact and possible clinical implications of these developmental changes on drug activity have not been fully elucidated. However, the differences observed between children and adults regarding the efficacy and safety of many psychotropics support the notion that developmental factors have a significant influence on the effects of psychotropic medications. For instance, it is possible that the apparent lack of efficacy of tricyclics in pediatric depression may be due to neurobiological differences between a child's brain and an adult's brain. Likewise, amphetamine-like stimulants are more likely to induce euphoria in adults than in children, and neuroleptics are more likely to trigger acute dystonic reactions in children than in adults.

Brain imaging techniques have been applied to enhance understanding of the possible mechanisms of action of psychotropics and to help identify possible markers of treatment response. Using proton magnetic resonance spectroscopy, Davanzo et al. (2001) found that clinical response during lithium treatment was accompanied by a reduction of the *myo*-inositol–creatinine ratio in the anterior cingulate in children with bipolar disorder. Another study demonstrated a decrease in caudate glutamatergic concentrations in children with obsessive-compulsive disorder (OCD) who were taking paroxetine (Rosenberg et al. 2000). Using magnetic resonance imaging, Szeszko et al. (2004) found a volume reduction in the amygdala during administration of paroxetine to children with OCD. Although these findings are preliminary and not yet applicable to the management of patients in current practice, they suggest it may someday be possible to understand how psychotropic drugs work.

Another area in rapid expansion is that of *pharmacogenomics,* the study of genes that influence drug effects. Thus far, the findings have found practical application mainly for predicting metabolism and pharmacokinetics, but research is under way to understand the interface between several genetic polymorphisms and clinical efficacy. A number of candidate genes, such as those coding for the dopamine transporter, dopamine type 4 and 5 receptors, and the enzymes dopamine β-hydroxylase and catechol *O*-methyltransferase, have been proposed as possible predictors of treatment response to stimulant medications (McGough 2005). The genetic influence on drug effects is complex, because multiple genes are likely to be involved in determining individual variability in pharmacodynamics expression. The practical appeal of this line of research is that it may eventually allow treatment to be tailored to individual patient characteristics.

Efficacy

Evidence of treatment efficacy in children is established primarily through controlled clinical trials. The theoretical framework of this methodology is the same as in adult psychopharmacology, but important differences apply to pediatric samples (Vitiello 2003a). One distinctive characteristic in pediatric samples is that collection of clinical information about both therapeutic and adverse effects of treatment often relies on input from adults and teachers, in addition to the child himself or herself. This is especially the case in the treatment of children who are young and/or who are experiencing cognitive disabilities or disruptive behavior disorders. This particular feature of pediatric pharmacology makes drug evaluations in both research and practice settings more complex and time-consuming than in adults. Clinicians must integrate information from a variety of sources and arrive at a coherent conclusion about treatment effects.

Several rating instruments have been developed and validated for assessing treatment effects on psychiatric symptoms and level of functioning in children. In the absence of biological markers of disease and treatment effects, the pharmacotherapist must rely on changes in clinical symptoms to gauge response. Although symptom rating scales have been introduced primarily for research purposes to quantify psychopathology at different points in time, they can and should be applied to routine clinical practice, because they help the clinician measure and document the patient condition prospectively. Population norms have been developed for many scales that rate ADHD, depression, and anxiety symptoms in children.

Assessment of ADHD typically involves use of parent and teacher questionnaires, such as the Conners' Parent Rating Scales Revised, the Conners' Teacher Rating Scales Revised, the IOWA Conners' Teacher Rating Scale, or the Swanson, Nolan, and Pelham Questionnaire. Some of these scales are available commercially (Conners et al. 1998), while others can be found in the scientific literature or at Internet sites (e.g., www.adhd.net). In the assessment of treatment effects in anxiety disorders, both rating instruments completed by the child or parent, such as the Screen for Child Anxiety Related Emotional Disorders (Birmaher et al. 1997) and the Multidimensional Anxiety Scale for Children (March et al. 1997), and rating scales completed by clinicians, such as the Pediatric Anxiety Rating Scale, are available (Research Units on Pediatric Psychopharmacology Anxiety Study Group 2002). Assessment of antidepressant treatment effects generally involves use of clinician-rated scales, in particular the Children's Depression Rating Scale, Revised (Poznanski and Mokros 1996), which has been used in most placebo-controlled trials of antidepressants in children and adolescents (Emslie et al. 1997; Treatment for Adolescents With Depression Study Team 2004). Self-administered scales, such as the Child Depression Inventory (Kovacs 1985) and the Beck Depression Inventory (Beck and Steer 1984), are commonly used in practice settings, especially with adolescents, but they have not been found in most studies to discriminate between antidepressant and placebo in clinical trials (Emslie et al. 2002). Recently, however, the self-rated Reynolds Adolescent Depression Scale (Reynolds 1987) was found to be sensitive to pharmacological treatment effects in adolescent depression (Treatment for Adolescents With Depression Study Team 2004). Scales of assessing behavior in children with cognitive disabilities are also available and have been used in autism clinical trials (Marshburn and Aman 1992; Research Units on Pediatric Psychopharmacology Autism Network 2002).

Several classes of medications (e.g., serotonin reuptake inhibitors in OCD, stimulants in ADHD) have been demonstrated to be effective in both children and adults, but important differences have also been documented. Most notably, none of the placebo-controlled trials of tricyclic antidepressants have established superiority of the active medication (Hazell et al. 1995), and among the SSRIs only fluoxetine has been identified as superior to placebo in more than one study (Emslie et al. 1997, 2002). It is difficult to determine if the failure to consistently demonstrate antidepressant efficacy for the other SSRIs is mainly due to intrinsic differences in pharmacological activity among these compounds (a difference that does seem to exist in adults) or, more likely, to variability in methods and implementation across studies (Kratochvil et al. 2006).

A growing body of research in child and adolescent psychiatry has enabled the development of evidence-based treatment algorithms. Treatment algorithms consist of step-by-step instructions on how to treat individual patients based on their symptoms and previous treatment history. Algorithms are therefore more detailed and specific than general treatment guidelines or practice parameters. Pediatric pharmacological algorithms have been developed for ADHD, depression, and other disorders (Emslie et al. 2004a; Pliszka et al. 2003).

The magnitude of treatment effect relative to a control is often expressed in standard deviation units using the effect size. One of the most common ways of computing an effect size is with Cohen's d or Hedge's g, which is the difference in outcome measure between the study groups divided by the pooled standard deviation (Rosenthal et al. 2000). Compared with a placebo condition, stimulants usually have a large effect size (≥ 0.8) in decreasing symptoms of ADHD (Greenhill et al. 2001). In trials that have detected a difference between SSRI and placebo, the SSRI had a moderate effect size (0.5–0.7) when used in the treatment of major depression (Emslie et al. 2002; Treatment for Adolescents With Depression Study Team 2004) or OCD (March et al. 1998; Pediatric OCD Treatment Study [POTS] Team 2004). However, meta-analyses of all available databases of clinical trials in pediatric depression indicate that the effect size of antidepressant medication versus placebo is small (0.26; 95% CI = 0.13–0.40) (Jureidini et al. 2004)—a finding that is consistent with adult data (Bech et al. 2000).

It should be stressed that the effect size is a purely mathematical computation to express a difference between means. As such, it is sometimes used to quantify the pre-post treatment difference within the same treatment group. When this approach is used, a large effect size often emerges because it includes the time effect. Because there is no control condition, and therefore treatment effect cannot be distinguished from mere time effect, the pre-post effect size has limited meaning and cannot be taken as an index of treatment effect.

In addition to effect size, it is also useful to express the strength of therapeutic benefit using the number needed to treat (NNT), which is the number of patients who need to be given the treatment in order to add one more improved patient to the number of those who are expected to improve with the control condition. Thus, in the Treatment for Adolescents With Depression Study, 61% of the fluoxetine-treated patients improved at the end of the 12-week treatment, as compared with 35% of the placebo patients (Treatment for Adolescents With Depression Study Team 2004). The NNT is 4 (i.e., 100/[61–35] or 100/26), which indicates that, on average, one will need to treat 4 patients in order to improve one patient more than would improve in the placebo condition. The smaller the NNT, the greater is the relative efficacy of the treatment. Clinical trials have shown that the NNTs of psychotropic medications, though variable across different studies, are often quite favorable and compare well with other nonpsychiatric drugs used in pediatrics.

Because most psychiatric conditions are chronic or recurrent in nature and symptoms tend to reemerge when treatment is discontinued, pharmacological treatment of child disorders is often prolonged. Until recently, few studies had addressed the long-term effectiveness of pharmacotherapy in child psychiatry. In the past few years, however, reports documenting the long-term effects of stimulants and antidepressants have begun to appear (Clarke et al. 2005; Emslie et al. 2004a; MTA Cooperative Group 2004; Research Units on Pediatric Psychopharmacology Autism Network 2005). More research is needed to test whether successful control of symptoms in the short term translates into better prognosis in the long term. This type of research poses many challenges from a methodological and implementational point of view. It is difficult to conduct long-term, randomized, controlled trials, but observational studies are usually insufficient for inferring causality.

Safety

Safety issues are paramount, especially in the treatment of children. Pharmacological treatment during a period when the organism undergoes marked developmental changes may result in toxicities not seen in adults. For example, prolonged administration of phenobarbital to young children to prevent recurrence of febrile seizures impairs their cognitive development (Farwell et al. 1990). The risk of valproic acid–induced hepatotoxicity is highest among children under the age of 2, and thereafter decreases with age (Bryant and Dreifuss 1996). Hepatotoxicity may be caused by a toxic metabolite, 4-ene-valproic acid, which is produced by CYP2C9 and CYP2A6 enzymes (Sadeque et al. 1997). Children are at higher risk of developing serious rash during treatment with lamotrigine, possibly because of a higher efficiency of CYP450 metabolism in children that may translate into higher levels of potentially toxic metabolites (Anderson 2002).

Another concern is that the administration of agents acting on neurotransmitter systems in rapid development may interfere with normal processes and result in unwanted long-lasting changes. The distal effects of early exposure to psychotropics have been investigated in animals. For example, administration of fluoxetine to newborn mice caused a transient inhibition of the serotonin transporter during early development and was associated with abnormal emotional behaviors in adult mice, such as reduced exploratory behavior and slower adaptation to novel environments or stimuli, which could be interpreted as signs of anxiety or depression (Ansorge et al. 2004). In another study, chronic administration of fluoxetine to young rats impaired dendritic growth and spine density in the hippocampus (Norrholm and Ouimet 2000). The relevance of these findings in animals to pediatric psychopharmacology remains unclear, but these findings raise the possibility that early exposure to psychotropics may have enduring effects on the brain.

A high level of suspicion is therefore warranted when treating children with medications, especially when the treatment is prolonged. Various types of adverse effects can occur (Vitiello et al. 2003). Some, such as rash or dystonias, emerge acutely after brief drug exposure, and others, such as tardive dyskinesia or metabolic syndrome, develop insidiously during treatment of chronic conditions. Some toxicities are related to drug dose and/or plasma concentrations, such as lithium-induced tremor, and others emerge after drug discontinuation, such as withdrawal dyskinesias. Adverse effects may be anticipated, such as well-known side effects of a medication (e.g., stimulant-induced anorexia), or unexpected, such as when fenfluramine-induced cardiotoxicity was first reported.

Like the evaluation of efficacy, assessment of safety in pediatric psychopharmacology depends in large part on adult monitoring and reporting. From the perspective of the clinician, identification of treatment-adverse effects is contingent on the level of detail with which the relevant information is elicited and classified. It has been shown that a very general and open-ended inquiry by the clinician to the child and parent during a medication management visit—such as "Any health problems since the last visit?"—will yield substantially less information about adverse effects than a detailed, body-system inquiry, such as "Any problems with your eyes? Ears? Throat? Breathing?" (Greenhill et al. 2004). Obviously, the latter method of eliciting adverse effects is much more time-consuming and labor-intensive than the former, and its feasibility in a busy clinical practice is questionable. Research is in progress to develop sensitive instruments to assess adverse events that could be easily administered in practice settings.

Over the years, more information has become available on the short- and long-term safety of psychotropic medications in children. Although limited by the fact that most of the studies have been observational in nature (i.e., without an internal control group), the available data provide some guidance to clinicians. Selected safety issues that pertain to commonly used psychotropics are as follows.

Amphetamine-like stimulants can cause a dose-related delay in physical growth, in both weight and height, and the exact mechanism of this effect is not fully understood. A 2-year follow-up of school-age children with ADHD indicated that children continuously treated with stimulant medications grew in height on average about 1.0 cm less during the first 14 months of treatment and about 0.87 cm less in the following 10 months compared with never-medicated children with ADHD, with similar differences found for weight (−2.8 kg in the first 14 months and −1.0 kg in the following 10 months) (MTA Cooperative Group 2004). Psychotropics other than stimulants, such as atomoxetine and SSRIs, have been found to decrease growth rate when given chronically for months, but the clinical significance of these effects is doubtful (Spencer et al. 2005). The effects of these agents on growth are considered to be transient, and there is no evidence that they influence final height and weight.

Because stimulant medications are drugs of potential abuse, concerns have been raised about the possibility that treatment in childhood may sensitize the brain and thus make substance abuse and dependence more likely in adolescence and adulthood. The feasibility of mounting randomized, well-controlled studies to address this issue is questionable, and researchers have relied on naturalistically treated samples. Most of these studies have not found an increased risk of substance abuse after treatment with stimulants (Biederman et al. 1999; Wilens et al. 2003).

Recent studies of stimulant medications in special populations have revealed interesting differences in tolerability across age and type of development. Preschool children with ADHD were found to have lower tolerability to methylphenidate, with a rate of intolerable adverse events of 9%, which is substantially greater than the 1% observed in school-age children (Greenhill et al. 2001, 2006; Wigal et al. 2006). Children ages 5–14 with ADHD symptoms in the context of autism or other pervasive developmental disorders have even greater sensitivity to methylphenidate, as indicated by an 18% treatment discontinuation rate due to intolerable adverse events (most commonly irritability) (Research Units on Pediatric Psychopharmacology Autism Network 2002).

The main safety concerns of typical neuroleptics relate to the risk for extrapyramidal side effects, especially tardive dyskinesia. The more recently introduced atypical antipsychotics have a more benign neurological profile but often induce substantial weight gain. For instance, after 6 months of treatment with risperidone at the mean total daily dose of about 2 mg, children ages 5–17 years of age showed an average weight gain of 5 kg, which is roughly twice the gain expected in normal growth (Research Units on Pediatric Psychopharmacology Autism Network 2005). Risperidone-induced weight gain in children is curvilinear and tends to decelerate with time (Martin et al. 2004), but the sustained increase in prolactin that accompanies the administration of this drug and the risk for metabolic syndrome are reasons for concern. The metabolic syndrome is characterized by obesity, hyperlipidemia, decreased glucose tolerance, and diabetes (Morrison et al. 2005).

Recently, antidepressant treatment in children and adolescent has been found to be associated with increased risk for certain suicide-related events, such as thoughts about suicide and suicidal attempts (Hammad et al. 2006). A similar link has been demonstrated in young adults. Even though a causal link between antidepressant use and suicide itself has not been proved, because suicidal thinking and attempts are not the same as completed suicide, careful monitoring for suicidality in youths treated with antidepressant medications is necessary (U.S. Food and Drug Administration 2005). The mechanisms through which antidepressants may trigger suicidality remain a matter of speculation. It is possible that some youths can become abnormally activated by the antidepressant and may display akathisia, agitation, anxiety, insomnia, and impulsivity. A recent analysis found that prepubertal children are more likely to show behavioral activation than adolescents or adults (Safer and Zito 2006).

Safety is a relative concept, and possible risks of pharmacotherapy must be weighed against possible risks of untreated psychopathology. Decisions about prescribing medications must also take into account the availability of effective nonpharmacological interventions. Although generally found to be less effective at decreasing symptoms of ADHD or depression in children and adolescents, psychotherapy can be considered in lieu of medication for mild depression or, in more severe cases, in combination with medications. Psychotherapy, used either sequentially (i.e., start first with psychotherapy, then add medication if insufficient) or in combination (i.e., start both psychotherapy and medication concurrently), may be able to reduce the medication dose needed to control symptoms. Consideration should be given to use psychosocial interventions as first-step treatment (Waschbusch and Pelham 2004), especially in the treatment of young children. In any case, careful monitoring of children who are receiving psychotropics and documentation of both positive and negative outcomes have emerged as critically important components of rational pharmacotherapy.

Ethical Aspects

Although children should have their condition explained to the extent they can reasonably understand, and, whenever possible, asked for assent to treatment, they cannot give legal permission for treatment. Parents are responsible for health care decisions involving their children. Moreover, parents are also instrumental in implementing pharmacotherapy by ensuring appropriate administration of prescribed medication and in reporting possible treatment-emergent adverse effects. Parental permission is also required for child participation in research.

Considering that psychopathology is a common cause of impairment and suffering in childhood, that psychotropics are of potential benefit, and that adult data cannot adequately inform pediatric care, child participation in research is the only rational approach to decreasing the burden of mental illness in children (Vitiello et al. 2003). Participation of children in research is subject to special regulations in addition to those required for adult research participation (U.S. Department of Health and Human Services 2005a, 2005b; U.S. Food and Drug Administration 2001, 2004).

Only scientifically sound research investigations that utilize valid methodology and are posited to add new knowledge about important health issues can be ethically acceptable. Pediatric research can be divided into two broad categories, based on whether the research does or does not present the prospect of direct benefit to the individual participant. *Prospect of direct benefit* means that each participant has the potential to derive a health benefit from participation. General acquisition of knowledge relevant to a child's condition does not satisfy the requirement of direct benefit. To be ethically acceptable, research with prospect of direct benefit must ensure a favorable balance between anticipated benefits and foreseeable harms. A study that tests the efficacy of a treatment intervention usually has potential for direct benefit to the research participants. In this case, the main criterion for determining if the study is ethically acceptable is the risk-benefit ratio. The presence of a placebo arm in randomized clinical trials is usually considered acceptable in child psychiatry conditions. Placebo does not equal absence of treatment and has been associated with substantial improvement, especially in the context of mood and anxiety disorders.

Pharmacological research that does not offer a prospect of direct benefit includes pharmacokinetics and pharmacodynamics studies. In order to examine the acceptability of a study in this category, it must be determined whether such a study has the potential for generating essential knowledge relevant to the research participant's disorder or condition. If the information that the study will acquire is not relevant to the child's disorder or condition (e.g., a pharmacokinetics study in healthy children who are at no increased risk for the condition being targeted by the treatment), the research can be conducted only if it entails no more than *minimal risk*. Minimal risk is defined as "risk for harm not greater than ordinarily encountered in daily life, or during routine physical or psychological examinations or tests" (Section 46.102[i]) (U.S. Department of Health and Human Services 2005a). The prevailing interpretation is that the daily life, exams, and tests of a normal child are to be used as reference, but precise quantification of risk in ordinary daily life is not easy and remains a matter of discussion (Wendler et al. 2005).

If the information that the study aims to acquire is relevant to the participant condition (e.g., the pharmacokinetics of a medication for ADHD being studied in children with ADHD), the research risk cannot be greater than a *minor increase of minimal risk*. A minor increase over minimal risk can be considered acceptable only if a) it presents "experiences to the subjects that are commensurate with those inherent in their actual or expected medical, dental, psychological, social, or educational situations," and b) the study has the potential to generate new knowledge considered of "vital importance" for understanding or treating the child's disorder or condition (U.S. Department of Health and Human Services 2005a).

Research that is not otherwise approvable on the basis of these criteria but that presents an opportunity to understand, prevent, or alleviate a serious problem affecting the health or welfare of children can be referred to the Secretary of Health for further review under Health and Human Services regulations at 45 CFR 46.407 (U.S. Department of Health and Human Services 2005a, 2005b) and to the U.S. Food and Drug Administration (FDA) for review under its regulations at 21 CFR 50 and 56 (U.S. Food and Drug Administration 2001). Studies in which psychotropic medications are given to normal children in order to better understand the medication's mechanisms of action on the brain usually fall into this category. Generally, nontherapeutic administration of a psychotropic drug would be considered to pose more than minimal risk. For example, a protocol for a brain magnetic resonance imaging study of healthy children age 9 and older receiving a single oral dose of dextroamphetamine was referred by the institutional review board of the National Institute of Mental Health in 2004 under the regulation at 45 CFR 46.407 (Couzin 2004). The study was reviewed and approved by the Pediatric Ethics Subcommittee of the FDA Pediatric Advisory Committee in September 2004. The reviewers determined that a single administration of 10 mg of dextroamphetamine to a child age 9 years or older entails more than minimal risk because the potential adverse effects are more than those expected in a routine visit to a doctor. But the risk is considered limited to a minor increase over minimal risk. That being the case, and because the study had the potential to generate critically important information on the brain effects of a commonly used medication in children, the research was approved (U.S. Food and Drug Administration 2004).

The process of informing parents and children about the aims, procedures, potential risks and benefits of research participation, the presence of alternative treatments, and the rights of research participants is critical for obtaining their informed permission and assent. In general, children age 7 and older are able to provide assent; this is often documented with an appropriate assent form in writing. One reported study systematically assessed the level of research knowledge among parents whose children had participated in a placebo-controlled clinical trial. The results showed that the large majority of parents had a very good understanding of both research procedures and participant rights (Vitiello et al. 2005).

Many public and private Web sites provide detailed information about child participation in research and the process of determining if a particular project is ethically acceptable (Children's Hospital Boston 2005; (U.S. Department of Health and Human Services, Office for Human Research Protections 2005).

Regulatory Aspects

Many drugs are prescribed to children for the treatment of conditions that are not included in the FDA-approved drug labeling, as summarized in Table 1–4. Use of a drug *off-label* is not in itself an inappropriate practice, because it is often supported by considerable empirical evidence and is consistent with treatment guidelines. However, it is important that parents be aware that a medication is going to be prescribed off-label before making treatment decisions for their child.

Since recognition in the mid-1990s of the widespread and increasing off-label use of medications in children, major initiatives have been initiated to increase pediatric research and thus acquire the necessary information for appropriate drug utilization in children. In 1997, the U.S. Congress passed the Food and Drug Administration Modernization Act, which provided financial incentives to pharmaceutical companies in return for conducting pediatric research (U.S. Congress 1997). Implementation of the patent exclusivity extension program started in June 1998. This legislation was then further expanded and extended until 2008 with the Best Pharmaceuticals for Children Act of 2002 (U.S. Congress 2002). The incentive (i.e., a 6-month extension in the

Table 1–4.   Pediatric indications approved by the U.S. Food and Drug Administration (FDA) and off-label use of selected psychotropic medications

Medication	FDA-approved indication	Relative child age	Off-label use
methylphenidate	ADHD	6 years and older	ADHD: under age 6 years
dexmethylphenidate	ADHD	6 years and older	ADHD: under age 6 years
amphetamine products	ADHD	3 years and older	
atomoxetine	ADHD	6 years and older	ADHD: under age 6 years
clonidine	Hypertension	12 years and older	ADHD: under age 12 years Tourette's disorder
guanfacine	None		ADHD: under age 12 years Tourette's disorder
imipramine	Enuresis	6 years and older	MDD: 6 years and older
fluoxetine	MDD	8 years and older	MDD: under age 8 years
	OCD	7 years and older	Other anxiety disorders: 6 years and older
sertraline	OCD	6 years and older	OCD, anxiety disorders: 6 years and older MDD: 6 years and older
citalopram	None		OCD, other anxiety disorders: 6 years and older MDD: 6 years and older
paroxetine	None		OCD, other anxiety disorders: 6 years and older MDD: 6 years and older
fluvoxamine	OCD	7 years and older	Other anxiety disorders: 6 years and older
venlafaxine	None		MDD: age 6 years and older
bupropion	None		MDD: age 6 years and older ADHD: age 6 years and older

Table 1–4.   Pediatric indications approved by the U.S. Food and Drug Administration (FDA) and off-label use of selected psychotropic medications (*continued*)

Medication	FDA-approved indication	Relative child age	Off-label use
haloperidol	Psychosis, Tourette's disorder, hyperactivity, severe behavioral problems, explosive hyperexcitability	3 years and older	
pimozide	Tourette's disorder	2 years and older	
atypical antipsychotics			
risperidone	None		Psychosis, aggression, self-injury, severe tantrums, mania, Tourette's disorder[a]
olanzapine	None		
quetiapine	None		
ziprasidone	None		
aripiprazole	None		
lithium	Bipolar disorder	12 years and older	Bipolar disorder: under age 12 years Aggression: age 6 years and older
anticonvulsants			
valproate	Epilepsy: since infancy		Mania, aggression
carbamazepine	Epilepsy: since infancy		Mania, aggression
oxcarbazepine	Epilepsy	4 years and older	Mania, aggression
lamotrigine	Epilepsy	2 years and older	Depression in bipolar disorder

Note.   ADHD=attention-deficit/hyperactivity disorder; MDD=major depressive disorder; OCD=obsessive-compulsive disorder.
[a]Possible off-label uses for all antipsychotics.

drug patent exclusivity) has substantially changed the approach of industry to pediatric pharmacology, including pediatric psychopharmacology. Both pharmacokinetics and clinical trials have been conducted in children under the additional exclusivity program. For instance, clinical trials have been conducted to test the efficacy of citalopram, sertraline, venlafaxine, and nefazodone in pediatric depression.

For medications that need pediatric data but that are already off-patent, the incentive of additional patent exclusivity cannot apply. For these cases, the Best Pharmaceuticals for Children Act established a program that, through a collaboration between the FDA and the National Institutes of Health (NIH), arranges for the necessary studies to be conducted with public funding. Accordingly, a contract to study lithium carbonate in children with mania was awarded by the NIH in 2005.

In addition, legislation to prevent the pediatric off-label use of future medications was enacted with the Pediatric Research Equity Act of 2003 (U.S. Congress 2003). This act provides the FDA with the authority to request that industry conduct pediatric studies of a drug even before its approval for adult use when there is a likelihood that the drug will also be prescribed to children.

Conclusions

Pediatric psychopharmacology is a field in rapid growth due to an expanding research base and active regulatory action. It is also the object of frequent debate and, at times, controversy in the media and among the general public. The therapeutic value of a number of psychotropics is now well documented in both the short and intermediate term (i.e., up to 12–24 months). Knowledge gaps remain in our understanding of the long-term impact of pharmacotherapy with respect to both efficacy and safety. The recent debate about the safety of SSRI antidepressants in children has highlighted the need for careful evaluation and monitoring of psychopharmacological treatment. One obvious implication is that practicing rational pharmacotherapy requires integration of knowledge at different levels, including developmental psychopathology, pharmacology, drug regulation, and bioethics, and a considerable investment of time on the part of the treating clinician and the child's parents.

Clinical Pearls

- Simply decreasing adult medication doses on the basis of child weight can result in undertreatment because of faster drug elimination in children.

- Assessing treatment effects and safety usually requires collection and integration of data from different informants (e.g., child, parent, teacher).

- Assaying for genetic polymorphism is currently considered not a routine procedure in the practice of child psychopharmacology, but it can be clinically useful in individual cases.

- Safety is paramount, and a high level of suspicion is warranted when treating children with medications, especially at the beginning of treatment, during long-term treatment, or when multiple medications are concomitantly prescribed.

- Younger children tend to be more sensitive to the adverse effects of medications.

- Children should have their condition explained to the extent they can reasonably understand and, whenever possible, asked for assent to treatment.

- Pediatric psychopharmacology is an area of active research, and clinicians should remain attuned to reports of new findings.

References

Anderson GD: Children versus adults: pharmacokinetics and adverse-effects differences. Epilepsia 43(suppl):53–59, 2002

Ansorge MS, Zhou M, Lira A, et al: Early life blockade of the 5-HT transporter alters emotional behavior in adult mice. Science 306:879–881, 2004

Axelson DA, Perel JM, Birmaher B, et al: Sertraline pharmacokinetics and dynamics in adolescents. J Am Acad Child Adolesc Psychiatry 41:1037–1044, 2002

Axelson DA, Perel JM, Birmaher B, et al: Platelet serotonin reuptake inhibition and response to SSRIs in depressed adolescents. Am J Psychiatry 162:802–804, 2005

Bech P, Cialdella P, Haugh MC, et al: Meta-analysis of randomized controlled trials of fluoxetine vs. placebo and tricyclics antidepressants in the short-term treatment of major depression. Br J Psychiatry 176:421–428, 2000

Beck AT, Steer RA: Internal consistencies of the original and revised Beck Depression Inventory. J Clin Psychol 140:1365–1367, 1984

Biederman J, Wilens T, Spencer T, et al: Pharmacotherapy of attention-deficit/hyperactivity disorder reduces the risk for substance use disorder. Pediatrics 104:e20, 1999

Birmaher B, Brent DA, Chiappetta L, et al: The Screen for Child Anxiety Related Emotional Disorders (SCARED): scale construction and psychometric characteristics. J Am Acad Child Adolesc Psychiatry 38:1230–1236, 1997

Bryant AE, Dreifuss FE: Valproic acid hepatic fatalities, III: I.S. experience since 1986. Neurology 46:465–469, 1996

Chambers CD, Johnson KA, Dick LM, et al: Birth outcomes in pregnant women taking fluoxetine. N Engl J Med 335:1010–1015, 1996

Children's Hospital Boston: Parents' guide to medical research. Available at: http://www.bostonchild.vitalconsent.com/bstnchld/index.html. Accessed December 1, 2005.

Chugani DC, Muzik O, Juhasz C, et al: Postnatal maturation of human GABAA receptors measured with positron emission tomography. Ann Neurol 49:618–626, 2001

Clarke DB, Birmaher B, Axelson D, et al: Fluoxetine for the treatment of childhood anxiety disorders: open-label, long-term extension to a controlled trial. J Am Acad Child Adolesc Psychiatry 44:1263–1270, 2005

Conners CK, Sitarenios G, Parker JD, et al: The revised Conners' Parent Rating Scale (CPRS-R): factor structure, reliability, and criterion validity. J Abnorm Child Psychol 26:257–268, 1998

Couzin J: Pediatric study of ADHD drug draws high-level public review. Science 305:1088–1089, 2004

Davanzo P, Thomas MA, Yue K, et al: Decreased anterior cingulate myo-inositol/creatine spectroscopy resonance with lithium treatment in children with bipolar disorder. Neuropsychopharmacology 24:359–369, 2001

Daviss WB, Perel JM, Rudolph GR, et al: Steady-state pharmacokinetics of bupropion SR in juvenile patients. J Am Acad Child Adolesc Psychiatry 44:349–357, 2005

DeWildt SN, Kearns GL, Leader JS, et al: Cytochrome P450 3A: ontogeny and drug disposition. Clin Pharmacokinet 37:485–505, 1999

Emslie GJ, Rush AJ, Weinberg WA, et al: A double-blind, randomized, placebo-controlled trial of fluoxetine in children and adolescents with depression. Arch Gen Psychiatry 54:1031–1037, 1997

Emslie GJ, Heiligenstein JH, Wagner KD, et al: Fluoxetine for acute treatment of depression in children and adolescents: a placebo-controlled, randomized clinical trial. J Am Acad Child Adolesc Psychiatry 41:1205–1215, 2002

Emslie GJ, Heiligenstein JH, Hoog SL, et al: Fluoxetine treatment for prevention of relapse of depression in children and adolescents: a double-blind, placebo-controlled study. J Am Acad Child Adolesc Psychiatry 43:1397–1405, 2004a

Emslie GJ, Hughes CW, Crimson ML, et al: A feasibility study of the childhood depression medication algorithm: the Texas Children's Medication Algorithm Project (CMAP). J Am Acad Child Adolesc Psychiatry 43:519–527, 2004b

Farwell JR, Lee YJ, Hirtz DG, et al: Phenobarbital for febrile seizures: effects on intelligence and on seizure recurrence. N Engl J Med 322:364–369, 1990

Findling RL, Reed MD, Myers C, et al: Paroxetine pharmacokinetics in depressed children and adolescents. J Am Acad Child Adolesc Psychiatry 38:952–959, 1999

Findling RL, Preskorn SH, Marcus RN, et al: Nefazodone pharmacokinetics in depressed children and adolescents. J Am Acad Child Adolesc Psychiatry 39:1008–1016, 2000

Findling RL, McNamara NK, Stansbrey RJ, et al: The relevance of pharmacokinetic studies in designing efficacy trials in juvenile major depression. J Child Adolesc Psychopharmacol 16:131–145, 2006

Greenhill LL, Swanson JM, Vitiello B, et al: Impairment and deportment responses to different methylphenidate doses in children with ADHD: the MTA titration trial. J Am Acad Child Adolesc Psychiatry 40:180–187, 2001

Greenhill LL, Vitiello B, Fisher P, et al: Comparison of increasingly detailed elicitation methods for the assessment of adverse events in pediatric psychopharmacology. J Am Acad Child Adolesc Psychiatry 43:1488–1496, 2004

Greenhill LL, Abikoff H, Chuang S, et al: Efficacy and safety of immediate-release methylphenidate treatment for preschoolers with ADHD. J Am Acad Child Adolesc Psychiatry 45:1284–1293, 2006

Hammad TA, Laughren T, Racoosin J: Suicidality in pediatric patients treated with antidepressant drugs. Arch Gen Psychiatry 63:332–339, 2006

Hazell P, O'Connell D, Heathcote D, et al: Efficacy of tricyclic drugs in treating child and adolescent depression: a meta-analysis. Br Med J 310:897–901, 1995

Jureidini JN, Doeke CJ, Mansfield PR, et al: Efficacy and safety of antidepressants for children for children and adolescents. Br Med J 328:879–883, 2004

Kovacs M: Children's Depression Inventory (CDI). Psychopharmacol Bull 21:995–998, 1985

Kratochvil CJ, Vitiello B, Walkup J, et al: SSRIs in pediatric depression: is the balance between benefits and risks favorable? J Child Adolesc Psychopharmacol 16:11–24, 2006

March JS, Parker JD, Sullivan K, et al: The Multidimensional Anxiety Scale for Children (MASC): factor structure, reliability, and validity. J Am Acad Child Adolesc Psychiatry 36:554–565, 1997

March JS, Biederman J, Wolkow R, et al: Sertraline in children and adolescents with obsessive-compulsive disorder: a multicenter randomized controlled trial. JAMA 280:1752–1756, 1998

Marshburn EC, Aman MG: Factor validity and norms for the Aberrant Behavior Checklist in a community sample of children with mental retardation. J Autism Dev Disord 22:357–373, 1992

Martin A, Scahill L, Anderson GM, et al: Weight and leptin changes among risperidone-treated youths with autism: 6-month prospective data. Am J Psychiatry 161:1125–1127, 2004

McGough JJ: Attention-deficit/hyperactivity disorder pharmacogenomics. Biol Psychiatry 57:1367–1373, 2005

Moore CM, Demopulos CM, Henry ME, et al: Brain-to-serum lithium ratio and age: an in vivo magnetic resonance spectroscopy study. Am J Psychiatry 159:1240–1242, 2002

Morrison JA, Friedman LA, Harlan WR, et al: Development of the metabolic syndrome in black and white adolescent girls: a longitudinal assessment. Pediatrics 116:1178–1182, 2005

MTA Cooperative Group: National Institute of Mental Health Multimodal Treatment Study of ADHD follow-up: changes in effectiveness and growth after the end of treatment. Pediatrics 113:762–769, 2004

Norrholm SD, Ouimet CC: Chronic fluoxetine administration to juvenile rats prevents age-associated dendritic spine proliferation in hippocampus. Brain Res 883:205–215, 2000

Pediatric OCD Treatment Study (POTS) Team: Cognitive-behavior therapy, sertraline, and their combination for children and adolescents with obsessive-compulsive disorder: the Pediatric OCD Treatment Study (POTS) randomized controlled trial. JAMA 292:1969–1976, 2004

Pliszka SR, Lopez M, Crimson ML, et al: A feasibility study of the children's medication algorithm project (CMAP) algorithm for the treatment of ADHD. J Am Acad Child Adolesc Psychiatry 42:279–287, 2003

Poznanski EO, Mokros HB: Manual for the Children's Depression Rating Scale–Revised. Los Angeles, CA, Western Psychological Services, 1996

Research Units on Pediatric Psychopharmacology Anxiety Study Group: The Pediatric Anxiety Rating Scale (PARS): development and psychometric properties. J Am Acad Child Adolesc Psychiatry 41:1061–1069, 2002

Research Units on Pediatric Psychopharmacology Autism Network: Risperidone in children with autism and serious behavioral problems. N Engl J Med 347:314–321, 2002

Research Units on Pediatric Psychopharmacology Autism Network: Risperidone treatment of autistic disorder: longer-term benefits and blinded discontinuation after 6 months. Am J Psychiatry 162:1361–1369, 2005

Reynolds WM: Professional Manual for the Reynolds Adolescents Depression Scale. Odessa, FL, Psychological Assessment Resources, 1987

Rho JM, Storey TW: Molecular ontogeny of major neurotransmitter receptor systems in the mammalian central nervous system: norepinephrine, dopamine, serotonin, acetylcholine, and glycine. J Child Neurol 16:271–279, 2001

Rosenberg DR, MacMaster FP, Keshavan MS, et al: Decrease in caudate glutamatergic concentrations in pediatric obsessive compulsive disorder patients taking paroxetine. J Am Acad Child Adolesc Psychiatry 39:1096–1103, 2000

Rosenthal R, Rosnow R, Rubin DB: Contrasts and Effect Sizes in Behavioral Research. Cambridge, England, Cambridge University Press, 2000

Sadeque AJM, Fisher MB, Korzekwa KR, et al: Human CYP2C9 and CYP2A6 mediate formation of the hepatoxin 4-ene-valproic acid. J Pharmacol Exp Therapeutics 283:698–703, 1997

Safer DJ, Zito JM: Treatment-emergent adverse events from selective serotonin reuptake inhibitors by age group: children vs. adolescents. J Child Adolesc Psychopharmacol 16:159–169, 2006

Sallee FR, DeVane CL, Ferrell RE: Fluoxetine-related death in a child with cytochrome P-450 2D6 genetic deficiency. J Child Adolesc Psychopharmacol 10:27–34, 2000

Sanz EJ, De-las-Cuevas C, Kiuru A, et al: Selective serotonin reuptake inhibitors in pregnant women and neonatal withdrawal syndrome: a database analysis. Lancet 365:482–487, 2005

Sauer JM, Ring BJ, Witcher JM: Clinical pharmacokinetics of atomoxetine. Clin Pharmacokinet 44:571–590, 2005

Spencer TJ, Newcorn JH, Kratochvil CJ, et al: Effects of atomoxetine on growth after 2-year treatment among pediatric patients with attention-deficit/hyperactivity disorder. Pediatrics 116:e74–e80, 2005

Stein MA, Sarampote CS, Waldman ID, et al: A dose-response study of OROS methylphenidate in children with attention-deficit/hyperactivity disorder. Pediatrics 112:e404, 2003

Swanson JM, Gupta S, Lam A, et al: Development of a new once-a-day formulation of methylphenidate for the treatment of attention-deficit/hyperactivity disorder: proof-of-concept and proof-of-product studies. Arch Gen Psychiatry 60:204–211, 2003

Swanson JM, Wigal SB, Wigal T, et al: A comparison of once-daily extended-release methylphenidate formulations in children with attention-deficit/hyperactivity disorder in the laboratory school (the Comacs Study). Pediatrics 113:e206–e216, 2004

Szeszko PR, MacMillan S, McMeniman M, et al: Amygdala volume reductions in pediatric patients with obsessive-compulsive disorder treated with paroxetine: preliminary findings. Neuropsychopharmacology 29:826–832, 2004

Treatment for Adolescents With Depression Study Team: The Treatment for Adolescents With Depression Study (TADS): short-term effectiveness and safety outcomes. JAMA 292:807–820, 2004

U.S. Congress: Food and Drug Administration Modernization Act. Public Law 105–115, 1997

U.S. Congress: Best Pharmaceuticals for Children Act (BPCA). Public Law 107–109, 2002

U.S. Congress: Pediatric Research Equity Act of 2003. Public Law 108–155, 2003

U.S. Department of Health and Human Services: Code of Federal Regulations, Title 45, Public Welfare, Part 46, Protection of Human Subjects, Subpart A: Basic HHS Policy for Protection of Human Research Subjects. Revised June 23, 2005. Washington, DC, U.S. Department of Health and Human Services, 2005a. Available at: http://www.dhhs.gov/ohrp/humansubjects/guidance/45cfr46.htm#subparta. Accessed December 6, 2005.

U.S. Department of Health and Human Services: Code of Federal Regulations, Title 45, Public Welfare, Part 46, Protection of Human Subjects, Subpart D: Additional Protections for Children Involved as Subjects in Research. Revised June 23, 2005. Washington, DC, U.S. Department of Health and Human Services, 2005b. Available at: http://www.dhhs.gov/ohrp/humansubjects/guidance/45cfr46.htm#subpartd. Accessed December 6, 2005.

U.S. Department of Health and Human Services, Office for Human Research Protections: Special Protections for Children as Research Subjects. Children Involved as Subjects in Research: Guidance on the HHS 45 CFR 46.407 ("407") Review Process. May 26, 2005. Rockville, MD, Office for Human Research Protections, U.S. Department of Health and Human Services, 2005. Available at: http://www.hhs.gov/ohrp/children/guidance_407process.html. Accessed December 1, 2005.

U.S. Food and Drug Administration: 21 CFR Parts 50 and 56. Additional safeguards for children in clinical investigations of FDA-regulated products. Federal Register 66:20589–20600, 2001. Available at: http://www.fda.gov/ohrms/dockets/98fr/042401a.pdf. Accessed November 28, 2005.

U.S. Food and Drug Administration: Summary Minutes of the Pediatric Ethics Subcommittee of the Pediatric Advisory Committee, September 10th, 2004. Rockville, MD, U.S. Food and Drug Administration, 2004. Available at: http://www.fda.gov/ohrms/dockets/ac/04/minutes/2004-4066m1_summary%20Minutes.pdf. Accessed November 29, 2005.

U.S. Food and Drug Administration: Medication guide about using antidepressants in children and teenagers. Rockville, MD, U.S. Food and Drug Administration, 2005. Available at: http://www.fda.gov/cder/drug/antidepressantsMG_template.pdf. Accessed November 29, 2005.

Vitiello B: Clinical trials methodology and design issues, in Child and Adolescent Psychopharmacology. Edited by Martin A, Scahill L, Charney D, et al. New York, Oxford University Press, 2003a

Vitiello B: Ethical considerations in psychopharmacological research involving children and adolescents. Psychopharmacology 171:86–91, 2003b

Vitiello B, Behar D, Malone R, et al: Pharmacokinetics of lithium carbonate in children. J Clin Psychopharmacol 8:355–359, 1988

Vitiello B, Riddle MA, Greenhill LL, et al: How can we improve the assessment of safety in child and adolescent psychopharmacology? J Am Acad Child Adolesc Psychiatry 42:634–641, 2003

Vitiello B, Aman MG, Scahill L, et al: Research knowledge among parents of children participating in a randomized clinical trial. J Am Acad Child Adolesc Psychiatry 44:145–149, 2005

Waschbusch DA, Pelham WE : Using stimulants in children with ADHD. Science 306:1473, 2004

Wendler D, Belsky L, Thompson KM, et al: Quantifying the federal minimal risk standard : implications for pediatric research without a prospect of direct benefit. JAMA 294:826–832, 2005

Wigal T, Greenhill LL, Chuang S, et al: Safety and tolerability of methylphenidate in preschool children with ADHD. J Am Acad Child Adolesc Psychiatry 45:1294–1303, 2006

Wilens TE, Cohen L, Biederman J, et al: Fluoxetine pharmacokinetics in pediatric patients. J Clin Psychopharmacol 22:568–575, 2002

Wilens TE, Faraone SV, Biederman J, et al: Does stimulant therapy of attention-deficit/hyperactivity disorder beget later substance abuse? A meta-analytic review of the literature. Pediatrics 111:179–185, 2003

Wong DF, Wagner HN, Darmals RF, et al: Effect of age on dopamine and serotonin receptors measured by positron tomography of the living human brain. Science 226:1393, 1984

2

Attention-Deficit/ Hyperactivity Disorder

Natalya Paykina, M.A.

Laurence Greenhill, M.D.

Attention-deficit/hyperactivity disorder (ADHD) is a frequently diagnosed behavioral condition (American Psychiatric Association 2000). The prevalence of ADHD has been estimated, in the U.S. National Health Interview Survey, to be 6.7% of all school-age children (Woodruff et al. 2004). This rate is close to the estimate of 7.5% found in an epidemiological survey of elementary and secondary school children in Minnesota (Barbaresi et al. 2002).

ADHD is a chronic disorder. Follow-up studies of school-age children diagnosed early with ADHD suggest that 60%–85% will continue to meet the full DSM-IV-TR criteria (American Psychiatric Association 2000) for the disorder throughout their teenage years (Barkley et al. 1990; Biederman et al. 1996). These data indicate that the condition does not disappear with the onset of puberty. It is estimated that 2% (Mannuzza et al. 1993) to 27% (Barkley et al. 2002) will continue to meet the criteria for the disorder into adult life. Epidemiological studies using a two-stage probability sample screen of 3,199 individuals ages 19–44 estimated the point prevalence of adult ADHD to be 4.4% (Kessler et al. 2006).

Medications of choice for ADHD are the psychostimulants (Greenhill et al. 2002a, 2002b), which include various preparations of methylphenidate and amphetamines. Long-duration stimulant oral preparations (Biederman et al. 2002; M. Wolraich, L.L. Greenhill, H. Abikoff, et al.: "Randomized Controlled Trial of OROS Methylphenidate Q.D. in Children With Attention-Deficit/Hyperactivity Disorder," unpublished paper, 2000), the stimulant transdermal patch (McGough et al. 2006), atomoxetine (Michelson et al. 2003), and the daytime alertness drug modafinil (Greenhill et al. 2006a) have been introduced within the last decade. These agents have been tested for efficacy in multisite, double-blind, randomized, parallel-design, placebo-controlled trials, and their safety has been monitored in longer-term open-label studies.

The prevalence of ADHD in school-age children may be gleaned from comprehensive reviews (Bauermeister et al. 1994; Bird et al. 1988; Szatmari 1992) and from epidemiological surveys conducted in the United States (Visser and Lesesne 2006) including Pittsburgh, Pennsylvania (Costello 1989); Puerto Rico (Bird et al. 1988); and the Great Smoky Mountain area of rural North Carolina (Costello et al. 2003). Similar research was conducted in other countries, such as Australia (Connell et al. 1982); Norway (Vikan 1985); East London (Taylor et al. 1991); the Netherlands (Verhulst et al. 1992); Ontario, Canada (Szatmari et al. 1989); Mannheim, Germany (Esser et al. 1996); and New Zealand (Anderson et al. 1987). Rates for ADHD range from 2.0% to 6.3% (Szatmari et al. 1989), but ADD (attention-deficit disorder) shows a wider range, between 2.2% and 12.6% (Velez et al. 1989). Selecting from families identified in the National Comorbidity Survey, Kessler et al. (2006) estimated the prevalence of ADHD to be 4.4% of adults ages 18–44 in the United States.

Diagnosis of ADHD

ADHD is a heterogeneous condition characterized by a persistent, developmentally inappropriate pattern of gross motor overactivity, inattention, and impulsivity that impairs academic, social, and family function. The condition was first described in the nineteenth century. The most recent definition of the disorder appears in DSM-IV-TR (American Psychiatric Association 2000), which subdivides it into three subtypes: predominately hyperactive-impulsive, predominately inattentive, and combined. The deficits in behavioral inhibition are thought by some investigators to disrupt the development of normal self-regulation (Barkley 1997). Two-thirds of young children with ADHD also meet criteria for other childhood psychiatric disorders, including anxiety, depressive, oppositional defiant, conduct, and mood disorders. These comorbid psychiatric conditions are thought to increase the impairment associated with ADHD.

Although ADHD has its onset in childhood, follow-up studies have found that 30%–50% of children with the disorder continue to experience impairment from its symptoms as adults. Although adults with ADHD may not meet all childhood symptom criteria necessary for the diagnosis, their symptoms continue to cause significant impairment. The National Comorbidity Survey Replication (Kessler et al. 2006) identified impairing ADHD symptoms in 4.5% of adults in the U.S. population, suggesting that considerable suffering continues to occur in adults who had childhood ADHD.

DSM-IV-TR requires the persistence of six or more symptoms of inattentiveness or hyperactivity/impulsivity for at least 6 months at a level that is maladaptive and exceeds the norm for the subject's age group. In addition, there is an age-at-onset criterion (before 7 years), a duration criterion (symptoms must have persisted more than 6 months), a pervasiveness criterion (the symptoms must cause impairment in more than one settings), and a differential diagnosis criterion (symptoms cannot be better explained by a different disorder).

Diagnostic Procedures

Guidelines for making the ADHD diagnosis in an office practice context have been published by the American Academy of Pediatrics (2001) and the American Academy of Child and Adolescent Psychiatry (AACAP) (Pliszka and AACAP Work Group on Quality Issues 2007). Because ADHD is so prevalent, the AACAP recommends that screening for ADHD should be part of any patient's mental health assessment. Such screening can be accomplished by having the practitioner ask questions about inattention, impulsivity, and hyperactivity, and whether such symptoms cause impairment. Alternatively, parents and teachers can be asked to fill out rating scales containing DSM-IV-TR symptoms of ADHD before the practitioner starts the first interview. A positive screen on a rating scale, however, does not constitute a definitive ADHD diagnosis.

A physical examination and medical history should be carried out during the diagnostic evaluation. If the patient's medical examination and history are unremarkable, no additional laboratory or neurological testing is required (Pliszka and AACAP Work Group on Quality Issues 2007). Similarly, no routine psychological testing is needed for the evaluation of ADHD, unless the patient's history suggests low achievement in reading, language, writing, or mathematics "relative to the patient's intellectual ability" beyond that accounted for by the ADHD symptoms themselves (Pliszka and AACAP Work Group on Quality Issues 2007).

The next diagnostic procedure includes an interview with the child or adolescent to determine if other psychiatric disorders are present that would better explain the symptoms causing impairment. Although it is helpful to interview a preschool- or school-age child with the parent present, older children and adolescents should be interviewed alone, because they are more likely to discuss symptoms of substance use, suicidal ideation or behavior, or depression with the parents absent.

Because a majority of children with ADHD also have at least one other Axis I psychiatric disorder (Biederman et al. 1991), the clinician should make inquiries about symptoms of oppositional defiant disorder, conduct disorder, depression, anxiety disorders, tic disorders, substance use disorders, and mania. Symptoms of these conditions can be captured by parent symptom checklists (e.g., Achenbach Child Behavior Checklist [Achenbach and Ruffle 2000]) and rating scales (e.g., SNAP-IV [revised Swanson, Nolan, and Pelham rating scale]; Collett et al. 2003). In addition, the clinician should obtain information about the family history, patient's prenatal history, developmental milestones, and medical history.

Diagnostic Controversy

ADHD diagnosis has been controversial because there are no confirmatory laboratory tests to corroborate that the diagnosis is accurate, and because the condition is treated with psychostimulants, medications deemed to be abusable by the U.S. Drug Enforcement Administration. ADHD diagnosis is further complicated because the criteria have been revised four times since 1970.

The most recent criteria appear in DSM-IV-TR (Table 2–1). ADHD covers two symptom domains (inattention and hyperactivity-impulsivity) and is subdivided into predominately inattentive, predominately hyperactive-impulsive, and combined subtypes. The DSM-IV-TR criteria for ADHD will be replaced by the DSM-V criteria, which are under development.

Because there is no laboratory test to confirm the disorder, the ADHD diagnosis must be established by history taken from multiple informants, including the child, the parents, and the teacher. The clinician should consider each of the major components of the DSM-IV-TR criteria: age at onset (before 7 years), requirement for impairment in a minimum of two settings, 6-month duration of symptoms, and a differential diagnosis that rules out other diagnostic conditions that can cause inattention, overactivity, or impulsivity. Confirmation depends on specific ADHD symptom criteria that encompass the type, duration, severity, and frequency of ADHD problems present. The clinician must confirm that the patient has at least six of nine ADHD symptoms in either or both inattention and hyperactivity-impulsivity symptom lists, answering "yes" only if the symptom occurs often (at least half the time). The symptoms must start in childhood and follow a chronic course.

Psychostimulant treatment is the most important factor in the controversy surrounding ADHD. Although psychostimulants are the most widely researched, clinically effective, and commonly prescribed treatments for ADHD, their use in children has become the focus of a major controversy. The controversy is related to their classification as drugs of abuse, which generates concern because the drugs are administered to young children for a condition that has no readily available laboratory test for validation of the diagnosis. At the 1998 Consensus Development Conference on ADHD sponsored by the National Institutes of Health (Kupfer et al. 2000), a panel concluded that stimulants are effective in reducing the defining pediatric ADHD symptoms in the short term, but that the controversy about their long-term use demands serious consideration. The panel, in its statement of consensus, noted a lack of evidence for the long-term benefits and safety; considerable risks of treatment; wide variation in prescribing practices among practitioners; and an absence of evidence regarding the appropriate ADHD diagnostic threshold above which the benefits of psychostimulant therapy outweigh the risks.

The CDC's conclusions were not as positive as those reached by the Council on Scientific Affairs of the American Medical Association. After re-

Table 2–1. DSM-IV-TR diagnostic criteria for attention-deficit/ hyperactivity disorder

A. Either (1) or (2):

(1) six (or more) of the following symptoms of **inattention** have persisted for at least 6 months to a degree that is maladaptive and inconsistent with developmental level:

Inattention

(a) often fails to give close attention to details or makes careless mistakes in schoolwork, work, or other activities

(b) often has difficulty sustaining attention in tasks or play activities

(c) often does not seem to listen when spoken to directly

(d) often does not follow through on instructions and fails to finish schoolwork, chores, or duties in the workplace (not due to oppositional behavior or failure to understand instructions)

(e) often has difficulty organizing tasks and activities

(f) often avoids, dislikes, or is reluctant to engage in tasks that require sustained mental effort (such as schoolwork or homework)

(g) often loses things necessary for tasks or activities (e.g., toys, school assignments, pencils, books, or tools)

(h) is often easily distracted by extraneous stimuli

(i) is often forgetful in daily activities

(2) six (or more) of the following symptoms of **hyperactivity-impulsivity** have persisted for at least 6 months to a degree that is maladaptive and inconsistent with developmental level:

Hyperactivity

(a) often fidgets with hands or feet or squirms in seat

(b) often leaves seat in classroom or in other situations in which remaining seated is expected

(c) often runs about or climbs excessively in situations in which it is inappropriate (in adolescents or adults, may be limited to subjective feelings of restlessness)

(d) often has difficulty playing or engaging in leisure activities quietly

(e) is often "on the go" or often acts as if "driven by a motor"

(f) often talks excessively

Impulsivity

(g) often blurts out answers before questions have been completed

(h) often has difficulty awaiting turn

(i) often interrupts or intrudes on others (e.g., butts into conversations or games)

Table 2–1. DSM-IV-TR diagnostic criteria for attention-deficit/
hyperactivity disorder *(continued)*

B. Some hyperactive-impulsive or inattentive symptoms that caused impairment
were present before age 7 years.

C. Some impairment from the symptoms is present in two or more settings (e.g., at
school [or work] and at home).

D. There must be clear evidence of clinically significant impairment in social,
academic, or occupational functioning.

E. The symptoms do not occur exclusively during the course of a pervasive
developmental disorder, schizophrenia, or other psychotic disorder and are not
better accounted for by another mental disorder (e.g., mood disorder, anxiety
disorder, dissociative disorder, or a personality disorder).

Code based on type:
  314.01 Attention-Deficit/Hyperactivity Disorder, Combined Type: if both
  Criteria A1 and A2 are met for the past 6 months
  **314.00 Attention-Deficit/Hyperactivity Disorder, Predominantly
  Inattentive Type:** if Criterion A1 is met but Criterion A2 is not met for
  the past 6 months
  **314.01 Attention-Deficit/Hyperactivity Disorder, Predominantly
  Hyperactive-Impulsive Type:** if Criterion A2 is met but Criterion A1 is not met
  for the past 6 months

  Coding note: For individuals (especially adolescents and adults) who currently
  have symptoms that no longer meet full criteria, "In Partial Remission" should be
  specified.

viewing hundreds of trials involving thousands of patients, the council concluded that "the risk-benefit ratio of stimulant treatment in ADHD must be
evaluated and monitored on an ongoing basis in each case, but in general is
highly favorable" (Goldman et al. 1998, p. 1106).

Treatment of ADHD

Fortunately, ADHD responds to both psychosocial and psychopharmacological treatments (Richters et al. 1995). Between 2% and 2.5% of all school-age
children in North America receive some pharmacological intervention for
hyperactivity (Bosco and Robin 1980), and more than 90% of those are treated

with the psychostimulant methylphenidate (Wilens and Biederman 1992). If all ADHD medication treatments are included, over 4 million people—which includes 2.5 million children younger than 18 years and 1.5 million older than 18 years—in the United States take pills every day to alleviate ADHD symptoms. Estimates (Swanson et al. 1995a) suggest that from 1990 to 1993, the number of outpatient visits for ADHD increased from 1.6 million to 4.2 million per year, and the amount of methylphenidate manufactured increased from 1,784 to 5,110 kg per year.

Psychostimulants produce a robust response, reducing core ADHD symptoms within 30 minutes of administration when the proper dose is given to a patient. This rapid and robust response explains, to some degree, why published drug research in the past four decades has focused mainly on studying stimulants (Vitiello and Jensen 1995). Rather than explore novel compounds, academic researchers have relied on either methylphenidate or amphetamines to study response patterns, adverse events, determination of "normalization" during drug treatment, and patient characteristics among nonresponders.

Stimulant Treatment

Psychopharmacological treatment of ADHD should begin with medications approved by the U.S. Food and Drug Administration (FDA) (Table 2–2). These medications have been tested for short-term efficacy and safety in at least two different randomized controlled trials (RCTs). Including generic preparations, 10 racemic (*d-,l-*) methylphenidate, 2 dexmethylphenidate, 2 dextroamphetamine, 3 mixed salts of amphetamine, and 1 atomoxetine medication have been approved for children, ages 6–12 (Table 2–2). Of these preparations, dexmethylphenidate, OROS methylphenidate, and atomoxetine have received a separate approval for ADHD treatment in adults.

Stimulants are highly effective in reducing ADHD symptoms. Meta-analyses of 62 three-month (or less) methylphenidate treatment RCTs revealed large effect sizes (SD = 0.8) when ratings were made by teachers and moderate effect sizes (SD = 0.5) when ratings were made by parents (Schachter et al. 2001). Six methylphenidate treatment RCTs involving adults with ADHD ($N = 140$) reported large effect sizes (0.9) when patients were rated by their physicians (Faraone et al. 2004).

Three groups of stimulants are currently approved by the FDA for ADHD treatment in the pediatric population. These medications are available in both brand and generic formulations: amphetamines (Adderall, Vyvanse, Dextrostat, and Dexedrine), methylphenidates (Concerta, Metadate ER, Metadate CD, methylphenidate, Methylin, Ritalin, Ritalin-SR, Ritalin LA, transdermal methylphenidate, and Focalin), and magnesium pemoline (Cylert). Their individual characteristics are described in Table 2–2. Dextroamphetamine and methylphenidate are structurally related to the catecholamines (dopamine and norepinephrine) (McCracken 1991). The term *psychostimulant* used for these compounds refers to their ability to increase CNS activity in some but not all brain regions.

Compared with placebo, psychostimulants have a significantly greater ability to reduce ADHD symptoms, such as overactivity (e.g., fidgetiness and off-task behavior during direct observation), and to eliminate behavior that disrupts the classroom (e.g., constant requests of the teacher during direct observation) (Jacobvitz et al. 1990). In experimental settings, stimulants have been shown to improve child behavior during parent–child interactions (Barkley and Cunningham 1979) and problem-solving activities with peers (Whalen et al. 1989). The behavior of children with ADHD has a tendency to elicit negative, directive, and controlling behavior from parents and peers (Campbell 1973). When these children are started on a regimen of stimulants, their mothers' rate of disapproval, commands, and control diminishes to the extent seen between mothers and their children who do not have ADHD (Barkley and Cunningham 1979; Barkley et al. 1984; Humphries et al. 1978). In the laboratory, stimulant-treated children with ADHD demonstrate major improvements during experimenter-paced continuous performance tests (Halperin et al. 1992), paired-associate learning, cued and free recall, auditory and reading comprehension, spelling recall, and arithmetic computation (Pelham and Bender 1982; Stephens et al. 1984). Some studies show correlations between methylphenidate plasma levels and performance on a laboratory task, but plasma levels rarely correlate with clinical response. Likewise, hyperactive conduct-disordered children and pre-adolescents show reductions in aggressive behavior when treated with stimulants, as observed in structured and unstructured school settings (Hinshaw 1991). Stimulants also can reduce the display of covert antisocial behaviors such as stealing and property destruction (Hinshaw et al. 1992).

Table 2–2. Medications used in the treatment of attention-deficit/hyperactivity disorder

Medication	Duration of action	Pediatric		Adult	
		Starting dose	Typical dose	Starting dose	Typical dose
Dexmethylphenidate					
Focalin (Novartis)	6 hours[a]	2.5 mg A.M.	5 mg bid	2.5 mg bid	10 mg bid
Focalin XR (Novartis)	8–12 hours; dual pulse	5 mg A.M.	10 mg A.M.	5 mg A.M.	20 mg A.M.
d,l-Methylphenidate					
Short-acting (immediate release)	3–5 hours				
Methylin Oral Solution (Mallinckrodt)		5 mg tid	10 mg tid	10 mg bid	20 mg tid
Methylin Chewable Tablets (Mallinckrodt)		5 mg tid	10 mg tid	10 mg bid	20 mg tid
Intermediate-acting	3–8 hours				
Metadate ER (Celltech)	Single pulse	10 mg bid	30 mg A.M.	10 mg bid	80 mg A.M.
Methylin ER (Mallinckrodt)	Single pulse	10 mg bid	30 mg A.M.	10 mg bid	80 mg A.M.
Ritalin-SR (Novartis)	Single pulse	20 mg A.M.	40 mg	20 mg A.M.	80 mg A.M.
Long-acting	8–12 hours				
Metadate CD (Celltech)	8–10 hours; dual pulse	10 mg A.M.	30 mg A.M.	20 mg A.M.	80 mg A.M.
Concerta (McNeil)	8–12 hours; ascending single pulse	18 mg A.M.	36 mg A.M.	18 mg A.M.	72 mg A.M.
Ritalin LA (Novartis)	8–10 hours; dual pulse	10 mg A.M.	30 mg A.M.	10 mg A.M.	80 mg A.M.
Daytrana (Shire)	10–12 hours; transdermal single pulse	10 mg patch qd×9 hours, off 15 hours	30 mg patch qd×9 hours, off 15 hours	10 mg patch qd×9 hours, off 15 hours	60 mg patch qd×9 hours, off 15 hours

Table 2–2. Medications used in the treatment of attention-deficit/hyperactivity disorder *(continued)*

Medication	Duration of action	Pediatric		Adult	
		Starting dose	Typical dose	Starting dose	Typical dose
d-Amphetamine					
Short-acting	4–6 hours				
Dextrostat generic		5 mg bid	10 mg bid	5 mg bid	15 mg bid
Dexedrine (GlaxoSmithKline)		5 mg bid	10 mg bid	5 mg bid	15 mg bid
Long-duration	6–8 hours				
Dexedrine Spansules (GlaxoSmithKline)		5 mg A.M.	15 mg A.M.	5 mg A.M.	30 mg A.M.
Amphetamine mixed salts					
Generic	4–6 hours	5 mg bid	10 mg bid	5 mg bid	15 mg bid
Adderall (Shire)		5 mg bid	10 mg bid	5 mg bid	10 mg bid
Adderall XR (Shire)	8–10 hours; dual pulse	5 mg A.M.	30 mg A.M.	5 mg A.M.	60 mg A.M.
Nonstimulant					
Atomoxetine (Eli Lilly)	24 hours	0.5 mg/kg/day, in divided doses (bid)	1.2 mg/kg/day, in divided doses (bid)	40 mg/day, in divided doses (bid)	100 mg/day, in divided doses (bid)

[a]Limited data.

No single theory explains the psychostimulant mechanism of action on the CNS that ameliorates ADHD symptoms. The theory that the drug's effect is based on a single neurotransmitter has been discounted (Zametkin and Rapoport 1987), as has the belief in the drug's ability to correct the ADHD child's under- or overaroused CNS (Solanto 1984). A two-part theory of stimulant action has been postulated (McCracken 1991), in which stimulants increase dopamine release, producing enhanced autoreceptor-mediated inhibition of ascending dopamine neurons, while simultaneously increasing adrenergic-mediated inhibition of the noradrenergic locus coeruleus via epinephrine activity. This theory awaits confirmation from basic research in animals and imaging studies in humans.

Brain imaging has reported few consistent psychostimulant effects on glucose metabolism. Although some studies in ADHD adults using positron emission tomography (PET) and ^{18}F-labeled fluorodeoxyglucose have shown that stimulants lead to increased brain glucose metabolism in the striatal and frontal regions (Ernst and Zametkin 1995), others (Matochik et al. 1993, 1994) have been unable to find a change in glucose metabolism during acute and chronic stimulant treatment.

Psychostimulants are thought to release catecholamines and block their reuptake. Methylphenidate, like cocaine, has affinity for the dopamine transporter (DAT), and DAT blockade is now regarded as the putative mechanism for psychostimulant action in the human CNS. PET scan data show that ^{11}C-labeled methylphenidate concentration in brain is maximal in striatum, an area rich in dopamine terminals where DAT resides (Volkow et al. 1995). These PET scans reveal a significant difference in the pharmacokinetics of ^{11}C]methylphenidate and ^{11}C]cocaine (Volkow et al. 1995). Although both drugs display rapid uptake into striatum, methylphenidate is cleared more slowly from brain. The authors speculate that this low reversal of binding to the DAT means that methylphenidate is not as reinforcing as cocaine and, therefore, does not lead to as much self-administration as cocaine. More recently, the same authors (Volkow et al. 2001) were able to show that therapeutic doses of oral methylphenidate significantly increase extracellular dopamine in the human brain: "DA decreases the background firing rates and increases signal-to-noise in target neurons[;] we postulate that the amplification of weak DA signals in subjects with ADHD by methylphenidate would enhance task-specific signaling, improving attention and decreasing distractibility" (p. 1).

One of the most important findings in the stimulant treatment literature is the high degree of short-term efficacy results for *behavioral* targets, with weaker effects shown for *cognition and learning*. Conners (personal communication, 1993) notes that 0.8, 1.0, and 0.9 effect sizes are reported for behavioral improvements in the Type 4 meta-analytic reviews of stimulant drug actions (Kavale 1982; Ottenbacher and Cooper 1983; Thurber and Walker 1983). These behavioral responses to stimulant treatment, when compared with placebo, resemble the treatment efficacy of antibiotics. Less powerful effects are found for laboratory measures of cognitive changes, in particular on the continuous performance task, for which the effect size was 0.6 and 0.5 for omissions and commissions, respectively, in a within-subject design (Milich et al. 1989); and 0.6 and 1.8 in a between-subject study (Schechter and Keuezer 1985).

Psychostimulants continue to show behavioral efficacy in the Type 1 RCTs published since 1985 (Table 2–3). These modern-day controlled trials have matured along with the field and now utilize multiple-dose conditions with multiple stimulants (Elia et al. 1991), parallel designs (Spencer et al. 1995), and a common definition of response as normalization (Abikoff and Gittelman 1985a; Rapport et al. 1994). These studies test psychostimulants in special ADHD populations, including adolescents (Klorman et al. 1990; Wilens et al. 2006), adults (Spencer et al. 1995), mentally retarded subjects (Horn et al. 1991), and ADHD subjects with comorbid anxiety disorders, internalizing disorders, and tic disorders (Gadow et al. 1995). As shown in Table 2–3, 70% of ADHD subjects respond to stimulants, whereas less than 13% respond to placebo (Greenhill et al. 2001).

Studies have also been conducted that attempt to evaluate stimulant nonresponders. Some drug trials (Douglas et al. 1988) report a 100% response rate in small samples in which multiple methylphenidate doses are used. Other results indicate that a trial involving two stimulants effectively lowers the nonresponse rate. Elia et al. (1991) reduced the 32% nonresponse rate of a single psychostimulant to less than 4% when two stimulants, dextroamphetamine and methylphenidate, were titrated sequentially in the same subject. However, if the sample includes children with comorbidity, the rate of medication nonresponse might be higher.

Finally, few studies have used the placebo discontinuation model, double-blind or single-blind, to determine if the child continues to respond to stimulants after 1 or more years of treatment. One study revealed that 80% of children

Table 2–3.   Controlled studies showing stimulant efficacy in attention-deficit/hyperactivity disorder (ADHD) drug treatments (N=3,125)

Study	N	Age range (years)	Design	Drug (dose)	Duration	Response	Comment
Abikoff and Gittelman 1985b	28	6–12	ADHD, controls	MPH (PB, 41 mg)	8 weeks	80.9%	Normalization in ADHD children
Barkley et al. 1989	74	6–13	Crossover (37 aggressive, 37 nonaggressive)	MPH (PB, 0.3, 0.5)	4 weeks	80%	Aggression responsive to MPH
Barkley et al. 1991	40	6–12	Crossover (23 ADHD, 17 ADHD-W)	MPH bid (5, 10, 15 mg bid); PB bid	6 weeks	ADHD, 95% ADHD-W, 76%	Few children with ADHD-W responded; need low dose
Castellanos et al. 1997	20	6–13	Crossover	MPH 45 mg bid DEX 22.5 mg bid	9 weeks	ADHD + TS	Dose-related tics at high doses
Douglas et al. 1988	19	7–13	Crossover	MPH (PB, 0.15, 0.3, 0.6)	2 weeks	100%	Linear dose-response relationships
Douglas et al. 1995	17	6–11	Crossover	MPH (0.3, 0.6, 0.9); PB	4 weeks	70% (behavior)	No cognitive toxicity at high doses; linear dose-response curves

Table 2–3. Controlled studies showing stimulant efficacy in attention-deficit/hyperactivity disorder (ADHD) drug treatments (N=3,125) *(continued)*

Study	N	Age range (years)	Design	Drug (dose)	Duration	Response	Comment
DuPaul and Rapport 1993	31	6–12	Crossover (31 ADHD, 25 controls)	MPH (20 mg); PB bid	6 weeks	78% (behavior) 61% (attention)	MPH can normalize classroom behavior; academics did not normalize in 25% of ADHD subjects
DuPaul et al. 1994	40	6–12	Crossover (12 high anxiety, 17 moderate anxiety, 11 low anxiety)	MPH (5, 10, 15 mg); PB single dose	6 weeks	High: 68% nortriptyline Moderate: 70% nortriptyline Low: 82% nortriptyline	25% of children with comorbid internalizing disorders deteriorated while taking medications; ADHD subjects with comorbid internalizing disorders less likely to experience normalization of behavior or to respond to MPH
Elia et al. 1991	48	6–12	Crossover	MPH (0.5, 0.8, 1.5); PB bid; DEX (0.25, 0.5, 0.75)	6 weeks	MPH: 79% DEX: 86%	Response rate for two stimulants: 96%

Table 2–3. Controlled studies showing stimulant efficacy in attention-deficit/hyperactivity disorder (ADHD) drug treatments (*N*=3,125) (*continued*)

Study	*N*	Age range (years)	Design	Drug (dose)	Duration	Response	Comment
Gadow et al. 1995	34	6–12	Crossover (ADHD + tic)	MPH (0.1, 0.3, 0.5); PB bid	8 weeks	MPH: 100%	No nonresponders in terms of behavior; M.D.'s motor tic ratings showed two minimal increases while subjects were taking drug; only effects over 8 weeks of treatment studied
Gillberg et al. 1997	62	6–12	Parallel	MAS (17 mg); PB bid	60 weeks	70%; 27%–40% improved	No dropouts, but only 25% placebo group at 15-month assessment
Greenhill et al. 2001	277	6–12	Parallel	Long-acting MPH; PB	3 weeks	70%	Mean total daily dose=40 mg; FDA registration
Greenhill et al. 2002	321	6–16	Parallel	MPH-MR (Metadate ER) (20, 60 mg) qd; PB tid	3 weeks	MPH-MR: 64% PB: 27%	Mean MPH-MR ER daily dose=40.7 mg (1.28 mg/kg/day)

Table 2–3. Controlled studies showing stimulant efficacy in attention-deficit/hyperactivity disorder (ADHD) drug treatments (N=3,125) (continued)

Study	N	Age range (years)	Design	Drug (dose)	Duration	Response	Comment
Greenhill et al. 2006a	165	3–5.5	Crossover	Immediate-release MPH (1.25, 2.5, 5, 7.5 mg) tid; PB tid	70 weeks	88%	Optimal immediate-release MPH dosage=14.22±8.1 mg/day (0.7±0.4 mg/kg/day); treatment effect sizes less than in school-age children
Greenhill et al. 2006b	97	6–17	Parallel	d-MPH-ER (Focalin LA) (5–30 mg) qd; PB	7 weeks	d-MPH-ER: 67.3% PB: 13.3%	Mean d-MPH-ER daily dose=24 mg
Klorman et al. 1990	48	12–18	Crossover	MPH tid (0.26); PB bid	6 weeks	MPH 60%	Less medical benefits for adolescents
Klein et al. 1997	84	6–15	Parallel	MPH bid (1.0)	5 weeks	MPH: 59%–78% PB: 9%–29%	MPH reduced ratings of antisocial behaviors

Table 2–3.   Controlled studies showing stimulant efficacy in attention-deficit/hyperactivity disorder (ADHD) drug treatments (N=3,125) (continued)

Study	N	Age range (years)	Design	Drug (dose)	Duration	Response	Comment
McGrough et al. 2006	97	6–17	Crossover	MPH transdermal system on 9 hours/day (12.5, 18.75, 25, 37.5 cm²); PB	2 weeks	79.8%	MPH transdermal system well tolerated and significantly more efficacious than PB
MTA Cooperative Group ("A 14-Month Randomized Clinical Trial of Treatment Strategies" 1999)	579	7–9	Parallel	MPH tid (<0.8)	4 weeks (14 months)	MPH: 77% DEX: 10% None: 13%	Titration trial for multisite multi-modal study; full study data for 288 subjects taking 38.7 mg MPH
Musten et al. 1997	31	4–6	Crossover	MPH bid (0.3, 0.5)	3 weeks	MPH > NA	MPH improves attention in preschoolers
Pelham et al. 1990	22	8–13	Crossover	MPH 10 mg bid; PB bid; DEX spansule 10 mg; PEM 56.25 mg qd	24 days	Stimulant: 68%	DEX spansule, PEM best for behavior; 27% did best with DEX, 18% with SR, 18% with PEM, and 5% with MPH bid

Table 2–3. Controlled studies showing stimulant efficacy in attention-deficit/hyperactivity disorder (ADHD) drug treatments (*N*=3,125) *(continued)*

Study	*N*	Age range (years)	Design	Drug (dose)	Duration	Response	Comment
Pelham et al. 1995	28	5–12	Crossover	PEM (18.75, 37.5, 75, 112.5 mg); PB od	7 weeks	PEM: 89% PB: 0%	PEM dosage of 37.5 mg/day or higher lasts 2–7 hours; efficacy and time course equal to those of MPH
Rapport et al. 1988	22	6–10	Crossover	MPH (PB, 5, 10, 15 mg)	5 weeks	72%	MPH response same in home and at school
Rapport et al. 1994	76	6–12	Crossover	MPH (5, 10, 15, 20 mg); PB bid	5 weeks	94% (behavioral) 53% (attention)	MPH normalizes behavior more than it does academic performance; higher doses better; linear dose-response curve
Schachar et al. 1997	91	6–12	Parallel	MPH (33.5 mg); PB bid	52 weeks	0.7 SD effect size	15% side effects: affective, overfocusing led to dropouts

Table 2–3. Controlled studies showing stimulant efficacy in attention-deficit/hyperactivity disorder (ADHD) drug treatments (N=3,125) (*continued*)

Study	N	Age range (years)	Design	Drug (dose)	Duration	Response	Comment
Spencer et al. 1995	23	18–60	Crossover	MPH (1 mg/kg/day)	7 weeks	MPH: 78% PB: 4%	MPH at 1 mg/kg/day led to improvement in adults equivalent to that seen in children
Swanson et al. 1998	29	7–14	Crossover	MAS (5, 10, 15, 20 mg; PB, MPH)	7 weeks	100%	Adderall peaks at 3 hours; MPH at 1.5 hours
Tannock et al. 1995a	40	6–12	Crossover	MPH 22 (0.3, 0.6); 17 ADHD-Anxiety	2 weeks	70%	Activity level better in both groups; working memory not improved in anxious children
Tannock et al. 1995b	28	6–12	Crossover	MPH (0.3, 0.6, 0.9); PB	2 weeks	70%	Effects on behavior: dose-response curve linear; but effects on response inhibition: U-shaped; suggests adjustment of dose on objective measures

Table 2–3.   Controlled studies showing stimulant efficacy in attention-deficit/hyperactivity disorder (ADHD) drug treatments (*N*=3,125) (*continued*)

Study	*N*	Age range (years)	Design	Drug (dose)	Duration	Response	Comment
Taylor et al. 1987	38	6–10	Crossover	MPH (PB, 0.2–1.4)	6 weeks	58%	Better response in children with severe ADHD symptoms
Whalen et al. 1989	25	6.3–12	Crossover	MPH (PB, 0.3, 0.5)	5 weeks	48%–72%	MPH helps, but does not normalize, peer status
Wigal et al. 2004	132	6–17	Parallel	d-MPH; d,l-MPH; PB bid	4 weeks	d-MPH: 67% d,l-MPH: 49%	Average d-MPH dose (18.25 mg) was as safe and effective as half of the average d,l-MPH dose (32.14 mg)
Wilens et al. 2006	177	13–18	Parallel	OROS-MPH (18, 36, 54, 72 mg) qd; PB	2 weeks	OROS-MPH: 52% PB: 31%	OROS-MPH well tolerated and effective in adolescents at total daily dose of up to 72 mg

Table 2–3. Controlled studies showing stimulant efficacy in attention-deficit/hyperactivity disorder (ADHD) drug treatments (*N*=3,125) (*continued*)

Study	*N*	Age range (years)	Design	Drug (dose)	Duration	Response	Comment
Wolraich et al. 2001	282	6–12	Parallel	OROS-MPH 36 mg; immediate-release MPH tid; PB	4 weeks	62%	Concerta rated effective by teachers and parents

Note.   Doses listed as mg/kg/dose, and medication is given twice daily, unless otherwise stated.
ADHD=attention-deficit/hyperactivity disorder; ADHD-W=attention-deficit disorder without hyperactivity; ANX=anxiety; DEX=dextroamphetamine; ER=extended release; FDA=U.S. Food and Drug Administration; MAS=mixed amphetamine salts (Adderall); MPH=methylphenidate; OROS-MPH= osmotic-release oral system formulation of methylphenidate; PB=placebo; PEM=pemoline.

with ADHD relapsed when switched, in a single-blind fashion, from methylphenidate to a placebo after 8 months of treatment (H. Abikoff, personal communication, 1994). Even so, these observations about the rare nonresponder do not address the rate of placebo response. More of the current industry-sponsored RCTs are parallel designs—an approach that can assess whether the placebo response emerges at some point over the entire drug trial. However, few treatment studies prescreen for placebo responders, so the percentage of actual medication responders in any sample of children with ADHD might be closer to 55%, not the 75%–96% often quoted. Furthermore, these estimates apply to group effects and do not inform the clinician about the individual patient.

Methylphenidate, Short-Acting Preparations

Pharmacokinetics.   Methylphenidate forms the active ingredient of the majority of stimulant medications prescribed in the United States. With the exception of the two dexmethylphenidate (Focalin and Focalin XR; methyl α-phenyl-2-piperidineacetate hydrochloride) products, methylphenidate is a racemic mixture composed of the *d-* and *l-threo* enantiomers. The *d-threo* enantiomer is more pharmacologically active than the *l-threo* enantiomer. Methylphenidate is thought to block the reuptake of dopamine into the presynaptic neuron in the CNS and increase the concentration of these neurotransmitters in the interneuronal space.

Methylphenidate absorption into the systemic circulation is rapid after the immediate-release tablet is swallowed, so that effects on behavior can be seen within 30 minutes. Plasma concentration reaches a peak by 90 minutes, with a mean half-life of about 3 hours and a 3- to 5-hour duration of action. Although children take one immediate-release dose just after breakfast, most will require a second dose at lunch (which for young children must be given by the school nurse), and a third dose just after school in the afternoon to prevent loss of effectiveness as well as rebound crankiness and tearfulness. Long-duration preparations have been developed in the past decade to overcome the need for multiple daily doses of methylphenidate, and these preparations are now the mainstay of practice.

Metabolism and excretion.   In humans, methylphenidate is metabolized extra-hepatically via de-esterification to α-phenylpiperidine acetic acid (PPA,

ritalinic acid), an inactive metabolite. About 90% of radiolabeled methylphenidate is recovered from the urine.

Dosage and administration.   Immediate-release tablets may be used to augment long-duration forms, such as OROS methylphenidate, in clinical practice
to provide a boost in the morning or to smooth withdrawal in the late afternoon. When used as the main ADHD treatment, immediate-release methylphenidate should be initiated at low morning doses, 5 mg for children and 10 mg
for adults. The dose should be increased every 3 days by adding noontime and
afternoon doses until the three-times-daily schedule is achieved. The dosage
should be increased through the recommended range up to 20 mg three times
daily, which is equivalent to a total daily dose (TDD) of 60 mg.

Efficacy: clinical trials.   Myriad RCTs (see Schachter et al. 2001 for meta-
analysis), in addition to a half-century of use in the community, have supported methylphenidate's safety and efficacy for ADHD treatment in youth
(Greenhill et al. 2002b; Pliszka and AACAP Work Group on Quality Issues
2007). Investigators for the National Institute of Mental Health (NIMH)
Multimodal Treatment Study of Children With ADHD (MTA) study identified immediate-release methylphenidate to be the most effective initial treatment strategy for their trial, in which 579 children, ages 7–10, with ADHD
combined-type were randomly assigned to receive methylphenidate alone,
behavior therapy alone, the combination of methylphenidate and behavior
therapy, or community care ("A 14-Month Randomized Clinical Trial of Treatment Strategies" 1999). A double-blind, placebo-controlled titration protocol
was used to titrate each MTA subject to their *best* immediate-release dose,
which was given according to a three-times-per-day dosing schedule (Greenhill et al. 1996, 2001). Similar methods were used in the NIMH Preschool
ADHD Treatment Study. This study employed a randomized clinical trial of
immediate-release methylphenidate in 165 preschool children with ADHD,
ages 3–5.5 years (Greenhill 2001). Both studies showed a response rate of
more than 75% among those exposed to methylphenidate. However, the mean
best immediate-release methylphenidate TDD varied by age, with preschoolers
doing best at a dosage of 14.4 ± 0.75 mg/day (0.75 mg/kg/day) and school-age
children in the MTA doing best at 31.2 ± 0.55 mg/day (0.95 mg/kg/day). Immediate-release effect sizes were greater in school-age children (1.2 for teachers,
and 0.8 for children at 30 mg/day) than in preschoolers (0.8 for teachers, and

0.5 for parents at 14 mg/day), but optimal total daily doses were higher in the former.

Adverse effects specifically associated with methylphenidate.   Short- and long-duration methylphenidate preparations demonstrate the same adverse-event profile during placebo-controlled randomized clinical trials. Adverse effects include delay in sleep onset, appetite loss, weight decrease, headache, abdominal pain, and new-onset tics. Other adverse effects reported as infrequent are nausea, abdominal pain, dryness of the throat, dizziness, palpitations, headache, akathisia, dyskinesia, and drowsiness. Rare but serious adverse events include angina, tachycardia, urticaria, fever, arthalgia, exfoliative dermatitis, erythema multiforme, and thrombocytopenic purpura. Also rare are tactile hallucinations (including formication), phobias of insects, leukopenia, anemia, eosinophilia, transient depression, sudden unexpected death, and hair loss. Neuroleptic malignant syndrome (NMS) has been reported very rarely and only when methylphenidate is used in combination with other drugs that are by themselves associated with NMS.

Drug–drug interactions.   Methylphenidate interacts with few medications. These include monoamine oxidase inhibitors (isocarboxazid, phenelzine, selegiline, and tranylcypromine), as well as antibiotics with monoamine oxidase–inhibiting activity (linezolid), leading to blood pressure elevations and an increase in methylphenidate serum concentrations. In addition, phenytoin, phenobarbital, tricyclic antidepressants, and warfarin increase the serum concentrations of methylphenidate. The effects of centrally acting antihypertensives (guanadrel, methyldopa, and clonidine) can be reduced by methylphenidate. NMS has been reported to occur in patients treated with both venlafaxine and methylphenidate.

Methylphenidate, Long-Duration Preparations

Despite the effectiveness of immediate-release methylphenidate, its short 3- to 5-hour duration of action necessitates midday dosing in school, which exposes children to peer ridicule. The short duration of action also requires administration by nonfamily members when children are attending after-school programs.

Long-duration methylphenidate preparations address these problems with a once-daily dosing format and have become a mainstay of clinical practice in the United States. (Biederman et al. 2002; Greenhill et al. 2002a, 2006c; McCracken et al. 2003; Pelham et al. 1999; Wolraich et al. 2001). Although most medications use methylphenidate as the active ingredient, the formulations differ in the number and shape of methylphenidate pulses they release into the blood circulation. The range of medications includes the older, single-pulse methylphenidate drugs such as Ritalin-SR; newer dual-pulse beaded methylphenidate products such as Metadate CD, Ritalin LA, and Focalin XR; and complex-release formulations such as OROS methylphenidate (Concerta).

Methylphenidate, single-pulse, sustained-release. Single-pulse, sustained-release methylphenidate formulations (Ritalin-SR and Metadate ER) are formulated in a wax-matrix preparation to prolong release. They display a slower onset of action than immediate-release methylphenidate, produce lower serum concentrations, and have a 6- to 8-hour duration of action (Birmaher et al. 1989). Clinicians regard these as less effective in practice than immediate-release or dual-pulse beaded methylphenidate or OROS methylphenidate preparations. To compensate for the reduced effectiveness of single-pulse, sustained-release methylphenidate, clinicians administer them twice daily or give them with an immediate-release tablet in the morning to compensate for the slow onset of action. Metadate ER and Methylin ER are referred to as *branded generics* because they are copies of Ritalin-SR.

Methylphenidate, beaded. The beaded methylphenidate products are an extended-release formulation with a bimodal release profile. In Ritalin LA, this profile is created by using a proprietary SODAS (Spheroidal Oral Drug Absorption System) technology involving a mixture of immediate-release and delayed-release beads. Products using SODAS technology (Ritalin LA and Focalin XR) may help young children who have difficulty swallowing pills. The capsule can be opened, and the tiny medication spheres can be sprinkled into applesauce.

Ritalin LA incorporates the SODAS technology, which encloses the active immediate-release methylphenidate into a bead. Each bead-filled Ritalin LA capsule contains half the dose as immediate-release methylphenidate beads and half as enteric-coated delayed-release beads, thus providing a two-pulse release system that mimics the use of immediate-release methylphenidate given in two doses 4 hours apart. In a single dose, Ritalin LA 10-, 20-, 30-, and 40-mg capsules provide the same amount of methylphenidate as twice-daily doses of 5, 10, 15, or 20 mg of the immediate-release preparation. Given once daily, Ritalin LA exhibits a lower second-peak concentration ($C_{max}2$), higher interpeak minimum concentrations, and less peak-to-peak trough fluctuations in serum concentration of methylphenidate than immediate-release methylphenidate tablets given 4 hours apart. This effect may be due to the earlier onset and more prolonged absorption of the delayed-release beads. The efficacy of Ritalin LA in ADHD treatment was established in one controlled trial involving 132 children, ages 6–12, who met DSM-IV (American Psychiatric Association 1994) criteria for ADHD.

Dexmethylphenidate (Focalin, Focalin XR)

Pharmacokinetics.   Dexmethylphenidate hydrochloride (Focalin) is the *d-threo*-enantiomer of racemic methylphenidate. The drug's plasma concentration increases rapidly after ingestion, reaching a maximum in the fasted state at about 1–1.5 hours postdose (Quinn et al. 2004; Wigal et al. 2004). Plasma levels of dexmethylphenidate are comparable to those achieved following single racemic immediate-release methylphenidate doses given as capsules in twice the total milligram amount.

Focalin XR is an extended-release formulation of dexmethylphenidate with a bimodal release that includes proprietary SODAS technology similar to that of Ritalin LA. Each bead-filled Focalin XR capsule contains half the dose as immediate-release beads and half as enteric-coated, delayed-release beads. In a single dose, Focalin XR 5, 10, and 20 mg capsules provide the same amount of dexmethylphenidate as Focalin at dosages of 2.5, 5, or 10 mg given twice daily. After administration of Focalin XR, the first peak was, on average, 45% higher in women, even though pharmacokinetic parameters for dexmethylphenidate after Focalin immediate-release tablets were similar for boys and girls.

Efficacy: clinical trials.   Dexmethylphenidate (5, 10, or 20 mg/day total dose), *d,l-threo*-methylphenidate hydrochloride (10, 20, or 40 mg/day total dose), and placebo, given twice daily, were compared in a multicenter, 4-week, parallel-group study of 132 patients (Keating and Figgitt 2002). Patients treated with dexmethylphenidate showed a statistically significant improvement in SNAP-ADHD teacher-rated symptom scores from baseline compared with patients who received placebo.

The effectiveness of Focalin XR was shown in a randomized, double-blind, placebo-controlled, parallel-group study of 103 pediatric patients, ages 6–17. Using mean change from baseline scores on teacher-rated Conners' ADHD/DSM-IV Scales (CADS-T), the study reported significantly greater decrease in ADHD scores for youth taking the active Focalin XR than for youth receiving placebo (Greenhill et al. 2006c). The drug's effectiveness for adult ADHD was reported in a 5-week, randomized, double-blind, parallel-group, placebo-controlled study of 221 adults, ages 18–60, who met DSM-IV criteria for ADHD on the DSM-IV Attention-Deficit/Hyperactivity Disorder Rating Scale (DSM-IV ADHD-RS). Signs and symptoms of ADHD were far fewer for adults taking 20-, 30-, and 40-mg daily doses than for those randomly assigned to receive placebo.

OROS Methylphenidate (Concerta)

Pharmacokinetics.   The OROS methylphenidate caplet utilizes an osmotic delivery system to produce ADHD symptom reduction for up to 12 hours (Swanson et al. 2004; Wolraich et al. 2001). The caplet is coated with immediate-release methylphenidate for rapid action. The long-duration component is delivered by an osmotic pump (OROS) that gradually releases the drug over a 10-hour period, producing a slightly ascending methylphenidate serum concentration curve. Taken once daily, it mimics the serum concentrations produced by taking immediate-release methylphenidate three times daily, but with less variation (Modi et al. 2000). Long-duration preparations containing the beaded dual-pulse technology have claimed greater efficacy than OROS methylphenidate for controlling ADHD symptoms in the early morning hours (Swanson et al. 2004).

Efficacy: clinical trials.   Two double-blind, placebo-controlled randomized clinical trials have tested the efficacy and safety of OROS methylphenidate compared with immediate-release methylphenidate for children with ADHD (Swanson et al. 2003; Wolraich et al. 2001). Another multisite trial showed Concerta's similar efficacy over placebo in adolescents when the upper limit of the dosage range of Concerta was extended to 72 mg/day (Wilens et al. 2006). The results show that once-daily dosing with OROS methylphenidate matches the robust reduction of ADHD symptoms for the active preparation and low placebo-response rates reported in the MTA study for methylphenidate. In addition, OROS methylphenidate has been demonstrated in a small study ($N=6$) to have a longer duration of effect in reducing ADHD-induced driving impairments in the evening than immediate-release methylphenidate given three times daily (Cox et al. 2004).

Special Methylphenidate Preparations

Methylin Chewable Tablets and Methylin Oral Solution are two forms of a short-duration branded methylphenidate generic that has been formulated for young children who have difficulty swallowing pills or capsules. Methylin Chewable Tablets show peak plasma methylphenidate concentrations in 1–2 hours (T_{max}), with a mean peak concentration (C_{max}) of 10 mg/mL after a 20 mg chewable tablet is taken. High-fat meals delay the peak by 1 hour (1.5 hours, fasted, and 2.4 hours, fed), which is similar to what is seen with an immediate-release methylphenidate tablet. Methylin Chewable Tablets are available in 2.5, 5, and 10 mg doses. Methylin oral solution is available in 5 mg/5 cc and 10 mg/5 cc strengths. There have been no large-scale clinical trials published in which Methylin Chewable Tablets or Methylin Oral Solution was used.

Transdermal Methylphenidate Preparations (Daytrana)

Methylphenidate is steadily absorbed after application of the transdermal patch, but the levels do not reach peak until 7–9 hours later, with no noticeable reduction of ADHD symptoms for the first 2 hours. Steady dosing with the patch results in higher peak methylphenidate levels than does equivalent doses of OROS methylphenidate, suggesting increased absorption. Duration of action for a 9-hour wear period is about 11.5 hours. A double-blind, placebo-controlled, crossover study conducted in a laboratory classroom showed significantly lower ADHD symptom scores and higher math test scores on active versus placebo patch for postdose hours 2 through 9 (McGough et al. 2006). Transdermal methylphenidate (Daytrana) appears to be as effective as other long-duration preparations, but adverse effects including anorexia, insomnia, and tics occur more frequently with the patch, and mild skin reactions are common.

Amphetamines

Pharmacokinetics.   As with methylphenidate, amphetamines are manufactured in the dextro isomer, as in dextroamphetamine (Dexedrine, Dextrostat) or in racemic forms, with mixtures of *d*- and *l*-amphetamine (Adderall or Adderall XR). Efficacy of these amphetamine products resembles the efficacy of the methylphenidate products in controlling overactivity, inattention, and impulsivity in patients with ADHD. Some children who experience severe adverse events associated with taking methylphenidate may respond without such problems when taking amphetamine products. Absorption is rapid, and the plasma levels of the drug peak 3 hours after oral administration. All the amphetamines are metabolized hepatically. Acidification of the urine increases urinary output of amphetamines (Greenhill et al. 2002b). Taking the medication with ascorbic acid or fruit juice decreases absorption, while alkalinizing agents such as sodium bicarbonate increase it (Vitiello 2006).

Effects of dextroamphetamine can be seen within 1 hour of ingestion, and the duration of action lasts up to 5 hours, which is somewhat longer than that of methylphenidate. Nevertheless, twice-daily administration is needed to extend the immediate-release preparation treatment throughout the school day.

Racemic Adderall and Adderall XR. Adderall and Adderall XR are amphetamine salt mixtures. Adderall XR is a dual-pulse capsule preparation that includes both immediate- and extended-release beads. There is no evidence that these mixed amphetamine salts offer any advantage over methylphenidate or dextroamphetamine, but some patients may respond to one and not to another.

Adverse Events Reported With Stimulants

Adverse events frequently reported during stimulant use include delay of sleep onset, headache, appetite decrease, and weight loss. Infrequently observed adverse effects include emotional lability and tics.

Standard Warnings

All stimulant products carry a warning in the package insert that the product should be used with care in patients with a history of drug dependence or alcoholism. In addition, there is a warning about sudden death that may be associated with preexisting cardiac abnormalities or other serious heart problems. For adults, the warning includes sudden death but also extends to stroke and myocardial infarction. Adults are also warned that they should be cautious about taking stimulants if they have preexisting hypertension, heart failure, recent myocardial infarction, or ventricular arrhythmia. Patients with preexisting psychotic and bipolar psychiatric illness are cautioned against taking stimulants because of their psychomimetic properties at high doses. Additionally, there is a warning about stimulants' ability to slow growth rates and lower the convulsive threshold in children.

Basis of Warnings About Serious, Unexpected Adverse Events Associated With Stimulant Use

Stimulant benefits have had to be weighed against reports of serious, unexpected adverse events in populations taking stimulants for ADHD treatment. These concerns arose from the FDA review of cardiovascular and psychiatric adverse events associated with approved stimulant medications. On June 30, 2005, the agency began this review by examining the passive surveillance reports associated with OROS methylphenidate (Concerta) (http://www.fda.gov/ohrms/dockets/ac/05/briefing/2005-4152b2_01_04_Concerta%20clin%20pharm.pdf). The review uncovered 135 adverse events, including 36 psychiatric adverse events and 20 cardiovascular events. In particular, the reports included 12 instances of tactile and visual hallucinations (classified under "psychosis") during OROS methylphenidate use—the same clinical phenomena seen in cases of alcoholic delirium. These OROS methylphenidate adverse event reports represent 135/1.3 million cases, and thus these events are rare and unexpected.

More worrisome were reports of 20 cases of sudden unexpected death (14 children and 6 adults) and 12 cases of stroke in patients taking mixed salts of amphetamine (Adderall XR). This led to Health Canada suspending the sales of Adderall XR (http://www.hc-sc.gc.ca/english/protection/warnings/2005/2005_01.html). Five patients had preexisting structural heart defects. The rest of the victims had "family histories of ventricular tachycardia, association of death with heat exhaustion, fatty liver, heart attack, and Type 1 diabetes." Pliszka notes that the rate of sudden, unexpected death is estimated to be 0.5 per 100,000 patient-years in patients taking mixed salts of amphetamine and 0.19 per 100,000 patient-years in patients taking methylphenidate, while the rate of sudden, unexpected death in the general population has been estimated at 1.3–1.6 per 100,000 patient-years (Liberthson 1996). However, patients with preexisting heart disease should be referred to a cardiologist before initiating stimulant treatment.

In summary, serious unexpected cardiac or psychiatric adverse events associated with taking stimulants are extremely rare. These rates are too low to prove a causal association with stimulants in patients with no history of previous heart disease. Routine electrocardiograms and echocardiograms are not indicated prior to starting stimulant treatment in patients with unremarkable medical histories and physical examinations.

Recommendations Concerning Cardiac Contraindications to Stimulant Use

It is advised that the physician prescribing stimulants first ask the patient and his or her family for a history of structural heart disease and whether they have previously consulted with a cardiologist. Known cardiac problems that raise a caution about using stimulants include tetralogy of Fallot, cardiac artery abnormalities, and obstructive subaortic stenosis. Clinicians should be alert if the patient has hypertension or complains of syncope, arrhythmias, or chest pain, because these may be indicators of hypertrophic cardiomyopathy. This condition has been associated with sudden, unexpected death.

Growth Slowdown

Growth slowdown is another infrequent psychostimulant adverse reaction. Psychostimulant-induced reduction in growth velocity has been the most consistently researched long-term side effect for this type of medication (Greenhill 1984). Even with the plethora of studies done in this area (Greenhill 1981), myriad methodological difficulties prevent an easy interpretation. Few studies employ the optimally necessary controls, which include untreated children with ADHD, a psychiatric control group, and an ADHD group receiving treatment with a class of medications other than stimulants. However, even these studies differ in the quality of compliance measures used and whether the children were taking stimulants on weekends or used the stimulants throughout the summer. One large controlled study (Gittelman-Klein et al. 1988) reported growth rate reductions among a subgroup of children, but growth may resume immediately when stimulant treatment is discontinued (Safer et al. 1975).

Most recently, growth slowdown for height and weight was reported for children with ADHD, ages 7–10, who were treated with methylphenidate at a mean dosage of 30 mg/kg/day in the MTA study (MTA Cooperative Group 2004). School-age children grew 1.0 cm less and gained 2.5 kg less than predicted from Centers for Disease Control and Prevention growth charts. Similar effects were observed for preschool children (Swanson et al. 2006), who grew 1.5 cm less height and gained 2.5 kg less weight than predicted while being treated with methylphenidate at a mean dosage of 14 mg/kg/day.

Safer and Allen (1973; Safer et al. 1972, 1975) first reported that treatment for 2 or more years with methylphenidate and dextroamphetamine could produce decrements in the rate of weight gain on age-adjusted growth rate charts. Dextroamphetamine, with a half-life of two to three times that of methylphenidate, produces more sustained effects on the rate of weight gain than methylphenidate, as well as suppressing mean sleep-related prolactin concentrations (Greenhill 1981). In methylphenidate-treated children with ADHD who were followed for 2–4 years, dose-related decreases in weight velocity were seen (Gittelman-Klein et al. 1988; Satterfield et al. 1979), with some tolerance of the suppressive effect developing in the second year (Satterfield et al. 1979). Hechtman et al. (1984) reported growth slowdown in untreated children with ADHD, suggesting that there may be differential growth in such children associated with the ADHD disorder itself. Spencer et al. (1996) detected similar differential growth for children with ADHD that could be associated with the disorder itself and not only with stimulant treatment.

The actual psychostimulant mechanism for any growth slowdown is unknown. Early theories blamed the drug's putative growth-suppressant action on its effects on growth hormone or prolactin, but research studies involving 13 children treated for 18 months with 0.8 mg/day of dextroamphetamine (Greenhill et al. 1981) and 9 children treated for 12 months with 1.2 mg/kg/day of methylphenidate (Greenhill et al. 1984) failed to demonstrate a consistent change in growth hormone release. The most parsimonious explanation for this drug effect is the medication's suppression of appetite, leading to reduced caloric intake. No study, however, has collected the standardized diet diaries necessary to track calories consumed by children with ADHD who are taking psychostimulants (Greenhill et al. 1981).

In any case, the growth effects of methylphenidate appear to be minimal. Satterfield et al. (1979) followed 110 children and found decreases in the rate of height growth during the first year of psychostimulant treatment, but this effect reversed during the second year of treatment. An initial growth loss during treatment was seen in 65 children followed to age 18, but these children caught up during adolescence and reached heights predicted from their parents' heights (Gittelman and Mannuzza 1988). These results confirm the observations by Roche et al. (1979) that psychostimulants have mild and transitory effects on weight and only rarely interfere with height acquisition. Height and weight should be measured at 6-month intervals during stimulant treatment and recorded on age-adjusted growth forms to determine the presence of a drug-related reduction in height or weight velocity. If such a decrement is discovered during maintenance therapy with psychostimulants, a reduction in dosage or change to another class of medication can be carried out.

Adverse Effects Associated With Discontinuation of Treatment With Stimulants

The most common adverse effects associated with discontinuation of stimulant treatment in controlled trials are twitching (motor or vocal tics), anorexia, insomnia, and tachycardia, with reported incident rates of approximately 1%.

Motor or vocal tics have been reported to occur in as many as 1% of children taking methylphenidate (Ickowicz et al. 1992). A controlled trial of children with ADHD and chronic tic disorder who were taking methylphenidate (Gadow et al. 1995) reported significant improvement in ADHD symptoms without consistent worsening or increase in tic frequency for all subjects. However, the TDD of methylphenidate used never exceeded 20 mg. These low doses and the short length of the 8-week study do not resemble the higher doses and longer treatment duration found in clinical practice, where tics may appear after several months of drug administration. Clinical literature has held that methylphenidate lowers the seizure threshold, although the treatment of patients with ADHD and seizures shows no change in seizure frequency (Klein 1995).

Contraindications to Stimulant Treatment

Several clinical conditions have been worsened by stimulant treatment. Florid psychosis, mania, concurrent substance abuse, Tourette's disorder, and eating disorders are common contraindications to stimulant use. More recently, structural cardiac lesions and hypertensive states have been added as reasons not to use stimulants to treat ADHD.

Stimulant Medications in Practice

In the mid-1990s, over 85% of psychostimulant prescriptions in the United States were written for methylphenidate (Safer et al. 1996; L. Williams, J. Swanson: "Some Aspects of the Efficacy and Safety of Clonidine in Children With ADHD," unpublished paper, 1996). The rate of methylphenidate prescription writing increased fourfold from 1990 to 1995. The drug's indications, pharmacology, adverse-effect profile, and usage directions are frequently highlighted in reviews (e.g., Dulcan 1990; Wilens and Biederman 1992). Methylphenidate has become the "first-line" psychostimulant for ADHD, followed by dextroamphetamine and atomoxetine (Richters et al. 1995). However, because of its liver toxicity, pemoline is no longer available in the United States. Within the group of stimulants, practitioners order methylphenidate first and dextroamphetamine second. The popularity of methylphenidate over dextroamphetamine as the first choice in psychostimulants is not supported by the literature, however. Dextroamphetamine and pemoline have identical efficacy to methylphenidate (Arnold et al. 1978; Elia et al. 1991; Pelham et al. 1990; Vyborova et al. 1984; Winsberg et al. 1974). Arnold and colleagues (2000) noted that of the 141 subjects in these studies, 50 responded better to dextroamphetamine, and only 37 responded better to methylphenidate.

Outpatient visits devoted to ADHD increased from 1.6 million per year in 1990 to 2 million visits (and 6 million stimulant drug prescriptions) in 1995 (Jensen et al. 1999). During those visits, 90% of the children were given prescriptions, 71% of which were for methylphenidate. Methylphenidate production in the United States increased from 1,784 to 5,110 kg during the same time period (Vitiello and Jensen 1997). It has been estimated that 2.8% of U.S. youth, ages 5–18, were prescribed stimulants in 1995 (Goldman et al. 1998). However, specific epidemiological surveys suggest that 12-month prescription rates for the school-age group, ages 6–12, may be higher, ranging from 6% in urban settings (Safer et al. 1996) to 7% in rural settings (Angold et al. 2000) and extending up to 10% in some communities (LeFever et al. 1999).

Psychostimulant use has increased fivefold since 1989, and this increase has raised concerns at the U.S. Drug Enforcement Administration—which regulates production of these drugs—about the risk of abuse and diversion. Increased use could be attributed to increases in ADHD prevalence, a change in the ADHD diagnosis, improved recognition of ADHD by physicians, broadened indications for use, or an increase in drug diversion and prescription for profit or abuse (Goldman et al. 1998). Analyses of managed-care data sets reveal a 2.5-fold increase in prescribing from 1990 to 1995 that can be accounted for by longer durations of treatment, inclusion of girls and patients with predominately inattention-ADHD subtype, and treatment of high school students (Safer et al. 1996). An epidemiologically based survey conducted in four communities found that only one-eighth of children diagnosed with ADHD received adequate stimulant treatment (Jensen et al. 1999); another survey, conducted in rural North Carolina, found that many school-age children taking stimulants did not meet DSM–IV criteria for ADHD (Angold et al. 2000).

Because of reports of hepatotoxicity during postmarketing surveillance by the FDA from 1975 to 1990, pemoline is no longer recommended as a first-line ADHD treatment (Burns et al. 1999). Sales of pemoline declined between 1996 and 1999, and it has been taken off most hospital formularies. Practitioners are advised to obtain informed consent using a form attached to the package insert prior to initiating treatment with pemoline and to monitor liver function via biweekly blood tests. Children with ADHD, especially those with needle phobias, may refuse the tests. Also, pemoline is more expensive than the other psychostimulants. For these reasons, practitioners are reluctant to prescribe it. However, pemoline is effective. A randomized clinical trial by Pelham et al. (1995) comparing four doses of once-daily pemoline with placebo showed a 72% rate of response for pemoline at a dosage of 37.5 mg/day.

Stimulant responsiveness or rates of side effects were originally thought to be affected by the presence of comorbid anxiety symptoms. Pliszka (1989) treated 43 ADHD subjects with methylphenidate (0.25–0.4 mg/kg and 0.45–0.70 mg/kg) and placebo for 4 weeks. The 22 ADHD subjects with comorbid anxiety symptoms showed less efficacy when active stimulant treatment was compared with placebo, as judged by teachers' global ratings, with no increase in side effects. This result might be explained by the strong placebo response in the group. Tannock et al. (1995a) reported findings from a treatment study involving 40 children with ADHD, some with ($N = 18$) and some without ($N = 22$) comorbid anxiety symptoms, in a double-blind, randomized, crossover design with three methylphenidate doses (0.3, 0.6, and 0.9 mg/kg). The two groups showed equal decreases in motor activity, but the group with comorbid anxiety did more poorly on a serial addition task and had a differential heart-rate response to methylphenidate. DuPaul et al. (1994) found that 40 children with ADHD and comorbid anxiety were less likely to respond to methylphenidate and showed more side effects for three methylphenidate doses (5, 10, and 15 mg) and placebo than children with ADHD and no comorbid anxiety. However, the study did not collect ratings for anxiety symptoms, so the direct effect of methylphenidate on such symptoms was not recorded.

Subsequent data do not support these early impressions. One controlled study (Gadow et al. 1995) that tested the methylphenidate effects in children with comorbid anxiety symptoms found equally good response in those with and those without the anxiety disorder. These divergent data leave open the question of whether comorbid anxiety symptoms predict poor response to stimulant treatment.

Predicting drug response in the individual child with ADHD is difficult. Although pretreatment patient characteristics (young age, low rates of anxiety, low severity of disorder, and high IQ) may predict a good response to methylphenidate on global rating scales (Buitelaar et al. 1995), most research shows that neurological, physiological, or psychological measures of functioning have not been identified as reliable predictors of response to psychostimulants (Pelham and Milich 1991; Zametkin and Rapoport 1987). Once a child responds, there has been no universally agreed-upon criterion for how much the symptoms must change before the clinician stops increasing the dose. Furthermore, there is no standard for the outcome measure. For example, should global ratings alone be used, or should they be combined with more "objective" academic measures, such as percentage of correct answers on completed lists of math problems? Some have advocated a 25% reduction of ADHD symptoms as a threshold, whereas others suggest that the dose continue to be adjusted until the child's behavior and classroom performance are normalized.

The concept of *normalization* has helped standardize the definition of a categorical responder across domains and studies. Studies now use normal classroom controls instead of just statistical significance to determine if the improvement from treatment is clinically meaningful. Treatment was noted to remove differences between children with ADHD and nonreferred classmates on measures of activity and attention (Abikoff and Gittelman 1985a), but not for positive peer nominations (Whalen et al. 1989). Further advances occurred when investigators used statistically derived definitions of clinically meaningful change during psychotherapeutic treatment (Jacobson and Truax 1991). Rapport et al. (1994) used this technique to calculate reliable change and normalization on the Conners' Abbreviated Teacher Rating Scale (ATRS) using national norms. They determined that a child's behavior would be considered normalized when his or her ATRS score fell closer to the mean of the normal population than to the mean of the ADHD population. Using this technique in a controlled trial of four methylphenidate doses in children with ADHD, Rapport et al. found that methylphenidate normalized behavior and, to a lesser extent, academic performance (94% and 53%). Similarly, DuPaul and Rapport (1993) found that methylphenidate normalized behavior for all children with ADHD treated but only 75% of the children for academic performance. In another study, DuPaul et al. (1994) reported that normalization in behavior and academic performance occurred less often when ADHD subjects had high levels of comorbid internalizing disorders. Swanson and colleagues (2001), applying this approach to the cumulative distribution curves on the SNAP parent and teacher behavior ratings at the end of the MTA study, found that 88% of children without ADHD, 68% of children with ADHD treated with medication plus behavior therapy, and 56% of children with ADHD treated with medication alone achieved symptom scores of 1 or less, which represent a *normal* response on those scales.

Limitations of Stimulant Treatment for ADHD

Although 3- to 7-month treatment studies carried out in groups of children with ADHD show impressive reductions in symptoms (for a review, see Schachar and Tannock 1993), clinicians must manage individual children with ADHD over years. When examined over periods greater than 6 months, children taking these medications fail to maintain academic improvement (Gadow 1983) or to improve the social problem-solving deficits that accompany ADHD. However, most long-term stimulant studies reporting lack of academic improvement have been uncontrolled, with many of the children followed not taking stimulants consistently, so it is not possible to draw conclusions about whether stimulant treatment reverses academic failure over time. In an authoritative review, Schachar and Tannock (1993) found that of the more than 100 controlled studies of stimulant efficacy in the literature, only 18 studies lasted as long as 3 months. Because the duration of ADHD treatment extends from first grade through college, there is growing interest in showing that stimulant treatment is effective over the long run.

In a dual-site multimodal treatment study (Abikoff et al. 2004) in which children were treated for more than 2 years, medication-alone treatment was as effective as combination treatment involving medication plus psychosocial interventions. However, this study did not include a no-medication group. Concern about drawing long-term conclusions from short-term benefits in the psychostimulant literature became one of the driving forces behind the implementation of the 14-month NIMH Multimodal Treatment Study of Children With ADHD ("A 14-Month Randomized Clinical Trial of Treatment Strategies" 1999; Richters et al. 1995). The study attempts to address long-term stimulant use by including a no-medication psychosocial treatment–only arm in a sample of 576 children with ADHD.

Other caveats have been expressed about psychostimulant use for ADHD treatment in children. First, if a single dose of a psychostimulant is administered in the morning, the behavioral benefits last only a few hours, during its absorption phase (Perel et al. 1991), and are often gone by the afternoon. Second, even with the new understanding about the relatively low rate of nonresponse (Elia et al. 1991), a small number of patients experience unmanageable side effects. Approximately 25% of children with ADHD are not helped by the first psychostimulant given or experience side effects so bothersome that meaningful dose adjustments cannot be made (DuPaul and Barkley 1990). Third, indications for choosing a particular psychostimulant and the best methods for adjusting the dose remain unclear, and these factors may prove confusing to the clinician and family. Although methylphenidate is regarded as the drug of choice for ADHD treatment, controlled treatment studies show no particular advantage of this medication over dextroamphetamine. Fourth, the credibility of many treatment studies is limited by methodological problems, including failure to control for prior medication treatment and inappropriately short washout periods.

In addition to the widely accepted short-term side effects of stimulants, more theoretical but still controversial concerns have been expressed. A few studies have reported problems with dissociation of cognitive and behavioral responses to methylphenidate (Sprague and Sleator 1977). Concerns have also been raised about children treated with stimulants who may develop negative self-attributions, coming to believe that they are incapable of functioning without the medication. In addition, investigators have sometimes found that stimulant effects may be influenced by the patient's IQ or age (Buitelaar et al. 1995; Pliszka 1989). It has been speculated that dose-response measures of academic performance in stimulant-treated children with ADHD may be influenced by state-dependent learning (Pliszka 1989; Swanson and Kinsbourne

1976). Finally, the possibility that stimulant medication response is related to the presence of minor physical anomalies, neurological soft signs, or metabolic or nutritional status has yet to be explored.

The practitioner may find it difficult to cull specific guidelines about dosing an individual patient from these studies involving large groups of children with ADHD. There is no universally agreed-upon method for dosing with these medications; some practitioners use the child's weight as a guideline (dose-by-weight method), and others titrate each child's response through the approved dose range until clinical response occurs or side effects limit further dose increases (stepwise-titration method). Rapport et al. (1989) showed that there is no consistent relationship between weight-adjusted methylphenidate doses and behavioral responses, calling into question the widely accepted practice in research of standardizing methylphenidate doses by weight adjustment. Dose response can be conceptualized as a simple linear function (Gittelman and Kanner 1986) in some children with ADHD and as a curvilinear pattern in others. These relationships may vary in the same child, with one type for cognitive performance and another type for behavioral domain (Sprague and Sleator 1977).

Adverse reactions to medications show the same variability and may appear unpredictable during different phases of the medication absorption or metabolic phases. Although long-term adverse reactions, such as inhibition of linear growth in children, have been shown to resolve by adulthood, no long-term, prospective studies have been published that show results of maintaining adolescents on psychostimulants through the critical period of the long bone epiphyses fuse. Therefore, more evidence remains to be gathered showing that continuously treated adolescents will reach the final height predicted from their parents' size (Greenhill 1981).

Nonstimulant Medication Treatments

Because of the controversy surrounding the use of scheduled drugs in children, clinicians and parents may prefer nonstimulant medications for the treatment of ADHD. Besides the controversy, other problems face the family with children using stimulants for ADHD. Short-acting stimulants require cooperation from school personnel for midday dosing, and this may not always be possible. Stimulants, which cause insomnia, cannot be given too late in the day. Methylphenidate's attention-enhancing effects, which last only 3–4 hours, are often needed in the late evening to help school-age children with their homework but may result in delayed sleep onset and insomnia. Adverse effects, including severe weight loss, headaches, insomnia, and tics, can also occur.

March et al. (1994) suggested that a nonstimulant may be used when there is an unsatisfactory response to two different stimulants; this is supported by the results of the studies of Elia et al. (1991). Other ADHD treatment parameters, as well as the Texas Children's Medication Algorithm Project, recommend the use of nonstimulants when stimulants cannot be used because of inadequate response, unwanted side effects, or parental preference (Pliszka et al. 2000).

Atomoxetine

Atomoxetine is a selective norepinephrine reuptake inhibitor. It is the first drug approved by the FDA to treat ADHD both in children and in adults because of its efficacy in RCTs (Michelson 2004; Michelson et al. 2001, 2002, 2003, 2004). Atomoxetine is neither a controlled substance nor a stimulant. It is rapidly absorbed, and peak serum concentrations occur in 1 hour without food and in 3 hours with food. The drug undergoes hepatic metabolism with cytochrome P450 2D6 isozyme (CYP2D6), and is then glucuronidated and excreted in urine. Plasma elimination half-life averages 5 hours for most patients. However, 5%–10% of patients have a polymorphism for the allele that codes for CYP2D6, and for them the half-life of atomoxetine can be as long as 24 hours. The pharmacodynamics differ from the pharmacokinetics in that the duration of action in reducing symptoms of ADHD is much longer than the pharmacokinetic half-life, so ADHD symptom can be managed with once-daily dosing. Atomoxetine also can be given in the evening, whereas stimulants cannot. It is valued as a treatment for patients who have not responded to or cannot tolerate stimulants, or for those who do not want treatment with a schedule II stimulant ("Atomoxetine [Strattera] for ADHD" 2003).

Efficacy.   Atomoxetine's effect size in reducing symptoms of ADHD was calculated to be 0.7, which indicates a medium effect size. This calculation was borne out in a double-blind, placebo-controlled treatment study by significantly higher response rates in patients who were randomly assigned to immediate-release stimulants (0.91) versus once-daily atomoxetine (0.62) (Faraone et al. 2003). In practice, some clinicians have been concerned by the low numbers of children with ADHD responding to atomoxetine.

Dosage and administration.   Atomoxetine is available in 10-, 18-, 25-, 40-, and 60-mg capsules. To limit adverse events, youth weighing 70 kg or less should have the medication started at 0.5 mg/kg/day in divided doses, with the dosage increased after 1 week to a target of 1.2 mg/kg/day. The maximum TDD is 1.4 mg/kg or 100 mg, whichever is less. Patients with hepatic dysfunction should take half the usual dose.

Drug interactions.   Atomoxetine and monoamine oxidase inhibitors should not be used together or within 2 weeks of each other. The initial dose of atomoxetine should not be increased rapidly if the patient is taking a potent CYP2D6 inhibitor, such as fluoxetine (Prozac).

Adverse events.   Somnolence, nausea, decreased appetite, and vomiting have occurred in children starting atomoxetine, particularly when the dose is increased from the initial to top levels within 3 days. Slow metabolizers displayed higher rates of decreased appetite. The FDA has added two warnings to the atomoxetine package insert instructions. The first warning, added on December 17, 2004, was based on reports of severe liver injury and jaundice in two patients (one adult and one child). The FDA warned that atomoxetine should be discontinued in patients who develop jaundice or have dark urine or who have laboratory evidence of liver injury. A second warning, added in September 29, 2005, was based on the report by Eli Lilly stating that 5 of 1,800 youth in atomoxetine trials spontaneously reported suicidal ideation, while none of the youth randomly assigned to placebo made such reports. The FDA required that atomoxetine's label carry a black box warning about its possible association with suicidality. It is noteworthy that both warnings are based on spontaneous reports, not systematically elicited adverse events.

Bupropion

Bupropion, an antidepressant with noradrenergic activity, has been reported to be effective for some ADHD symptoms in placebo-controlled trials (Casat et al. 1989; Clay et al. 1988; Simeon et al. 1986). Barrickman et al. (1995) reported that bupropion was equivalent to methylphenidate in the treatment of 15 children with ADHD, who showed equal improvements from both medications on the Clinical Global Impression Scale, Conners' teacher and parent rating scales, and Continuous Performance Test, as well as ratings of anxiety and depression. The study showed an order effect that suggested a carryover from one drug condition to the next. Also, subjects were not assigned to receive placebo in the crossover, so the study was not placebo controlled. The multisite, double-blind, placebo-controlled trial of bupropion revealed that teachers could detect a reduction of ADHD symptoms at a significant level but that parents could not (Conners et al. 1996). This finding suggests that bupropion is a second-line agent for ADHD treatment.

Clonidine and Guanfacine

Clonidine is an α_2 presynaptic receptor agonist indicated for adult hypertension. The drug has been touted as a nonstimulant treatment for aggressive children with ADHD, although much of its popularity among practitioners and families for ADHD treatment may be based on its sedating effects, which are useful for countering stimulant-related insomnia (Wilens et al. 1994). However, in a review, Swanson et al. (1995b) found a fivefold increase in physicians writing clonidine prescriptions for children with ADHD from 1990 to 1995. Safety and efficacy issues have not been addressed for this age group. Only one small controlled study of 10 children with ADHD (Hunt et al. 1985) suggests that clonidine may be effective for ADHD treatment, showing results of reduction in hyperactivity and aggression. Another review (L. Williams, J. Swanson, "Some Aspects of the Efficacy and Safety of Clonidine in Children With ADHD," unpublished paper, 1996) shows that publications mention only 124 clonidine-treated children, 42 with ADHD, 74 with Tourette's disorder, and 8 with early infantile autism. Improvements averaged 22.9% for parent ADHD ratings in the five published studies of ADHD children.

Connor conducted a pilot study comparing methylphenidate, clonidine, or their combination in 24 children with ADHD and comorbid aggression and either oppositional defiant disorder or conduct disorder (Connor et al. 2000). Although all groups showed improvement, the group taking clonidine showed a decrease in fine motor speed. Connor et al. (1999), in reviewing this clonidine study and others in a meta-analysis, concluded that clonidine has a moderate effect size of 0.56 on ADHD symptoms in children and adolescents with comorbid conduct disorder, developmental delay, and tic disorders.

Although Connor concluded that clonidine may be an effective second-tier treatment for ADHD symptoms, its clinical use is associated with many side effects. This finding was seconded by reports coming into the FDA's MedWatch postmarketing surveillance system, in which 23 children treated simultaneously with clonidine and methylphenidate were reported for drug reactions, including heart rate and blood pressure abnormalities. Among that group, 4 experienced severe adverse events, including death (Swanson et al. 1995b).

Guanfacine, a similar α_2 presynaptic agonist, has been studied in two open trials involving 23 children (Chappell et al. 1995; Hunt et al. 1995), but no efficacy or safety data are available. On the basis of the results of unpublished Phase III clinical trials, a New Drug Application (NDA) was submitted to the FDA in August 2006 for an extended-release formulation of guanfacine for the treatment of ADHD in children and adolescents.

Modafinil

Modafinil is a nonstimulant with no cardiovascular effects that is used for narcolepsy treatment. It also has been used off-label for ADHD treatment. Its mechanism of action has not been determined. Some claim it may inhibit sleep-promoting neurons by blocking norepinephrine uptake ("New Indications for Modafinil" 2004). It was found to be equivalent to 600 mg of caffeine (approximately six cups of coffee) in maintaining alertness and performance in sleep-deprived healthy adults (Wesensten et al. 2002). A recent report of Stevens-Johnson syndrome in a child and visual hallucinations emerged from large sponsor-supported registration trials, after which the manufacturer withdrew their application to the FDA for a new indication for use in ADHD.

Selective Serotonin Reuptake Inhibitors

Selective serotonin reuptake inhibitors (SSRIs) enjoy a reputation for high efficacy and low adverse effects reported in adults with major depressive disorder. Castellanos found no signs of efficacy for SSRIs in the treatment of ADHD in children in the seven studies (68 children) he reviewed (X. Castellanos, "SSRIs in ADHD," unpublished paper, 1996).

Monitoring Treatment

The AACAP practice parameter for ADHD (Pliszka and AACAP Work Group on Quality Issues 2007) recommends that during a psychopharmacological intervention for ADHD, the patient should be monitored for treatment-emergent side effects. The effectiveness of regular monthly visits and dose adjustments based on tolerability and lingering ADHD symptoms was shown in the MTA study ("A 14-Month Randomized Clinical Trial of Treatment Strategies" 1999). Those assigned the medication management by NIMH protocol had significantly lower ADHD symptom scores than those followed by the providers in the community. When compared, the children in the MTA study had five times the rate of appointments, feedback from the teacher to the provider, and higher mean methylphenidate TDDs.

Monitoring can be done through direct visits between patient and provider, by phone calls with the patient and family, or even by e-mail contact. Teacher input should be sought at least once in the fall and once in the spring for ADHD patients attending primary, middle, or high school. Monitoring should follow a predetermined plan that is worked out with the patient and, if the patient is a child, with the parents as well. Generally, the schedule of monitoring visits is weekly during the initial dose adjustment phase, then monthly for the first few months of maintenance. After that, the visits can be regularly scheduled but less frequent. During the monitoring visit, the clinician should collect information on the exact dose used and the schedule according to which the stimulants were administered, including times of days. The clinician should ask about skipped doses. Questions about the common and less common and acute and long-term side effects should be raised by the clinician. At that point, the family and clinician should agree on whether the patient should continue taking the stimulant at the same dose or whether the dose should be changed. A new prescription should be written and a new appointment scheduled. The patient should leave the visit with a prescription, a plan for administration, possibly a schedule for intervisit phone contact, and the new appointment date.

The practitioner and family should agree on the pattern of stimulant treatment. One choice lies between the continuous daily administration of stimulant medications or treatment only for school days, with the patient not taking the drug on weekends and holidays. Those patients with more impairing ADHD symptoms will benefit from treatment with stimulants 365 days per year. Patients should have their need for continued treatment with stimulant medication verified once per year through a brief period of medication discontinuation. The discontinuation period should be planned for a part of the school year when testing is not in progress.

Strategies for maintaining adherence to treatment is a key monitoring component. These include the option to adjust stimulant doses to reduce treatment-emergent adverse events. When a treatment-emergent adverse event appears, the practitioner would do well to assess the impairment induced. Some adverse events may not interfere with the child's health or cause significant interruption of routine. If the adverse event worsens, then dose reduction is indicated. If the dose reduction alleviates the adverse event but leads to worsening of the ADHD symptoms, the clinician may want to consider switching the patient to another stimulant.

The AACAP practice parameter (Pliszka and AACAP Work Group on Quality Issues 2007) suggests that adjunctive pharmacotherapy can be used to deal with a troublesome adverse event when the stimulant treatment is particularly helpful. Patients with stimulant-induced delay of sleep onset may benefit from antihistamines, clonidine, or a bedtime dose (3 mg) of melatonin (Tjon Pian Gi et al. 2003). Gadow et al. (1999) found that children with ADHD and comorbid tic disorders often show a decrease in tic frequency when they begin taking a stimulant.

Choice of Medication

An international consensus statement (Kutcher et al. 2004), the AACAP ADHD practice parameter for ADHD (Pliszka and AACAP Work Group on Quality Issues 2007), the Texas Children's Medication Algorithm Project (Pliszka et al. 2006), and the American Academy of Pediatrics (2001) all recommend stimulant medications as the first line of treatment for ADHD. Direct comparisons of methylphenidate and atomoxetine in a double-blind, randomized, multisite trial (Buitelaar et al. 2007; Michelson et al. 2004; Newcorn et al. 2006) have shown a decided benefit for methylphenidate and confirm the meta-analysis by Faraone et al. (2003) that suggested methylphenidate had a larger effect size (0.91) than atomoxetine (0.62). However, atomoxetine might take precedence if the family has an aversion to stimulants or the patient has comorbid anxiety or chronic motor tics or is an adolescent or adult with a substance abuse problem.

According to the AACAP practice parameters, treatment should begin with either an amphetamine- or methylphenidate-based stimulant in long-duration formulation. The specific drug chosen can be based on its rapidity of onset, duration of action, and effectiveness for the specific patient in treatment. Short-acting stimulants can be used at first for small children and/or preschoolers if there is no long-acting preparation available in a low-enough dose. Dual-pulse methylphenidate and amphetamine products (Table 2–2) have strong effects in the morning and early afternoon, but the effects wear off by late afternoon. These drugs work best for children with academic problems at the beginning and middle of the school day, for those whose appetite is strongly suppressed, or for those whose sleep onset is delayed during stimulant treatment. Because transdermal stimulants are reported to have a higher-than-average number of adverse events, orally administered stimulants should be used first. Atomoxetine should be employed only if the family does not want treatment with a controlled substance or if the patient fails full-dose-range trials of both a long-duration methylphenidate and a long-duration amphetamine formulation.

The AACAP practice parameter for ADHD (Pliszka and AACAP Work Group on Quality Issues 2007) wisely points out that none of the extant practice guidelines should be interpreted as justification for requiring that a patient experience treatment failure (or adverse events) with one agent before allowing the trial of another.

Conclusions

Psychostimulant medications have become a mainstay in the American treatment of ADHD primarily based on their proven efficacy during short-term controlled studies. In fact, the majority of children with ADHD will respond to either methylphenidate or dextroamphetamine, so nonresponders are rare (Elia et al. 1991). Although the long-term response of children with ADHD to psychostimulants has not been examined in a controlled study much longer than 24 months (Jacobvitz et al. 1990), anecdotal reports suggest that children relapse when their medication is withdrawn and respond when it is restarted. Optimal treatment involves initial titration to an optimal dose, followed by regular appointments, and a clinician who remains in regular contact with the teacher or school (Greenhill et al. 2001).

The effects of psychostimulants are rapid, dramatic, and normalizing. The risk of long-term side effects remains low, and no substantial impairments have emerged to lessen the remarkable therapeutic benefit-risk ratio of these medications. More expensive and demanding treatments, including behavior modification and cognitive-behavioral therapies, have, at best, only equaled psychostimulant treatment. The combination of behavioral and medication therapies is only slightly more effective than medication alone in reducing ADHD symptoms ("A 14-Month Randomized Clinical Trial of Treatment Strategies" 1999). The NIMH MTA Follow-Up Study will test whether combined treatment results in better long-term functioning and decreased appearance of comorbid conditions than monomodal treatment with psychostimulants alone.

Psychostimulant treatment research has also flourished, but there is ample opportunity for more studies. Not all patients respond to psychostimulants, and this is particularly true in patients with comorbid psychiatric disorders. It is also important to determine medication effects on the acquisition of social skills in children with ADHD (Hinshaw 1991). The aim of the new psychopharmacological studies will be to target populations with comorbid disorders (e.g., children with ADHD and comorbid anxiety disorder) and to examine differential responses to medications in these patients versus those without additional psychiatric diagnoses.

Clinical Pearls

• ADHD is characterized by a persistent, developmentally inappropriate pattern of gross motor overactivity, inattention, and impulsivity that impairs academic, social, and family functioning. The disorder has three subtypes: predominately hyperactive/impulsive, predominately inattentive, and combined. The patient must experience at least six of nine symptoms in either or both the inattention and hyperactivity/impulsivity symptom lists, giving positive endorsement only if the symptom occurs often (at least half of the time). The symptoms must start in childhood and have a chronic course. Two-thirds of young children with ADHD also meet criteria for other childhood psychiatric disorders, including anxiety, depressive, oppositional defiant disorder, conduct disorder, and mood disorders.

• Because of the high prevalence of ADHD, screening for ADHD should be included in routine mental health assessments. This can be accomplished by asking questions about inattention, impulsivity, and hyperactivity, and whether such symptoms cause impairment.

- ADHD responds to both psychosocial and psychopharmacological treatments. Medication treatment should begin with either an amphetamine or a methylphenidate-based stimulant in a long-duration formulation. The specific drug chosen can be based on its rapidity of onset, duration of action, and effectiveness in the specific patient under treatment. Short-acting stimulants can be used at first for small children and/or preschoolers if there is no long-acting preparation available in a low-enough dose. Dual-pulse methylphenidate and amphetamine products have strong effects in the morning and early afternoon, but the effects wear off by late afternoon. Because transdermal stimulants are reported to have higher-than-average number of adverse events, orally administered stimulants should be used first. Atomoxetine should only be employed if the family does not want treatment with a controlled substance, or if the patient fails full-dose range trials of both long-duration methylphenidate and long-duration amphetamine formulation.

- Psychostimulants produce a robust response, reducing core ADHD symptoms within 30 minutes of administration when the proper dose is given to a patient. One of the most important findings in the stimulant treatment literature is the high degree of short-term efficacy for *behavioral* targets, with weaker effects for cognition and learning.

- There is no universally agreed-upon method for dosing with stimulants; some practitioners use the child's weight as a guideline (*dose-by-weight* method), and others titrate each child's response through the approved dose range until clinical response occurs or side effects limit further dose increases (*stepwise-titration* method).

- Methylphenidate is the active ingredient of the majority of stimulant medications. Its absorption into the systemic circulation is rapid, with the effects on behavior seen within 30 minutes of medication administration. Because of the short, 3- to 5-hour duration of action, multiple dosing is usually required. Long-duration preparations have been developed, and they are now the mainstay of practice. Their main difference from short-acting forms is in the number and shape of the methylphenidate pulses released into the blood circulation. They include older single-pulse methylphenidate drugs, such as Ritalin SR; newer dual-pulse beaded methylphenidate products, such as Metadate CD, Ritalin LA, and Focalin-XR; as well as complex-release formulations, such as OROS-MPH (Concerta). Special preparations such as Methylin Chewable and Methylin Solution are short-duration, branded methylphenidate generics formulated for young children who cannot swallow pills or capsules. Transdermal methylphenidate (Daytrana) appears to be as effective as other long-duration methylphenidate preparations, but it is associated with more frequent adverse events.

- Amphetamines are manufactured in the dextro isomer, as in dextroamphetamine (Dexedrine, Dextrostat), or in racemic forms with mixtures of *d*- and *l*-amphetamine (Adderall or Adderall XR). Efficacy of these amphetamine products resembles that of the methylphenidate products for controlling overactivity, inattention, and impulsivity. Some children who experience severe adverse events associated with methylphenidate may respond without such problems when taking amphetamines. The duration of action of amphetamines is somewhat longer than that of methylphenidate. Nevertheless, twice-daily administration is needed to extend the immediate-release preparation treatment throughout the day.

- Short- and long-duration stimulant preparations demonstrate the same adverse events, including delay in sleep onset, appetite loss, weight decrease, headache, abdominal pain, and new-onset tics. Infrequent adverse effects include nausea, abdominal pain, dryness of the throat, dizziness, palpitation, headache, akathisia, dyskinesia, and drowsiness. Rare serious adverse events include angina, tachycardia, urticaria, fever, arthralgia, exfoliative dermatitis, erythema multiforme, and thrombocytopenic purpura. Also rare are tactile hallucinations, including formication, phobias of insects, leukopenia, anemia, eosinophilia, transiently depressed mode, sudden unexpected death, and hair loss. Several clinical conditions can be worsened by stimulant treatment, including florid psychosis, mania, concurrent substance abuse, Tourette's disorder, and eating disorders.

- All stimulant products carry a warning in the package insert that they should be used with care in patients with a history of drug dependence or alcoholism. In addition, there is a warning about sudden death that may be associated with preexisting cardiac abnormalities or other serious heart problems. In clinical practice, routine electrocardiograms and echocardiograms are not indicated prior to starting treatment in patients with unremarkable medical history and physical examination. It is advised that the clinician ask the patient and his or her family about a history of structural heart disease. Clinicians should be alert if the patient has hypertension or complains of syncope, arrhythmias, or chest pain.

- Growth slowdown is another infrequent psychostimulant adverse reaction. The growth effects of methylphenidate appear to be minimal and reversible. Dextroamphetamine, with a half-life two to three times that of methylphenidate, produces more sustained effects on weight velocity than methylphenidate. The actual psychostimulant mechanism for any growth slowdown is unknown. The most parsimonious explanation for this drug effect is the medication's suppression of appetite, leading to a reduced caloric intake. Height and weight should be measured at 6-month intervals during treatment and recorded on age-adjusted growth forms to determine the presence of reduction in height and weight velocity. If such a decrement is present, a reduction in dosage or change to another class of medication can be implemented.

- Nonstimulant treatment may be used when there is an unsatisfactory response to two different stimulants. It is also recommended when stimulants cannot be used because of inadequate response, unwanted side effects, or parental preference. Atomoxetine is a selective norepinephrine reuptake inhibitor that can be administered once-daily. In practice, some clinicians have been concerned by low numbers of ADHD children responding to atomoxetine. Somnolence, nausea, decreased appetite, and vomiting have occurred in children starting atomoxetine, particularly when the dose is increased from the initial to top levels within 3 days. Slow metabolizers displayed higher rates of decreased appetite. The FDA added two warnings to the atomoxetine package insert instructions. The first warning instructs patients developing jaundice or dark urine to stop atomoxetine; the second is a black box warning about a possible association of atomoxetine with suicidality.

- Other nonstimulants include bupropion and clonidine as second-line agents for ADHD treatment. Clonidine has been touted as a nonstimulant treatment for aggressive children with ADHD. Although much of its popularity among practitioners and families may be based on its sedating effects useful for counteracting stimulant-related insomnia, its clinical use is associated with many side effects.

- Modafinil is a nonstimulant with no cardiovascular effects that is used for narcolepsy treatment. It has been used off-label for ADHD treatment. The mechanism of action has not been determined. Recent reports of Stevens-Johnson syndrome and visual hallucinations emerged from large sponsor-supported registration trials, after which the manufacturer withdrew their application to the FDA for a new indication for use in ADHD.

- Optimal treatment involves initial titration to optimize dose, followed by regular appointments and the clinician's remaining in regular contact with the teacher or school. The patient should be monitored for treatment-emergent side effects. The monitoring can be done through direct visits between patient and healthcare provider, by phone calls with the patient and family, or even by e-mail contact. Teacher input should be sought at least once in the fall and once in the spring for patients attending primary, middle, or high school.

- Monitoring should follow a predetermined plan that is worked out with the patient and, if the patient is a child, with the parents as well. Generally, the schedule of monitoring visits is weekly during the initial dose adjustment phase, and then monthly for the first few months of maintenance. After that, the visits can be regularly scheduled but less frequent.

References

Abikoff H, Gittelman R: Hyperactive children treated with stimulants: is cognitive training a useful adjunct? Arch Gen Psychiatry 42:953–961, 1985a

Abikoff H, Gittelman R: The normalizing effects of methylphenidate on the classroom behavior of ADHD children. J Abnorm Child Psychol 13:33–44, 1985b

Abikoff H, Hechtman L, Klein RG, et al: Symptomatic improvement in children with ADHD treated with long-term methylphenidate and multimodal psychosocial treatment. J Am Acad Child Adolesc Psychiatry 43:802–811, 2004

Achenbach TM, Ruffle TM: The Child Behavior Checklist and related forms for assessing behavioral/emotional problems and competencies. Pediatr Rev 21:265–271, 2000

American Academy of Pediatrics, Subcommittee on Attention-Deficit/Hyperactivity Disorder and Committee on Quality Improvement: Clinical practice guideline: treatment of the school-aged child with attention-deficit/hyperactivity disorder. Pediatrics 108:1033–1044, 2001

American Psychiatric Association: Diagnostic and Statistical Manual of Mental Disorders, 4th Edition. Washington, DC, American Psychiatric Association, 1994

American Psychiatric Association: Diagnostic and Statistical Manual of Mental Disorders, 4th Edition, Text Revision. Washington, DC, American Psychiatric Association, 2000

Anderson JC, Williams S, McGee R, et al: DSM-III disorders in preadolescent children: prevalence in a large sample from the general population. Arch Gen Psychiatry 44:69–76, 1987

Angold A, Erkanli A, Egger HL, et al: Stimulant treatment for children: a community perspective. J Am Acad Child Adolesc Psychiatry 39:975–984, 2000

Arnold LE: Methylphenidate vs amphetamine: comparative review. Journal of Attention Disorders 3:200–211, 2000

Arnold LE, Christopher J, Huestis R, et al: Methylphenidate vs. dextroamphetamine vs. caffeine in minimal brain dysfunction: controlled comparison by placebo washout design with Bayes' analysis. Arch Gen Psychiatry 35:463–473, 1978

Atomoxetine (Strattera) for ADHD. Med Lett Drugs Ther 45:11–12, 2003

Barbaresi W, Katusic SK, Colligan RC, et al: How common is attention-deficit/hyperactivity disorder? Incidence in a population-based birth cohort in Rochester, Minn. Arch Pediatr Adolesc Med 156:217–224, 2002

Barkley R: ADHD and the Nature of Self-Control. New York, Guilford, 1997

Barkley RA, Cunningham CE: The effects of methylphenidate on the mother-child interactions of hyperactive children. Arch Gen Psychiatry 36:201–208, 1979

Barkley RA, Karlsson J, Strzelecki E, et al: Effects of age and Ritalin dosage on the mother-child interactions of hyperactive children. J Consult Clin Psychol 52:750–758, 1984

Barkley RA, McMurray MB, Edelbrock CS, et al: The response of aggressive and non-aggressive ADHD children to two doses of methylphenidate. J Am Acad Child Adolescent Psychiatry 28:873–881, 1989

Barkley RA, Fischer M, Edelbrock CS, et al: The adolescent outcome of hyperactive children diagnosed by research criteria, I: an 8-year prospective follow-up study. J Am Acad Child Adolesc Psychiatry 29:546–557, 1990

Barkley RA, DuPaul GJ, McMurray MB: Attention deficit disorder with and without hyperactivity: clinical response to three dose levels of methylphenidate. Pediatrics 87:519–531, 1991

Barkley RA, Fischer M, Smallish L, et al: The persistence of attention-deficit/hyperactivity disorder into young adulthood as a function of reporting source and definition of disorder. J Abnorm Psychol 111:279–289, 2002

Barrickman LL, Perry PJ, Allen AJ, et al: Bupropion versus methylphenidate in the treatment of attention-deficit hyperactivity disorder. J Am Acad Child Adolesc Psychiatry 34:649–657, 1995

Bauermeister JJ, Canino G, Bird H: Epidemiology of disruptive behavior disorders. Child Adolesc Psychiatr Clin N Am 3:177–194, 1994

Biederman J, Newcorn J, Sprich S: Comorbidity of attention-deficit/hyperactivity disorder with conduct, depressive, anxiety, and other disorders. Am J Psychiatry 148:564–577, 1991

Biederman J, Faraone S, Milberger S, et al: A prospective 4-year follow-up study of attention-deficit hyperactivity and related disorders. Arch Gen Psychiatry 53:437–446, 1996

Biederman J, Lopez FA, Boellner SW, et al: A randomized, double-blind, placebo-controlled, parallel-group study of SLI381 (Adderall XR) in children with attention-deficit/hyperactivity disorder. Pediatrics 110:258–266, 2002

Bird HR, Canino G, Rubio-Stipec M, et al: Estimates of the prevalence of childhood maladjustment in a community survey in Puerto Rico: the use of combined measures. Arch Gen Psychiatry 45:1120–1126, 1988

Birmaher B, Greenhill LL, Cooper TB, et al: Sustained release methylphenidate: pharmacokinetic studies in ADHD males. J Am Acad Child Adolesc Psychiatry 28:768–772, 1989

Bosco J, Robin S: Hyperkinesis: prevalence and treatment, in Hyperkinetic Children: The Social Ecology of Identification and Treatment. Edited by Whalen C, Henker B. New York, Academic Press, 1980

Buitelaar JK, Van der Gaag RJ, Swaab-Barneveld H, et al: Prediction of clinical response to methylphenidate in children with attention-deficit hyperactivity disorder. J Am Acad Child Adolesc Psychiatry 34:1025–1032, 1995

Buitelaar JK, Michelson D, Danckaerts M, et al: A randomized, double-blind study of continuation treatment for attention-deficit/hyperactivity disorder after 1 year. Biol Psychiatry 61:694–699, 2007

Burns BJ, Hoagwood K, Mrazek PJ: Effective treatment for mental disorders in children and adolescents. Clin Child Family Psychol Rev 2:199–254, 1999

Campbell S: Mother-child interaction in reflective, impulsive, and hyperactive children. Dev Psychol 8:341–349, 1973

Casat CD, Pleasants DZ, Schroeder D, et al: Bupropion in children with attention deficit disorder. Psychopharmacol Bull 25:198–201, 1989

Castellanos FX, Giedd JN, Elia J, et al: Controlled stimulant treatment of ADHD and comorbid Tourette's syndrome: effects of stimulant and dose. J Am Acad Child Adolesc Psychiatry 36:589–596, 1997

Chappell PB, Riddle MA, Scahill L, et al: Guanfacine treatment of comorbid attention-deficit hyperactivity disorder and Tourette's syndrome: preliminary clinical experience. J Am Acad Child Adolesc Psychiatry 34:1140–1146, 1995

Clay T, Gualtieri C, Evans P, et al: Clinical and neurophysiological effects of the novel antidepressant bupropion. Psychol Bull 24:143–148, 1988

Collett BR, Ohan JL, Myers KM: Ten-year review of rating scales, V: scales assessing attention-deficit/hyperactivity disorder. J Am Acad Child Adolesc Psychiatry 42:1015–1037, 2003

Connell H, Irvine L, Rodney J: Psychiatric disorder in Queensland primary school children. Aust Paediatr J 18:177–180, 1982

Conners CK, Casat CD, Gualtieri CT, et al: Bupropion hydrochloride in attention deficit disorder with hyperactivity. J Am Acad Child Adolesc Psychiatry 35:1314–1321, 1996

Connor DF, Fletcher KE, Swanson JM: A meta-analysis of clonidine for symptoms of attention-deficit hyperactivity disorder. J Am Acad Child Adolesc Psychiatry 38:1551–1559, 1999

Connor DF, Barkley RA, Davis HT: A pilot study of methylphenidate, clonidine, or the combination in ADHD comorbid with aggressive oppositional defiant or conduct disorder. Clin Pediatr 39:15–25, 2000

Costello EJ: Child psychiatric disorders and their correlates: a primary care pediatric sample. J Am Acad Child Adolesc Psychiatry 28:851–855, 1989

Costello EJ, Mustillo S, Erkanli A, et al: Prevalence and development of psychiatric disorders in childhood and adolescence. Arch Gen Psychiatry 60:837–844, 2003

Cox DJ, Merkel RL, Penberthy JK, et al: Impact of methylphenidate delivery profiles on driving performance of adolescents with attention-deficit/hyperactivity disorder: a pilot study. J Am Acad Child Adolesc Psychiatry 43:269–275, 2004

Douglas VI, Barr RG, Amin K, et al: Dose effects and individual responsivity to methylphenidate in attention deficit disorder. J Child Psychol Psychiatry 29:453–475, 1988

Douglas VI, Barr RG, Desilets J, et al: Do high doses of stimulants impair flexible thinking in attention-deficit hyperactivity disorder? J Am Acad Child Adolesc Psychiatry 34:877–885, 1995

Dulcan M: Using psychostimulants to treat behavior disorders of children and adolescents. J Child Adolesc Psychopharmacol 1:7–20, 1990

DuPaul GJ, Barkley RA: Medication therapy, in Attention-Deficit Hyperactivity Disorder: A Handbook for Diagnosis and Treatment, 2nd Edition. Edited by Barkley RA. New York, Guilford, 1990, pp 573–612

DuPaul GJ, Rapport MD: Does methylphenidate normalize the classroom performance of children with attention deficit disorder? J Am Acad Child Adolesc Psychiatry 32:190–198, 1993

DuPaul GJ, Barkley RA, McMurray MB: Response of children with ADHD to methylphenidate: interaction with internalizing symptoms. J Am Acad Child Adolesc Psychiatry 33:894–903, 1994

Elia J, Borcherding BG, Rapoport JL, et al: Methylphenidate and dextroamphetamine treatments of hyperactivity: are there true nonresponders? Psychiatry Res 36:141–155, 1991

Ernst M, Zametkin A: The interface of genetics, neuroimaging, and neurochemistry in attention-deficit hyperactivity disorder, in Psychopharmacology: The Fourth Generation of Progress, 4th Edition. Edited by Bloom F, Kupfer D. New York, Raven, 1995, pp 1643–1652

Esser G, Schmidt M, Woerner W: Epidemiology and course of psychiatric disorders in school-age children: results of a longitudinal study. J Child Psychol Psychiatry 31:243–253, 1996

Faraone SV, Spencer TJ, Aleardi M, et al: Comparing the efficacy of medications used for ADHD using meta-analysis. Presentation at the 156th annual meeting of the American Psychiatric Association, San Francisco, CA, May 17–22, 2003

Faraone SV, Spencer T, Aleardi M, et al: Meta-analysis of the efficacy of methylphenidate for treating adult attention-deficit/hyperactivity disorder. J Clin Psychopharmacol 24:24–29, 2004

A 14-month randomized clinical trial of treatment strategies for attention-deficit/hyperactivity disorder. The MTA Cooperative Group. Multimodal Treatment Study of Children With ADHD. Arch Gen Psychiatry 56:1073–1086, 1999

Gadow KD: Effects of stimulant drugs on academic performance in hyperactive and learning disabled children. J Learn Disabil 16:290–299, 1983

Gadow KD, Sverd J, Sprafkin J, et al: Efficacy of methylphenidate for attention-deficit hyperactivity disorder in children with tic disorder. Arch Gen Psychiatry 52:444–455, 1995

Gadow KD, Sverd J, Sprafkin, J, et al: Long-term methylphenidate therapy in children with comorbid attention-deficit hyperactivity disorder and chronic multiple tic disorder. Arch Gen Psychiatry 56:330–336, 1999

Gillberg C, Melander H, von Knorring AL, et al: Long-term stimulant treatment of children with attention-deficit hyperactivity disorder symptoms: a randomized, double-blind, placebo-controlled trial. Arch Gen Psychiatry 54:857–864, 1997

Gittelman R, Kanner A: Psychopharmacotherapy, in Psychopathological Disorders of Childhood, 3rd Edition. Edited by Quay H, Werry J. New York, Wiley, 1986, pp 455–495

Gittelman R, Mannuzza S: Hyperactive boys almost grown up: methylphenidate effects on ultimate height. Arch Gen Psychiatry 45:1131–1134, 1988

Gittelman-Klein R, Landa B, Mattes JA, et al: Methylphenidate and growth in hyperactive children. Arch Gen Psychiatry 45:1127–1130, 1988

Goldman L, Genel M, Bazman R, et al: Diagnosis and treatment of attention-deficit/hyperactivity disorder. JAMA 279:1100–1107, 1998

Greenhill LL: Stimulant-relation growth inhibition in children: a review, in Strategic Interventions for Hyperactive Children. Edited by Gittelman M. Armonk, NY, M E Sharpe, 1981, pp 39–63

Greenhill LL: Stimulant related growth inhibition in children: a review, in The Psychobiology of Childhood. Edited by Shopsin B. New York, SP Medical & Scientific Books, 1984, pp 135–157

Greenhill LL: Preschool ADHD Treatment Study (PATS): science and controversy. The Economics of Neuroscience 3:49–53, 2001

Greenhill LL, Puig-Antich J, Chambers W, et al: Growth hormone, prolactin, and growth responses in hyperkinetic males treated with d-amphetamine. J Am Acad Child Adolesc Psychiatry 20:84–103, 1981

Greenhill LL, Puig-Antich J, Novacenko H, et al: Prolactin, growth hormone and growth responses in boys with attention deficit disorder and hyperactivity treated with methylphenidate. J Am Acad Child Adolesc Psychiatry 23:58–67, 1984

Greenhill LL, Abikoff HB, Arnold LE, et al: Medication treatment strategies in the MTA study: relevance to clinicians and researchers. J Am Acad Child Adolesc Psychiatry 35:1304–1313, 1996

Greenhill LL, Swanson JM, Vitiello B, et al: Impairment and deportment responses to different methylphenidate doses in children with ADHD: the MTA titration trial. J Am Acad Child Adolesc Psychiatry 40:180–187, 2001

Greenhill LL, Findling RL, Swanson JM: A double-blind, placebo-controlled study of modified-release methylphenidate in children with attention-deficit/hyperactivity disorder. Pediatrics 109:E39, 2002a

Greenhill LL, Pliszka S, Dulcan MK, et al, American Academy of Child and Adolescent Psychiatry: Practice parameter for the use of stimulant medications in the treatment of children, adolescents, and adults. J Am Acad Child Adolesc Psychiatry 41 (2, suppl):26S–49S, 2002b

Greenhill LL, Biederman J, Boellner SW, et al: A randomized, double-blind, placebo-controlled study of modafinil film-coated tablets in children and adolescents with attention-deficit/hyperactivity disorder. J Am Acad Child Adolesc Psychiatry 45:503–511, 2006a

Greenhill LL, Kollins S, Abikoff H, et al: Efficacy and safety of immediate-release methylphenidate treatment for preschoolers with ADHD. J Am Acad Child Adolesc Psychiatry 45:1284–1293, 2006b

Greenhill LL, Muniz R, Ball RR, et al: Efficacy and safety of dexmethylphenidate extended-release capsules in children with attention-deficit/hyperactivity disorder. J Am Acad Child Adolesc Psychiatry 45:817–823, 2006b

Halperin JM, Matier K, Bedi G, et al: Specificity of inattention, impulsivity, and hyperactivity to the diagnosis of attention-deficit hyperactivity disorder. J Am Acad Child Adolesc Psychiatry 31:190–196, 1992

Hechtman L, Weiss G, Perlman T: Hyperactives as young adults: past and current substance abuse and antisocial behavior. American Journal of Orthopsychology 54:415–425, 1984

Hinshaw S: Effects of methylphenidate on aggressive and antisocial behavior. Proceedings of the American Academy of Child and Adolescent Psychiatry 7:31–32, 1991

Hinshaw S, Heller T, McHale JP: Covert antisocial behavior in boys with attention-deficit hyperactivity disorder: external validation and effects of methylphenidate. J Consult Clin Psychol 60:274–281, 1992

Horn WF, Ialongo NS, Pascoe JM, et al: Additive effects of psychostimulants, parent training, and self-control therapy with ADHD children. J Am Acad Child Adolesc Psychiatry 30:233–240, 1991

Humphries T, Kinsbourne M, Swanson J: Stimulant effects on cooperation and social interaction between hyperactive children and their mothers. J Child Psychol Psychiatry 19:13–22, 1978

Hunt RD, Minderaa RB, Cohen DJ: Clonidine benefits children with attention deficit disorder and hyperactivity: report of a double-blind placebo-crossover therapeutic trial. J Am Acad Child Adolesc Psychiatry 24:617–629, 1985

Hunt RD, Arnsten AF, Asbell MD: An open trial of guanfacine in the treatment of attention-deficit hyperactivity disorder. J Am Acad Child Adolesc Psychiatry 34:50–54, 1995

Ickowicz A, Tannock R, Fulford P, et al: Transient tics and compulsive behaviors following methylphenidate: evidence from a placebo controlled double blind clinical trial. Presented at the 39th Annual Meeting of the American Academy of Child and Adolescent Psychiatry, Washington, DC, October 1992

Jacobson NS, Truax P: Clinical significance: a statistical approach to defining meaningful change in psychotherapy research. J Consult Clin Psychol 59:12–19, 1991

Jacobvitz D, Sroufe LA, Stewart M, et al: Treatment of attentional and hyperactivity problems in children with sympathomimetic drugs: a comprehensive review. J Am Acad Child Adolesc Psychiatry 29:677–688, 1990

Jensen PS, Kettle L, Roper MT, et al: Are stimulants overprescribed? Treatment of ADHD in four U.S. communities. J Am Acad Child Adolesc Psychiatry 38:797–804, 1999

Kavale K: The efficacy of stimulant drug treatment for hyperactivity: a meta-analysis. J Learn Disabil 15:280–289, 1982

Keating GM, Figgitt DP: Dexmethylphenidate. Drugs 62:1899–1904, 2002

Kessler R, Adler L, Barkley R, et al: The prevalence and correlates of adult ADHD in the United States: results from the National Comorbidity Survey Replication. Am J Psychiatry 4:716–723, 2006

Klein RG: The role of methylphenidate in psychiatry. Arch Gen Psychiatry 52:429–433, 1995

Klein RG, Abikoff H, Klass E, et al: Clinical efficacy of methylphenidate in conduct disorder with and without attention deficit hyperactivity disorder. Arch Gen Psychiatry 54:1073–1080, 1997

Klorman R, Brumaghim JT, Fitzpatrick PA, et al: Clinical effects of a controlled trial of methylphenidate on adolescents with attention deficit disorder. J Am Acad Child Adolesc Psychiatry 29:702–709, 1990

Kupfer DJ, Baltimore RS, Berry DA, et al: National Institutes of Health Consensus Development Conference Statement: diagnosis and treatment of attention-deficit/hyperactivity disorder (ADHD). J Am Acad Child Adolesc Psychiatry 39:182–193, 2000

Kutcher S, Aman M, Brooks SJ, et al: International consensus statement on attention-deficit/hyperactivity disorder (ADHD) and disruptive behaviour disorders (DBDs): clinical implications and treatment practice suggestions. Eur Neuropsychopharmacol 14:11–28, 2004

LeFever GB, Dawson KV, Morrow AL: The extent of drug therapy for attention deficit-hyperactivity disorder among children in public schools. Am J Public Health 89:1359–1364, 1999

Liberthson RR: Current concepts: sudden death from cardiac causes in children and young adults. N Engl J Med 334:1039–1044, 1996

Mannuzza S, Klein RG, Bessler A, et al: Adult outcome of hyperactive boys: educational achievement, occupational rank, and psychiatric status. Arch Gen Psychiatry 50:565–576, 1993

March J, Conners CK, Erhardt D, et al: Pharmacotherapy of attention-deficit hyperactivity disorder. Ann Drug Ther 2:187–213, 1994

Matochik JA, Nordahl TE, Gross M, et al: Effects of acute stimulant medication on cerebral metabolism in adults with hyperactivity. Neuropsychopharmacology 8:377–386, 1993

Matochik JA, Liebenauer LL, King AC, et al: Cerebral glucose metabolism in adults with attention deficit hyperactivity disorder after chronic stimulant treatment. Am J Psychiatry 151:658–664, 1994

McCracken JT: A two-part model of stimulant action on attention-deficit hyperactivity disorder in children. J Neuropsychiatry Clin Neurosci 3:201–209, 1991

McCracken JT, Biederman J, Greenhill LL, et al: Analog classroom assessment of a once-daily mixed amphetamine formulation, SLI381 (Adderall XR), in children with ADHD. J Am Acad Child Adolesc Psychiatry 42:673–683, 2003

McGough JJ, Wigal SB, Abikoff H, et al: A randomized, double-blind, placebo-controlled, laboratory classroom assessment of methylphenidate transdermal system in children with ADHD. J Atten Disord 9:476–485, 2006

Michelson D: Results from a double-blind study of atomoxetine, OROS methylphenidate, and placebo. Presented at the 51st Annual Meeting of the American Academy of Child and Adolescent Psychiatry, Washington, DC, October 2004

Michelson D, Faries D, Wernicke J, et al: Atomoxetine in the treatment of children and adolescents with attention-deficit/hyperactivity disorder: a randomized, placebo-controlled, dose-response study. Pediatrics 108(5):E83, 2001

Michelson D, Allen AJ, Busner J, et al: Once-daily atomoxetine treatment for children and adolescents with attention deficit hyperactivity disorder: a randomized, placebo-controlled study. Am J Psychiatry 159:1896–1901, 2002

Michelson D, Adler L, Spencer T, et al: Atomoxetine in adults with ADHD: two randomized, placebo-controlled studies. Biol Psychiatry 53:112–120, 2003

Michelson D, Buitelaar JK, Danckaerts M, et al: Relapse prevention in pediatric patients with ADHD treated with atomoxetine: a randomized, double-blind, placebo-controlled study. J Am Acad Child Adolesc Psychiatry 43:896–904, 2004

Milich R, Licht BG, Murphy DA, et al: Attention-deficit hyperactivity disordered boys' evaluations of and attributions for task performance on medication versus placebo. J Abnorm Psychol 98:280–284, 1989

Modi NB, Wang B, Noveck RJ, et al: Dose-proportional and stereospecific pharmacokinetics of methylphenidate delivered using an osmotic, controlled-release oral delivery system. J Clin Pharmacol 40:1141–1149, 2000

MTA Cooperative Group: National Institute of Mental Health Multimodal Treatment Study of ADHD follow-up: changes in effectiveness and growth after the end of treatment 37. Pediatrics 113:762–769, 2004

Musten LM, Firestone P, Pisterman S, et al: Effects of methylphenidate on preschool children with ADHD: cognitive and behavioral functions. J Am Acad Child Adolesc Psychiatry 36:1407–1415, 1997

New indications for modafinil (Provigil). Med Lett Drugs Ther 46:34–35, 2004

Newcorn J, Michelson D, Kratochvil C, et al: Low-dose atomoxetine for maintenance treatment of attention-deficit/hyperactivity disorder. Pediatrics 118:e1701–e1706, 2006

Ottenbacher KJ, Cooper HM: Drug treatment of hyperactivity in children. Dev Med Child Neurol 25:358–366, 1983

Pelham W, Bender ME: Peer relationships in hyperactive children: description and treatment, in Advances in Learning and Behavioral Disabilities. Edited by Gadow KD, Bialer I. Greenwich, CT, JAI Press, 1982, pp 365–436

Pelham WE, Milich R: Individual differences in response to Ritalin in classwork and social behavior, in Ritalin: Theory and Patient Management. Edited by Greenhill LL, Osman B. New York, Mary Ann Liebert, 1991, pp 203–222

Pelham WE, Greenslade KE, Vodde-Hamilton M, et al: Relative efficacy of long-acting stimulants on children with attention deficit-hyperactivity disorder: comparison of standard methylphenidate, sustained-release methylphenidate, sustained-release dextroamphetamine, and pemoline. Pediatrics 86:226–237, 1990

Pelham WE, Swanson JM, Furman MB, et al: Pemoline effects on children with ADHD: a time-response by dose-response analysis on classroom measures. J Am Acad Child Adolesc Psychiatry 34:1504–1513, 1995

Pelham WE, Aronoff HR, Midlam JK, et al: A comparison of Ritalin and Adderall: efficacy and time-course in children with attention-deficit/hyperactivity disorder. Pediatrics 103:E43, 1999

Perel JM, Greenhill LL, Curran S, et al: Correlates of pharmacokinetics and attentional measures in methylphenidate treated hyperactive children. Clin Pharmacol Ther 49:160–161, 1991

Pliszka SR: Effect of anxiety on cognition, behavior, and stimulant response in ADHD. J Am Acad Child Adolesc Psychiatry 28:882–887, 1989

Pliszka SR, AACAP Work Group on Quality Issues: Practice parameter for the assessment and treatment of attention-deficit/hyperactivity disorder. J Am Acad Child Adolesc Psychiatry 46(7):894–921, 2007

Pliszka SR, Greenhill LL, Crismon ML, et al: The Texas Children's Medication Algorithm Project: report of the Texas Consensus Conference Panel on Medication Treatment of Childhood Attention-Deficit/Hyperactivity Disorder, part II: tactics. Attention-deficit/hyperactivity disorder. J Am Acad Child Adolesc Psychiatry 39, 920–927, 2000

Pliszka SR, Crismon ML, Hughes CW, et al: The Texas Children's Medication Algorithm Project: revision of the algorithm for pharmacotherapy of attention-deficit/hyperactivity disorder. J Am Acad Child Adolesc Psychiatry 45:642–657, 2006

Quinn D, Wigal S, Swanson J, et al: Comparative pharmacodynamics and plasma concentrations of d-threo-methylphenidate hydrochloride after single doses of d-threo-methylphenidate hydrochloride and d,l-threo-methylphenidate hydrochloride in a double-blind, placebo-controlled, crossover laboratory school study in children with attention-deficit/hyperactivity disorder. J Am Acad Child Adolesc Psychiatry 43:1422–1429, 2004

Rapport MD, DuPaul GJ, Kelly KL: Attention deficit hyperactivity disorder and methylphenidate: the relationship between gross body weight and drug response in children. Psychopharmacol Bull 25:285–290, 1989

Rapport MD, Denney C, DuPaul GJ, et al: Attention deficit disorder and methylphenidate: normalization rates, clinical effectiveness, and response prediction in 76 children. J Am Acad Child Adolesc Psychiatry 33:882–893, 1994

Rapport MD, Stoner G, DuPaul GJ, et al: Attention deficit disorder and methylphenidate: a multilevel analysis of dose-response effects on children's impulsivity across settings. J Am Acad Child Adolesc Psychiatry 27:60–69, 1988

Richters JE, Arnold LE, Jensen PS, et al: NIMH collaborative multisite Multimodal Treatment Study of Children with ADHD: background and rationale. J Am Acad Child Adolesc Psychiatry 34:987–1000, 1995

Roche AF, Lipman RS, Overall JE, et al: The effects of stimulant medication on the growth of hyperactive children. Pediatrics 63:847–849, 1979

Safer DJ, Allen RP: Factors influencing the suppressant effects of two stimulant drugs on the growth of hyperactive children. Pediatrics 51:660–667, 1973

Safer D, Allen R, Barr E: Depression of growth in hyperactive children on stimulant drugs. N Engl J Med 287:217–220, 1972

Safer DJ, Allen RP, Barr E: Growth rebound after termination of stimulant drugs. J Pediatr 86:113–116, 1975

Safer DJ, Zito JM, Fine EM: Increased methylphenidate usage for attention deficit disorder in the 1990s. Pediatrics 98:1084–1088, 1996

Satterfield JH, Cantwell DP, Schell A, et al: Growth of hyperactive children treated with methylphenidate. Arch Gen Psychiatry 36:212–217, 1979

Schachar RJ, Tannock R: Childhood hyperactivity and psychostimulants: a review of extended treatment studies. J Child Adolesc Psychopharmacol 3:81–97, 1993

Schachar RJ, Tannock R, Cunningham C, et al: Behavioral, situational, and temporal effects of treatment of ADHD with methylphenidate. J Am Acad Child Adolesc Psychiatry 36:754–763, 1997

Schachter HM, Pham B, King J, et al: How efficacious and safe is short-acting methylphenidate for the treatment of attention-deficit disorder in children and adolescents? A meta-analysis. Can Med Assoc J 165:1475–1488, 2001

Schechter M, Keuezer E: Learning in hyperactive children: are there stimulant-related and state-dependent effects? J Clin Pharmacol 25:276–280, 1985

Simeon JG, Ferguson HB, Van Wyck FJ: Bupropion effects in attention deficit and conduct disorders. Can J Psychiatry 31:581–585, 1986

Solanto MV: Neuropharmacological basis of stimulant drug action in attention deficit disorder with hyperactivity: a review and synthesis. Psychol Bull 95:387–409, 1984

Spencer T, Wilens T, Biederman J, et al: A double-blind, crossover comparison of methylphenidate and placebo in adults with childhood-onset attention-deficit hyperactivity disorder. Arch Gen Psychiatry 52:434–443, 1995

Spencer TJ, Biederman J, Harding M, et al: Growth deficits in ADHD children revisited: evidence for disorder-associated growth delays? J Am Acad Child Adolesc Psychiatry 35:1460–1469, 1996

Sprague RL, Sleator EK: Methylphenidate in hyperkinetic children: differences in dose effects on learning and social behavior. Science 198:1274–1276, 1977

Stephens RS, Pelham WE, Skinner R: State-dependent and main effects of methylphenidate and pemoline on paired-associate learning and spelling in hyperactive children. J Consult Clin Psychol 52:104–113, 1984

Swanson J, Kinsbourne M: Stimulant-related state-dependent learning in hyperactive children. Science 192:1354–1357, 1976

Swanson J, Flockhart D, Udrea D, et al: Clonidine in the treatment of ADHD: questions about the safety and efficacy. J Child Adolesc Psychopharmacol 5:301–305, 1995a

Swanson J, Lerner M, Williams L: More frequent diagnosis of attention deficit-hyperactivity disorder. N Engl J Med 333:944, 1995b

Swanson JM, Wigal S, Greenhill LL, et al: Analog classroom assessment of Adderall in children with ADHD. J Am Acad Child Adolesc Psychiatry 37:519–526, 1998

Swanson JM, Kraemer HC, Hinshaw SP, et al: Clinical relevance of the primary findings of the MTA: success rates based on severity of ADHD and ODD symptoms at the end of treatment. J Am Acad Child Adolesc Psychiatry 40:168–179, 2001

Swanson J, Gupta S, Lam A, et al: Development of a new once-a-day formulation of methylphenidate for the treatment of attention-deficit/hyperactivity disorder: proof-of-concept and proof-of-product studies. Arch Gen Psychiatry 60:204–211, 2003

Swanson J, Wigal SB, Wigal T, et al: A comparison of once-daily extended-release methylphenidate formulations in children with attention-deficit/hyperactivity disorder in the laboratory school (the Comacs Study). Pediatrics 113:e206–e216, 2004

Swanson J, Greenhill L, Wigal T, et al: Stimulant-related reductions of growth rates in the PATS. J Am Acad Child Adolesc Psychiatry 45:1304–1313, 2006

Szatmari P: The epidemiology of attention-deficit hyperactivity disorders. Child and Adolescent Psychiatric Clinics 1:361–371, 1992

Szatmari P, Offord DR, Boyle MH: Ontario Child Health Study: Prevalence of attention deficit disorder with hyperactivity. J Child Psychol Psychiatry 30:219–230, 1989

Tannock R, Schachar R, Logan R: Methylphenidate and working memory: differential effects in attention-deficit hyperactivity disorder (ADHD) with and without memory. American Academy of Child and Adolescent Psychiatry Scientific Proceedings of the Annual Meeting, 9, 42, 1993

Tannock R, Ickowicz A, Schachar R: Differential effects of methylphenidate on working memory in ADHD children with and without comorbid anxiety. J Am Acad Child Adolesc Psychiatry 34:886–896, 1995a

Tannock R, Schachar R, Logan G: Methylphenidate and cognitive flexibility: dissociated dose effects in hyperactive children. J Abnorm Child Psychol 23:235–266, 1995b

Taylor E, Sandberg S, Thorley G, et al: The epidemiology of childhood hyperactivity, in Child Psychiatry. Edited by Taylor E, Rutter M. London, Oxford University Press, 1991, pp 1–122

Taylor E, Schachar R, Thorley G, et al: Which boys respond to stimulant medication? A controlled trial of methylphenidate in boys with disruptive behaviour. Psychol Med 17:121–143, 1987

Thurber S, Walker CE: Medication and hyperactivity: a meta-analysis. J Gen Psychol 108:79–86, 1983

Tjon Pian Gi CV, Broeren JP, Starreveld JS, et al: Melatonin for treatment of sleeping disorders in children with attention deficit/hyperactivity disorder: a preliminary open label study. Eur J Pediatr 162:554–555, 2003

Velez CN, Johnson J, Cohen P: A longitudinal analysis of selected risk factors for childhood psychopathology. J Am Acad Child Adolesc Psychiatry 28:861–864, 1989

Verhulst F, Eussen M, Berden G: Pathways of problem behaviors from childhood to adolescence. J Am Acad Child Adolesc Psychiatry 32:388–392, 1992

Vikan A: Psychiatric epidemiology in a sample of 1510 ten-year-old children, I: prevalence. J Child Psychol Psychiatry 26:55–75, 1985

Visser SN, Lesesne CA: Mental health in the United States: prevalence of diagnosis and medication treatment for attention-deficit/hyperactivity disorder: United States, 2003. MMWR 54:842–847, 2006

Vitiello B: Research in child and adolescent psychopharmacology: recent accomplishments and new challenges. Psychopharmacology (Berl), Epub, 2006

Vitiello B, Jensen PS: Developmental perspectives in pediatric psychopharmacology. Psychopharmacol Bull 31:75–81, 1995

Vitiello B, Jensen PS: Medication development and testing in children and adolescents: current problems, future directions. Arch Gen Psychiatry 54:871–876, 1997

Volkow ND, Ding YS, Fowler JS, et al: Is methylphenidate like cocaine? Studies on their pharmacokinetics and distribution in the human brain. Arch Gen Psychiatry 52:456–463, 1995

Vyborova L, Nahunek K, Drtilkova I, et al: Intra-individual comparison of 21-day application of amphetamine and methylphenidate in hyperkinetic children. Act Nerv Super (Praha) 26:268–269, 1984

Wesensten NJ, Belenky G, Kautz MA, et al: Maintaining alertness and performance during sleep deprivation: modafinil versus caffeine. Psychopharmacology (Berl) 159:238–247, 2002

Whalen CK, Henker B, Buhrmester D, et al: Does stimulant medication improve the peer status of hyperactive children? J Consult Clin Psychol 57:545–549, 1989

Wigal S, Swanson JM, Feifel D, et al: A double-blind, placebo-controlled trial of dex-methylphenidate hydrochloride and d,l-threo-methylphenidate hydrochloride in children with attention-deficit/hyperactivity disorder. J Am Acad Child Adolesc Psychiatry 43:1406–1414, 2004

Wilens TE, Biederman J: The stimulants. Psychiatr Clin North Am 15:191–222, 1992

Wilens TE, Biederman J, Spencer T: Clonidine for sleep disturbances associated with attention-deficit hyperactivity disorder. J Am Acad Child Adolesc Psychiatry 33:424–426, 1994

Wilens TE, McBurnett K, Bukstein O, et al: Multisite controlled study of OROS methylphenidate in the treatment of adolescents with attention-deficit/hyperactivity disorder. Arch Pediatr Adolesc Med 160:82–90, 2006

Winsberg BG, Press M, Bialer I, et al: Dextroamphetamine and methylphenidate in the treatment of hyperactive-aggressive children. Pediatrics 53:236–241, 1974

Wolraich ML, Greenhill LL, Pelham W, et al: Randomized, controlled trial of OROS methylphenidate once a day in children with attention-deficit/hyperactivity disorder. Pediatrics 108:883–892, 2001

Woodruff TJ, Axelrad DA, Kyle AD, et al: Trends in environmentally related childhood illnesses. Pediatrics 113:1133–1140, 2004

Zametkin AJ, Rapoport JL: Neurobiology of attention deficit disorder with hyperactivity: where have we come in 50 years? J Am Acad Child Adolesc Psychiatry 26:676–686, 1987

3

Disruptive Behavior Disorders and Aggression

Natoshia Raishevich, B.A.

Elizabeth Pappadopulos, Ph.D.

Peter S. Jensen, M.D.

Disruptive behavior disorders (DBDs)—oppositional defiant disorder (ODD), conduct disorder (CD), and disruptive behavior disorder not otherwise specified (DBD-NOS)—are among the most common and debilitating psychiatric ailments in children and adolescents (Bambauer and Connor 2005; Kazdin 1995). Various amounts of verbal and physical aggression often accompany each of these disorders. However, it should be noted that symptoms of aggression are often present in children with disorders across the array of *Diagnostic and Statistical Manual of Mental Disorders* (DSM) psychiatric disorders (American Psychiatric Association 2000), even when such children do not meet diagnostic criteria for a DBD. Given the public health importance of aggression and its salience to impairment, the conceptualization of DBDs and their response to treatment interventions require a comprehensive understanding of aggression, its impact, prevalence, and presentation across the DBD spectrum.

An emerging literature suggests that aggression can be categorized by two discrete subtypes: proactive aggression and reactive aggression (Dodge and Coie 1987). Proactive aggression is instrumental or deliberate, and occurs without provocation. Reactive aggression is an emotive form of aggression and attributes hostile intent to others. These categories have also been described in the medical literature as *controlled-instrumental-predatory aggression* to denote the proactive form, and *impulsive-hostile-affective aggression* to signify the reactive form (Vitiello and Stoff 1997).

These two forms of aggression and their relationship to the DBDs remain to be fully understood. This conceptual gap is largely a result of the failure to take aggressive subtypes into account in the assessment and treatment studies of DBDs. Instead, research trials tend to globally target symptoms of physical aggression as opposed to proactive or reactive aggression in the treatment of DBDs (Volavka and Citrome 1999). Because the medical literature has largely failed to discriminate between these two types of aggression, the potential clinical benefits of treatment of different forms of aggression have not yet been fully addressed (Pappadopulos et al. 2006).

Some investigators have suggested that different subtypes of aggression may respond better to various forms of intervention (Gillberg and Hellgren 1986). As we discuss further in this chapter, youth with CD and impulsive aggression may be greatly benefited by pharmacotherapy (Connor et al. 2004; Jensen et al. 2007; Steiner et al. 2003; Vitiello and Stoff 1997; Vitiello et al. 1990). Yet it is unclear whether the psychopharmacological agents that have been proved efficacious in the treatment of CD actually ameliorate symptoms of proactive aggression (Jensen et al. 2007). Therefore, future randomized controlled trials (RCTs) may benefit from including a reliable measure of aggression that distinguishes between the aggressive subtypes (Brown et al. 1996), which may be used to help further refine treatment decisions. In this review we address what is currently known about the treatment of DBDs and aggression and note where aggression has or has not been explicitly studied as a part of these conditions.

Epidemiology

Oppositional Defiant Disorder and Aggression

Oppositional defiant disorder is defined as a consistent pattern of defiance, disobedience, and hostility toward various authority figures and adults and persists for at least 6 months (American Psychiatric Association 2000) (Table 3–1). To meet diagnostic criteria for ODD, the youth must exhibit at least four of the following behaviors: losing his or her temper, arguing with adults, refusing to comply with authority figures, deliberately doing things to annoy other people, blaming others for his or her mistakes, being easily annoyed by others, being angry or resentful, and being spiteful or vindictive. To qualify for a diagnosis of ODD, the presenting behaviors must occur more frequently than is developmentally appropriate and must lead to a significant impairment in functioning. Approximately 2%–16% of children in the United States meet the criteria for ODD (American Psychiatric Association 2000).

Of note, ODD is only marginally predictive of proactive aggression (Lahey et al. 1998). This relationship, to the extent it is present, may be related to the diagnostic criteria of ODD that specify *spiteful behaviors* and *deliberate* attempts to annoy other people (American Psychiatric Association 2000). On the other hand, there may be numerous features of the disorder that may be indicative of verbal forms of reactive aggression, such as losing one's temper, being easily annoyed by others, arguing with adults, and being angry or resentful. Perhaps the relationship between aggressive subtypes and ODD diagnostic criteria suggest that there may be as-yet-undefined ODD subtypes, one of which may be a marker or precursor to more explicit, impulsive aggressive behaviors, whereas one or more other types might be related to more willful oppositional behaviors. This possibility should be explored in future research.

Conduct Disorder

Conduct disorder occurs in 6%–16% of males and 2%–9% of females (American Psychiatric Association 2000). CD is defined as a persistent pattern of maladaptive behavior in which the rights of others and/or societal norms are violated (American Psychiatric Association 2000) (Table 3–2). These behaviors fall into four main categories: aggressive behavior toward people or animals, destruction of property, deceitfulness or theft, and serious violations

Table 3–1.   DSM-IV-TR diagnostic criteria for oppositional defiant disorder

A.   A pattern of negativistic, hostile, and defiant behavior lasting at least 6 months, during which four (or more) of the following are present:

   (1)   often loses temper

   (2)   often argues with adults

   (3)   often actively defies or refuses to comply with adults' requests or rules

   (4)   often deliberately annoys people

   (5)   often blames others for his or her mistakes or misbehavior

   (6)   is often touchy or easily annoyed by others

   (7)   is often angry and resentful

   (8)   is often spiteful or vindictive

  Note: Consider a criterion met only if the behavior occurs more frequently than is typically observed in individuals of comparable age and developmental level.

B.   The disturbance in behavior causes clinically significant impairment in social, academic, or occupational functioning.

C.   The behaviors do not occur exclusively during the course of a psychotic or mood disorder.

D.   Criteria are not met for conduct disorder, and, if the individual is age 18 years or older, criteria are not met for antisocial personality disorder.

of societal norms or rules. Just as with ODD, it is possible that the features of this behavioral disorder may correspond either to impulsive aggression or to proactive aggressive behaviors. Although some evidence suggests that proactive aggression, rather than reactive aggression, is a significant predictor of CD (Vitaro et al. 1998), this is an area in need of further study. In addition, other features of CD, such as truancy and theft, or early versus late onset, may indicate quite a different clinical course, but these issues also remain in need of further study.

Differential Diagnosis

Cases in which the youth meets some but not all of the criteria for either ODD or CD and experiences significant impairment suggest that a diagnosis of DBD-NOS may be appropriate (American Psychiatric Association 2000) (Table 3–3).

Table 3–2. DSM-IV-TR diagnostic criteria for conduct disorder

A. A repetitive and persistent pattern of behavior in which the basic rights of others or major age-appropriate societal norms or rules are violated, as manifested by the presence of three (or more) of the following criteria in the past 12 months, with at least one criterion present in the past 6 months:

Aggression to people and animals

(1) often bullies, threatens, or intimidates others

(2) often initiates physical fights

(3) has used a weapon that can cause serious physical harm to others (e.g., a bat, brick, broken bottle, knife, gun)

(4) has been physically cruel to people

(5) has been physically cruel to animals

(6) has stolen while confronting a victim (e.g., mugging, purse snatching, extortion, armed robbery)

(7) has forced someone into sexual activity

Destruction of property

(8) has deliberately engaged in fire setting with the intention of causing serious damage

(9) has deliberately destroyed others' property (other than by fire setting)

Deceitfulness or theft

(10) has broken into someone else's house, building, or car

(11) often lies to obtain goods or favors or to avoid obligations (i.e., "cons" others)

(12) has stolen items of nontrivial value without confronting a victim (e.g., shoplifting, but without breaking and entering; forgery)

Serious violations of rules

(13) often stays out at night despite parental prohibitions, beginning before age 13 years

(14) has run away from home overnight at least twice while living in parental or parental surrogate home (or once without returning for a lengthy period)

(15) is often truant from school, beginning before age 13 years

B. The disturbance in behavior causes clinically significant impairment in social, academic, or occupational functioning.

C. If the individual is age 18 years or older, criteria are not met for antisocial personality disorder.

Table 3–2.   DSM-IV-TR diagnostic criteria for conduct disorder *(continued)*

Code based on age at onset:

312.81   Conduct Disorder, Childhood-Onset Type: onset of at least one criterion characteristic of conduct disorder prior to age 10 years

312.82   Conduct Disorder, Adolescent-Onset Type: absence of any criteria characteristic of conduct disorder prior to age 10 years

312.89   Conduct Disorder, Unspecified Onset: age at onset is not known

Specify severity:

  Mild: few if any conduct problems in excess of those required to make the diagnosis **and** conduct problems cause only minor harm to others

  Moderate: number of conduct problems and effect on others intermediate between "mild" and "severe"

  Severe: many conduct problems in excess of those required to make the diagnosis **or** conduct problems cause considerable harm to others

As noted earlier, aggression is relatively common across an array of psychiatric disorders, including major depression, bipolar disorder, attention-deficit/hyperactivity disorder (ADHD), postraumatic stress disorder (PTSD), and psychosis (Jensen et al. 2007). Aggression is also notable among youth with a primary diagnosis within the autism spectrum disorders. Thus, the high co-occurrence of aggression along with other mental disorders appears to have important implications in the management and treatment of a broad range of mental disorders in youth (Pappadopulos et al. 2003), not just the DBDs.

Course and Outcome

The occurrence of a DBD and/or aggressive behaviors in youth may lead to the subsequent development of other mental disorders. For example, a diagnosis of ODD may precede a diagnosis of CD. Loeber et al. (1993) found that youth who were diagnosed with ODD had a 43% chance of eventually developing CD. However, it should be noted that the emergence of CD does not necessarily mitigate or supersede a diagnosis of ODD; in fact, it is more common for ODD symptoms to persist even after full CD symptoms emerge.

One of the most serious outcomes of CD and other DBDs is the emergence of antisocial personality disorder. Studies indicate that 70%–90% of youth with CD will also develop antisocial personality disorder in adulthood (Loeber et al. 2002, 2003).

Table 3–3.   DSM-IV-TR description of disruptive behavior disorder not otherwise specified

This category is for disorders characterized by conduct or oppositional defiant behaviors that do not meet the criteria for conduct disorder or oppositional defiant disorder. For example, include clinical presentations that do not meet full criteria either for oppositional defiant disorder or conduct disorder, but in which there is clinically significant impairment.

DSM-IV-TR (American Psychiatric Association 2000) categorizes antisocial personality disorder as a disregard for the rights of others, along with at least three of the following symptoms: disregard for the safety of oneself or others, failure to adhere to societal norms, impulsivity, irresponsibility, deceitfulness, lack of remorse, and physically aggressive behaviors. Antisocial personality disorder is also categorized by poor treatment outcomes, including an increased likelihood to commit violent acts or engage in illegal behaviors (Loeber et al. 2002). Thus, antisocial personality disorder, like CD, is linked by its diagnostic criteria to aggression. Proactive aggression, in and of itself, has also been shown to be related to later maladjustment (Dodge 1991). In addition, the clinical presentation of antisocial personality disorder may encompass features of reactive aggression, though this has been less well studied. Regardless of the primary psychiatric condition or nature of the aggressive behaviors, these ailments are often accompanied by poor treatment outcome and the need for longer and more intensive treatment (Mannuzza et al. 1993, 1998; Werry 1997).

In general, the prognosis for DBDs is especially poor if the youth fails to respond to behavioral interventions, which are often considered the first line of treatment for behavioral disorders and/or symptoms of aggression. Because of the limitations of current psychotherapeutic interventions, however, a growing body of literature has focused on the outcomes of psychopharmacological treatment of aggressive symptoms in youth with DBDs (Connor et al. 1999, 2002; dosReis et al. 2003; Pappadopulos et al. 2003; Schur et al. 2003; Steiner et al. 2003), which is the focus of this chapter.

Rationale and Justification for Psychopharmacological Treatment

As reviewed in subsequent sections of this chapter, psychotropic agents may be beneficial for the treatment of DBDs and/or aggression in youth. However, given the highly overlapping nature of DBDs and the aggressive subtypes with other conditions such as ADHD or bipolar disorder, decisions about which psychopharmacological treatments are appropriate depend on which "underlying" conditions are present. Not surprisingly then, the literature is sometimes unclear about whether psychotropic interventions are targeting a specific DBD or aggressive symptoms that may nor may not be co-occurring with other disorders. Although this distinction is often unclear, current research on the treatment efficacy of varying psychotropic agents does offer evidence and a preliminary framework to determine optimal use of psychopharmacological agents in the treatment of aggression and DBDs in youth.

Issues in Study Design and Interpretation

Treatment efficacy is most rigorously established through *randomized controlled trials,* which are defined as studies in which participants are randomly assigned to differing treatment conditions, including administration of psychopharmacological agents, behavioral interventions, and/or placebo. These conditions are used to compare treatment outcomes among groups.

As RCTs of psychotropic agents continue to emerge, the systematic evaluation of treatment outcomes across all of the studies becomes necessary. One useful and objective technique to compare efficacy between RCTs is through the evaluation of reported effect sizes (Pappadopulos et al. 2006). Comparing effect sizes allows for a broadband comparison across studies involving RCTs. Thus, we will use effect sizes as a comparative measure in the following review of treatment studies. However, because effect sizes are not necessarily sensitive to other factors, such as treatment duration, side effects, and number of studies or participants, we also review the efficacy of the various agents in terms of the *strength of evidence,* grading the overall strength of evidence of each agent in three hierarchical levels (Jensen et al. 1999; Jobson and Potter 1995; Vitiello and Stoff 1997). *Level A* denotes the highest level of empirical support, as demonstrated by two or more RCTs showing the agent's efficacy. *Level B* constitutes moderate support for a given agent, evidenced by at least one RCT with or without data from open trials and case studies. *Level C* is assigned to those agents that indicate evidence is based only on expert opinion, case studies, open-label trials, or only data from adult samples. A fourth level, *Level D,* is reserved for instances in which trials have been done but in which findings have been negative.

Below, we principally review key RCTs, as well as safety information, on the major classes of psychopharmacological agents that have been studied to manage aggression and/or DBDs in youth. These classes include atypical antipsychotics, typical antipsychotics, stimulants, mood stabilizers, α_2 agonists, and beta-blockers. Please note that we do not attempt to review all RCTs for each class of agents; rather, we seek to provide an overview of several key RCTs for each agent. When RCTs are not available, we provide other sources of evidence, such as open-label or uncontrolled trials, in order to assess the efficacy of a particular class of agents.

Atypical Antipsychotics: Review of Treatment Studies

Risperidone

Short-Term

Risperidone is currently the most extensively studied medication in the treatment of aggression in youth, with RCTs testing short- and long-term benefits of this agent in behaviorally disordered and/or aggressive youth. These studies include larger-scale, multisite trials and small-scale RCTs.

Two industry-sponsored, multisite RCTs were conducted in parallel to test the efficacy of risperidone in the treatment of aggressive symptoms and/or DBDs in youth with low-normal or subaverage intelligence. The first RCT evaluated 118 children (ages 5–12) with subaverage intelligence and a primary diagnosis of DBD, including ODD, CD, or DBD-NOS (Aman et al. 2002). Risperidone-treated youth experienced significant reduction in aggressive symptoms as measured by the Conduct Problem subscale of the Nisonger Child Behavior Rating Form (NCBRF) compared with subjects receiving placebo, with an effect size of 0.7. The second industry-sponsored study achieved comparable results in an identically designed RCT (Snyder et al. 2002).

Several smaller trials have yielded similar results. For example, Findling et al. (2000) demonstrated significant reductions in aggressive behaviors as measured by the Rating of Aggression Against People and/or Property (RAAPP) scale in a sample of 20 youth with CD (ages 5–15) receiving outpatient treatment. Similar gains were noted in an RCT that specifically targeted symptoms of severe aggression during a 6-week trial of 38 inpatient adolescents with subaverage intelligence and DBDs (Buitelaar et al. 2001). Their aggressive symptoms were measured by the Clinical Global Impression (CGI) Severity of Illness subscale and the Aberrant Behavior Checklist (ABC). Moreover, during the 2-week washout trial following the 6 weeks of treatment, the risperidone group experienced a statistically significant worsening of aggressive behaviors as measured by the CGI Severity of Illness subscale, the ABC, and the modified Overt Aggression Scale (OAS-M).

The efficacy of risperidone in the treatment of aggressive symptoms has also been documented in an 8-week, double-blind RCT of 101 autistic youth (McCracken et al. 2002). Risperidone treatment was associated with significant reductions in aggression as indicated by scores on the ABC and Clinical Global Impressions (CGI) scale within 4 weeks of receiving treatment. Moreover, a significant treatment-by-time interaction effect indicated that the risperidone group continued to improve through weeks 4–8, while the placebo group deteriorated.

Unfortunately, many of these studies are limited in that they involve atypical samples (e.g., inpatient, low/subaverage intelligence, and pervasive developmental disorders). Furthermore, the aforementioned trials were designed to evaluate short-term treatment outcome. As such, these findings may not be generalizable to the treatment of chronic aggression in youth. Similarly, it is less likely that serious adverse effects would occur during the relatively brief course of these studies. Therefore, other studies must document if adverse effects emerge more frequently with long-term use. In spite of these limitations, available data suggest that risperidone appears to be effective in the short-term treatment of aggressive symptoms and/or behavioral disorders in youth. For specific dosage information pertaining to the effective use of risperidone in the treatment of aggression in youth, see Table 3–4.

Long-Term and Maintenance

In addition to the evidence for short-term efficacy for symptoms of aggression and/or DBDs, emerging evidence suggests that risperidone may also be beneficial in the long-term maintenance of treatment gains. In one study of long-term efficacy (Reyes et al. 2006a), 335 youth ages 5–17 who had responded

Table 3–4. Selected agents prescribed for treatment of aggressive youth with disruptive behavior disorders

Class	Generic name	Trade name	Typical dosage
Antipsychotics, atypical	risperidone	Risperdal	1–4 mg/day
	clozapine	Clozaril	150–600 mg/day
	quetiapine	Seroquel	100–600 mg/day
	olanzapine	Zyprexa	2.5–20 mg/day
	aripiprazole	Abilify	2.5–15 mg/day
	ziprasidone	Geodon	40–160 mg/day
Antipsychotics, typical	thioridazine	Mellaril	25–400 mg/day
	haloperidol	Haldol	0.5–10 mg/day
Stimulants	methylphenidate	Ritalin, Ritalin LA, Ritalin-SR, Metadate, Metadate CD, Metadate ER, Methylin, Methylin ER	15–60 mg/day
		Concerta	18–72 mg/day
	mixed amphetamine salts	Adderall	10–40 mg/day
	dextroamphetamine	Dexedrine	10–40 mg/day
Mood stabilizers	lithium, lithium carbonate	Eskalith, Lithobid	10–30 mg/kg/day[a]
	valproic acid	Depakene, Depakote	15–60 mg/kg/day[b]
	carbamazepine	Tegretol	10–20 mg/kg/day[c]
Alpha2 agonists	clonidine	Catapres	0.025–0.4 mg/day
	guanfacine	Tenex	0.5–4 mg/day
Beta-blockers	nadolol	Corgard	20–200 mg/day
	propranolol	Inderal	2–8 mg/kg/day

Note. See Jensen et al. 2004 and Martin et al. 2003 for additional information.
[a]Lithium doses optimally adjusted based on blood levels, 0.6–1.1 mEq/L. [b]Valproic acid doses optimally adjusted based on blood levels 50–125 µg/L.
[c]Carbamazepine doses optimally adjusted based on blood levels, 4–14 µg/L.

to open-label risperidone treatment over 12 weeks were then blindly and randomly assigned to receive 6 additional months of either a continuation of risperidone or placebo. On average, aggressive symptoms, as measured by the NCBRF, a measure of both proactive and reactive aggressive behaviors, documented longer treatment maintenance periods in the risperidone group. Significant symptom recurrence occurred after 119 days in 25% of patients in the risperidone group and in 47.1% of patients in the placebo group. It should be noted that the results indicate more than half the placebo group did not experience a recurrence of symptoms. Therefore, psychopharmacological discontinuation may be a plausible treatment option for some youth with symptoms of aggression and/or DBD. Moreover, Reyes et al. (2006a) also reported significant treatment gains in hyperactive, compliant, and adaptive social behaviors in the risperidone group as compared with the placebo group. After the completion of this yearlong study, an additional yearlong, open-label expansion study was conducted involving 48 responders, and maintenance of the original treatment gains was again demonstrated (Reyes et al. 2006b). Overall, these studies suggest that risperidone may be efficacious in the treatment of DBDs and/or aggression in children for a cumulative period of 2 years.

Findings from the studies by Reyes et al. (2006a, 2006b) are also supported by other yearlong, open-label trials assessing the sustained safety and efficacy of risperidone in youth of subaverage intelligence with symptoms of aggression and other disruptive behaviors (Aman et al. 2004; Croonenberghs et al. 2005; Turgay et al. 2002). In general, across these yearlong, open-label, follow-on studies of initial RCTs, youth maintained treatment gains reported in the initial waves of the study (see preceding section on short-term effectiveness of risperidone). Of particular interest within the aggressive subtype literature, there was a highly significant decrease in the secondary outcome measure (the Vineland Adaptive Behavior Scales), which is used to assess physical aggression and emotional outbursts (Turgay et al. 2002). Therefore, preliminary evidence appears to indicate the utility of risperidone in the treatment of impulsive aggression.

Furthermore, some evidence has documented the efficacy of long-term use of risperidone in aggressive youth who have a primary diagnosis of autism or other pervasive developmental disorders. In the Research Units on Pediatric Psychopharmacology follow-up study (Research Units on Pediatric Psychopharmacology Autism Network 2005), two-thirds of patients maintained behavioral improvements for 6 months following the initial study, when youth were reassigned to receive either risperidone or placebo. It should be noted, however, that 37.5% of youth who had taken risperidone in the original study did not relapse even while taking placebo in the follow-up report. Similarly, Troost et al. (2005) studied 36 children with an autism spectrum disorder (5–17 years old) who had symptoms of severe aggression or self-injurious behavior. These youth were initially placed on an 8-week, open-label trial of risperidone. Those that responded continued treatment for another 16 weeks, and then a double-blind discontinuation (*n*=24), consisting of either 3 weeks of tapering and 5 weeks of placebo or continued use of risperidone, was carried out. The findings indicated that only 25% of patients who continued taking risperidone relapsed, versus 66.67% of youth who switched to placebo. Thus, both studies suggest that risperidone was more efficacious than placebo in preventing relapse, but both studies also imply that at least a subset of initially treated children may not relapse when their risperidone is switched to placebo, suggesting that considerations for medication discontinuation may be appropriate for children who have done well for a substantial period of time.

Overall, there is increasing evidence to suggest that risperidone is efficacious in the long-term treatment of aggressive symptoms and/or behavioral disorders in youth. However, the literature is limited in that it primarily focuses on samples of youth with low-normal or subaverage intelligence and/or autism.

Olanzapine

Several studies of olanzapine indicate preliminary success as a treatment in the management of aggressive disorders in youth. In a study by Stephens et al. (2004), 10 children with Tourette's syndrome and aggression were treated in single-blind fashion (after a 2-week placebo run-in) with olanzapine over 8 weeks. The authors demonstrated significant reductions in both aggressive symptoms and tic severity, as assessed with standard rating scales. One open-label trial of olanzapine documented significant behavioral improvement in children, adolescents, and adults, which was observed within the first several weeks of treatment (Potenza et al. 1999). Similarly, a case report by Horrigan et al. (1997) concluded that olanzapine was associated with decreased aggression toward people and property and a decreased number of explosive outbursts in youth. Even though these reports suggest that olanzapine may have a role in treating aggression and/or DBDs, firm conclusions about the potential efficacy of olanzapine cannot be reached without further studies.

Clozapine

To date, no RCTs have evaluated the efficacy of clozapine in the treatment of aggressive symptoms in children or adults. However, there are several case studies that suggest clozapine is an effective treatment for aggression in adult samples (Rabinowitz et al. 1996; Volavka and Citrome 1999). Significant reductions in physical and verbal aggression were observed in 75 adults with schizophrenia during 6 months of treatment. There have been few studies that have evaluated clozapine's effectiveness in the treatment of aggression in youth (Chalasani et al. 2001; Kranzler et al. 2005). In a chart review of six children and adolescents with schizophrenic disorders, violent episodes were significantly reduced and global functions improved significantly (Chalasani et al. 2001). Similarly, a recent open-label study by Kranzler et al. (2005) indicated that clozapine yielded significant pre-post benefits in patients with treatment-refractory schizophrenia and aggression. Nonetheless, additional research is needed in order to assess the efficacy of clozapine in the treatment of aggression and/or behavioral disorders in youth (see Table 3–4 for dosage information).

Other Atypical Antipsychotics

Currently, no data are available with regard to the efficacy of other atypical antipsychotic agents, including quetiapine, ziprasidone, and aripiprazole, in their ability to manage aggressive symptoms in youth. Therefore, additional research is needed to further assess the comparative efficacy of other atypical antipsychotics. This research may be especially beneficial in treatment planning for behaviorally disordered and/or aggressive youth in light of the reported efficacy of the other atypical antipsychotics (principally risperidone) that have been extensively studied. Moreover, it would be of great clinical relevance to assess the different side-effect profiles of the various atypicals to meet the need for a wider array of safe and effective therapeutic agents in the management of aggressive symptoms and/or behavioral disorders in youth.

Benefits of Atypical Antipsychotics

Overall, atypical antipsychotics have a notably large effect size (mean effect size = 0.9) on aggression that generally increases with the length of the study (Table 3–5). However, it should be noted that apart from risperidone, as discussed below, there is little evidence on the efficacy of atypical antipsychotics in the treatment of aggressive symptoms and/or behavioral disorders in youth. Risperidone may be the most appropriate treatment option, compared with the other atypical antipsychotics, because of the number of RCTs supporting its efficacy (Table 3–6).

Furthermore, risperidone is noted for its efficacy as both a monotherapy and in combination with other agents, and may also be associated with fewer extrapyramidal symptoms (EPS) over the long term, compared with typical antipsychotics. As a result of the potential for decreased adverse side effects in child and adolescent samples, risperidone has largely replaced conventional antipsychotics in the treatment of aggression in youth (Connor et al. 2001; McConville and Sorter 2004).

Risks of Atypical Antipsychotics

Although the adverse effects of atypical antipsychotics may be milder than typical antipsychotics, studies have indicated that atypical antipsychotic agents are nonetheless associated with mild to moderate side effects, including EPS, somnolence, headache, increases in prolactin levels, and increases in weight (Aman et al. 2004; Snyder et al. 2002). Of particular importance to pediatric care providers, youth treated with these agents appear to experience significantly greater weight gain than adults using atypical antipsychotics, even at low doses (Sikich et al. 2004). Less commonly reported problems in youth may include type 2 diabetes and cardiac rhythm abnormalities, but more studies may be necessary to address concerns about these possible side effects (Schur et al. 2003). In children and adolescents, long-term risks that are typically associated with atypical antipsychotic use also include withdrawal, tardive dyskinesia, parkinsonism, and neuroleptic malignant syndrome. See Table 3–7 for additional information on the potential side effects of atypical antipsychotics.

Because atypical antipsychotics are associated with an array of serious side effects, the U.S. Food and Drug Administration (FDA) has required that these agents carry warning labels to specifically indicate their potential risk for

Table 3–5.   Effect sizes of various psychotropic agents for the treatment of aggression and/or disruptive behavioral disorders in youth

Agent	Effect size	Total N across studies
Atypical antipsychotics	0.9	875
Risperidone	0.9	875
Typical antipsychotics	0.7	136
Haloperidol	0.8	53
Thioridazine	0.35	30
Stimulants	0.78	1,057
Methylphenidate	0.9	844
Mood stabilizers	0.4	217
Lithium	0.5	195
Alpha$_2$ agonists	0.5	42
Clonidine	1.1	8
Guanfacine	0.4	34
Beta-blockers	ND	ND
Mean effect size	0.56	

Note.   See Pappadopulos et al. 2006 for additional information. ND= no data.

increased weight gain and disruption of metabolic functioning (Stigler et al. 2004; U.S. Food and Drug Administration 2005). Given the knowledge of side effect concerns and the increasing rates at which atypicals are being prescribed to youth with symptoms of aggression (Olfson et al. 2006), additional studies are necessary to examine the safety of atypical antipsychotics in the treatment of aggression in youth.

Typical Antipsychotics: Review of Treatment Studies

Haloperidol

Prior to the emergence of atypical psychotics, conventional antipsychotic agents were considered first-line in the treatment of aggression and/or behav-

Table 3–6. Efficacy levels of various psychotropic agents for the treatment of aggression and/or disruptive behavioral disorders in youth

Class	Agent	Short-term efficacy	Long-term efficacy
Atypical antipsychotics	risperidone	A	A
	olanzapine	C	ND
	clozapine	C	ND
	quetiapine	ND	ND
	ziprasidone	ND	ND
	aripiprazole	ND	ND
Typical antipsychotics	haloperidol	A	B
	thioridazine	A	B
Stimulants	methylphenidate	A	B
	dextroamphetamine	B	ND
	pemoline	B	ND
Mood stabilizers	lithium	A	C
	divalproex	A	C
	carbamazepine	C	ND
Alpha$_2$ agonists	clonidine	A	ND
	guanfacine	B	ND
Beta-blockers	nadolol	C	ND

Note. A = highest level of empirical support, two or more randomized controlled trials (RCTs); B = moderate support by at least one RCT plus or minus data from open trials and case studies; C = support based only on expert opinion, case studies, or open-label trials; ND = no data.

ioral disorders in youth (for a review, see Campbell et al. 1999). Notably, haloperidol was considered an effective means to treat aggression. For example, in a double-blind study of treatment-resistant inpatient youth (ages 5.2–12.9 years) with CD, a significant reduction in aggressive symptoms was seen during the course of the study (Campbell et al. 1984). On the other hand, a double-blind, placebo-controlled study of haloperidol in the treatment of aggression in adolescents of subaverage intelligence found that the treatment only led to moderate behavioral improvements (Aman et al. 1989). Interestingly, haloperidol was considered most effective in treating youth with aggres-

Table 3–7.   Common and serious side effects for various classes of psychopharmacological agents

Class	Common side effects	Serious side effects
Atypical antipsychotics	Insomnia, agitation, extrapyramidal symptoms, headache, anxiety, rhinitis, constipation, nausea/vomiting, dyspepsia, dizziness, tachycardia, somnolence, increased dream activity, dry mouth, diarrhea, weight gain, visual disturbance, sexual dysfunction, hyperprolactinemia, menstrual irregularities	Hypotension, severe syncope (rare), extrapyramidal symptoms, severe tardive dyskinesia, neuroleptic malignant syndrome, hyperglycemia, severe diabetes mellitus, seizures (rare), priapism (rare), stroke, transient ischemic attack
Typical antipsychotics	Extrapyramidal symptoms, tardive dyskinesia, akathisia, insomnia, anxiety, drowsiness, lethargy, weight changes, anticholinergic effects, gynecomastia, breast tenderness, galactorrhea, menstrual irregularities, injection site reaction (depot), elevated prolactin levels	Neuroleptic malignant syndrome, tardive dyskinesia, pneumonia, arrhythmia, hypotension, hypertension, seizures, jaundice, hyperpyrexia, heat stroke, dystonia
Stimulants	Nervousness, insomnia, abdominal pain, nausea, anorexia, motor tics, headache, palpitations, dizziness, blurred vision, tachycardia, weight loss, fever, depression, transient drowsiness, dyskinesia, angina, rash, urticaria, blood pressure changes	Growth suppression (long term), seizures, dependency, abuse, arrhythmia, leukopenia (rare), thrombocytopenic purpura (rare), toxic psychosis (rare), Tourette's syndrome (rare), exfoliative dermatitis (rare), erythema multiforme (rare), neuroleptic malignant syndrome (rare), cerebral arteritis (rare), hepatotoxicity (rare)

Table 3–7. Common and serious side effects for various classes of psychopharmacological agents *(continued)*

Class	Common side effects	Serious side effects
Mood stabilizers	Enuresis, fatigue, ataxia, increased thirst, nausea, vomiting, urinary frequency, gastrointestinal upset, sleepiness, and weight gain (Bassarath 2003; Malone et al. 2000)	Disruption in hepatic, hematological, and metabolic functioning (Cummings and Miller 2004)
Alpha$_2$ agonists	Drowsiness and dizziness (Cantwell et al. 1997), dry mouth, irritability, dysphoria, rebound hypertension (Martin et al. 2003)	Syncope (rare) (Cantwell et al. 1997), hypotension (rare) (Martin et al. 2003)
Beta-blockers	Sedation, mild hypotension, lowered heart rate, bronchoconstriction, dizziness, sleep disruption (Riddle et al. 1999)	Hypoglycemia (in patients with diabetes), growth-hormone regulation issues (Riddle et al. 1999)

Note. See Center for the Advancement of Children's Mental Health, Office of Mental Health, manuscript in preparation, for further information. Side effects for specific medications may vary within classes; specific details of differences among specific agents can be found elsewhere (Connor et al. 2001; Pappadopulos et al. 2003; Weiner 1996).

sive symptoms of irritability, thereby suggesting that haloperidol may be useful in the treatment of reactive aggression in youth (Campbell et al. 1999) (see Table 3–4 for dosage information).

Thioridazine

Several early studies of thioridazine suggest its efficacy in managing aggressive symptoms in youth. For example, an RCT of thioridazine demonstrated modest clinical improvements in symptoms of aggression in youth (Aman et al. 1991) and led to a reduction in hyperactivity and conduct problems. Although thioridazine has shown superiority over placebo for treatment of youth meeting criteria for ADHD, it also may be less effective in maintaining treatment gains (Gittelman-Klein et al. 1976). Specifically, thioridazine appeared to be less effective at week 12 than at week 4 of the treatment (see Table 3–4 for dosage information).

Benefits of Typical Antipsychotics

Early studies suggested that low doses of typical antipsychotics were effective for managing aggressive behaviors in youth with a moderate effect size (mean = 0.7) (Table 3–5) (Pappadopulos et al. 2006). Typical antipsychotics may also be beneficial when the aggressive youth experiences comorbid psychotic disorder (Table 3–6).

Risks of Typical Antipsychotics

Available evidence indicates that typical antipsychotics can produce debilitating side effects in youth (Table 3–7), including an increased occurrence of EPS and tardive dyskinesia (Connor et al. 2001; McConville and Sorter 2004). On the basis of available knowledge, the risks associated with typical antipsychotics may outweigh the benefits of prescribing these agents in the treatment of aggression in youth. Therefore, typical antipsychotics should not be used to treat aggressive symptoms and/or DBDs in youth prior to a trial in which an atypical agent is used (Pappadopulos et al. 2003). In specific instances, however, if the patient is being treated with an atypical agent, emergent problems with weight gain or diabetes may warrant case-by-case use of typical antipsychotics.

Stimulants: Review of Treatment Studies

Methylphenidate

Short-Term

To date, a growing number of short-term RCTs have provided evidence for the efficacy of methylphenidate and other stimulants in the treatment of aggression and DBDs in youth. For example, one meta-analysis of 28 studies occurring over the past 30 years examined the efficacy of stimulants on covert and overt aggressive behavior in ADHD, with largely promising findings with regard to short-term efficacy (Connor et al. 2002). Moreover, it appears that the treatment of aggression with methylphenidate and other stimulants has a substantial treatment effect that is independent from effects on core ADHD symptoms in AHDH/aggressive youth.

For example, one RCT of methylphenidate in 18 children with ADHD found significant improvement in aggressive behaviors and symptoms of hyperactivity and inattention (Bukstein and Kolko 1998). Moreover, notable improvements in peer relations were also demonstrated. Similarly, an RCT testing the efficacy of methylphenidate in 84 children with CD with or without ADHD found significant reductions in core behaviors associated with CD, independent of the effects of the children's ADHD symptoms (Klein et al. 1997).

Long-Term and Maintenance

Several reports from the National Institute of Mental Health (NIMH) Multi-modal Treatment Study of Children With ADHD (MTA) study have explored longer-term treatment for youth experiencing comorbid impulsive aggression and ADHD. For example, the MTA's 14-month follow-up indicated that stimulants (principally methylphenidate) not only alleviated core symptoms of ADHD but also reduced the secondary symptoms of ODD and aggression in youth ("A 14-Month Randomized Clinical Trial of Treatment Strategies" 1999), as rated on the Swanson, Nolan, and Pelham, Version IV (SNAP-IV) scale (Swanson et al. 2001). However, symptoms of aggression and oppositionality that are present along with internalizing disorders, such as depression or anxiety, may improve most with psychopharmacological treatment that is combined with a behavioral intervention (Jensen et al. 2001). Overall, the evidence suggests that methylphenidate may be efficacious in treating aggressive symptoms associated with DBDs and ADHD.

Other Stimulants

Although methylphenidate is the most commonly prescribed stimulant for the treatment of ADHD and co-occurring aggressive symptoms, some evidence suggests that other stimulants may also be efficacious in the treatment of youth with comorbid symptoms of aggression and ADHD (see also Chapter 2, "Attention-Deficit/Hyperactivity Disorder," in this manual). These agents include a combination of methylphenidate and amphetamine mixed salts, and a combination of methylphenidate, dextroamphetamine (Dexedrine), and pemoline (Cylert) (Pappadopulos et al. 2004). Given the small number of studies available for evaluation, however, it is unclear whether the efficacy of the other stimulants on the treatment of aggression is comparable to that of methylphenidate.

Benefits of Stimulants

Stimulants are recommended as a first-line treatment in youth with comorbid ADHD and aggression (Pappadopulos et al. 2006). The rationale for stimulant use in the management of aggressive symptoms of ADHD or behavior disorder is based on the number of controlled trials demonstrating its efficacy and its large overall effect size (effect size=0.78–0.84) (Tables 3–5 and Table 3–6) (Connor et al. 2002; Pappadopulos et al. 2006). Therefore, the use of stimulants may be an appropriate treatment option for the management of aggression in youth in instances of comorbidity with the DBDs and other psychiatric disorders that are also typically treated with stimulants ("A 14-Month Randomized Clinical Trial of Treatment Strategies" 1999). In contrast to earlier concerns regarding stimulant usage, MTA data also suggest that stimulant use is effective in treating ADHD, even among youth who present with co-occurring symptoms of mania and aggression (Galanter et al. 2004). Stimulant treatment also appears to yield improvements in global functioning and social interaction (Bukstein and Kolko 1998; "A 14-Month Randomized Clinical Trial of Treatment Strategies" 1999; Swanson et al. 2001).

Risks of Stimulants

Despite their efficacy, stimulants are associated with several adverse effects, including insomnia, reduced appetite, stomachache, headache, and dizziness. Stimulants have also been linked to long-term adverse effects, including height and weight suppression (Lisska and Rivkees 2003). MTA analyses support the potential for a growth-suppression effect in youth who were systematically treated with stimulants. However, findings are also consistent with the interpretation that growth is merely delayed as opposed to reduced, compared with youth who are not taking stimulant medications (MTA Cooperative Group 2004). Further long-term follow-up studies must address the lingering questions.

Of note, the FDA has recently recommended that stimulants be labeled with a black box warning that indicates their potential for adverse cardiac effects in children (U.S. Food and Drug Administration 2006). Although the possibility of causing adverse cardiac effects remains unproven, caution should be taken in prescribing stimulants to youth with preexisting heart conditions. See Table 3–7 for additional information pertaining to the potential adverse effects associated with stimulant usage.

Mood Stabilizers: Review of Treatment Studies

Lithium

Most existing literature on the efficacy of mood stabilizers in the treatment of aggression in youth has focused on the use of lithium in patients with CD. Overall, these results suggest that lithium is associated with reduction in aggressive behavior in youth with CD (Campbell et al. 1995; Malone et al. 2000). For example, in one RCT, inpatient children with a primary diagnosis of CD received either lithium or placebo (Campbell et al. 1995). Lithium was associated with reduction in aggressive behaviors across several standardized measures, including the Children's Psychiatric Rating Scale. More recently, an RCT comparing lithium and placebo among 40 youth with CD found improvements in aggressive behaviors, as measured by the Overt Aggression Scale (OAS), for those treated with lithium versus placebo (Malone et al. 2000).

Overall, lithium has been shown to reduce bullying, fighting, and temper outbursts in severely aggressive, inpatient youth with CD (Campbell et al. 1984, 1995; Carlson et al. 1992; Malone et al. 2000). This evidence implies that lithium may have an important role in the treatment of reactive or affective aggression in youth. But the necessity of frequent monitoring and blood draws associated with this treatment, as well as its potential for side effects, may render it a second-line choice after pharmacological agents such as the atypical antipsychotics (Pappadopulos et al. 2003) (see Table 3–4 for dosage information).

Divalproex

Some evidence indicates that divalproex is effective in reducing aggressive symptoms and/or behavioral disorders in youth. For example, one RCT of divalproex in incarcerated male youth demonstrated improvement in impulse control when given high doses of the agent; moreover, global improvements among the subjects, as measured by the CGI Scale (Steiner 2003), were also noted. Similarly, another trial found that divalproex was associated with a reduction in aggressive symptoms in youth with CD (Donovan et al. 2000, 2003). Evidence also suggests that divalproex may be especially beneficial to youth who present with explosive and severe aggression (Donovan et al. 1997), as well as for treating impulsive aggression symptoms in youth with pervasive developmental disorders (Hollander et al. 2001). Last, a 12-week, open-label trial of divalproex sodium in 25 youth with bipolar disorder indicated a significant reduction in aggressive symptoms as measured by the Overt Aggression Scale (Saxena et al. 2006). Therefore, preliminary evidence suggests that divalproex may be efficacious in treating youth with an array of psychiatric disorders, including CD and bipolar disorder, whose behavior is characterized by severe impulsive aggression (see Table 3–4 for dosage information).

Carbamazepine

The use of carbamazepine and other mood stabilizers/anticonvulsants in the treatment of aggressive disorders has increased twofold over the past decade (Hunkeler et al. 2005). Preliminary research indicates that carbamazepine produces statistically significant decreases in aggressiveness and explosiveness in youth, with a moderate effect size (Evans et al. 1987; Kafantaris et al. 1992; Pappadopulos et al. 2006). On the other hand, countervailing evidence suggests that carbamazepine does not differ from placebo in reducing aggression in youth (Cueva et al. 1996). Thus, the results are inconclusive with regard to the efficacy of carbamazepine (see Table 3–4 for dosage information).

Benefits of Mood Stabilizers

In general, mood stabilizers appear to be beneficial in the treatment of aggression in youth with behavior disorders. Overall, the mean effect size for mood stabilizers appears to be moderate (0.4, see Table 3–5) (Pappadopulos et al. 2006). These agents may be a suitable alternative for cases in which the youth does not respond to the more rigorously tested atypical antipsychotics or stimulants.

Lithium, in particular, can be considered an evidence-based treatment in aggressive behaviors in youth with DBDs (Table 3–6). Moreover, lithium should be considered as the first-line treatment option for severe aggressive symptoms in youth who have received a primary diagnosis of a mood disorder, such as bipolar disorder. Lithium may also be a suitable treatment option when the youth has a sole diagnosis of CD in addition to showing severe aggressive symptoms, given that RCTs have demonstrated its efficacy in treating CD among children and adolescents..

Overall, the current evidence largely supports mood stabilizers' efficacy in the treatment of reactive aggression in youth with CD. However, because many of the symptoms of CD correspond to proactive aggression, additional research is needed to determine whether either subtype of aggression responds differentially to mood stabilizers.

Risks of Mood Stabilizers

To date, studies pertaining to mood stabilizers in the treatment of aggression in youth have been limited, in that they have measured short-term treatment outcomes. Therefore, it is possible that certain adverse effects may not become evident during the limited duration of these studies, but may appear in trials spanning longer periods. Furthermore, these studies have also been limited in scope, given that they have largely relied on inpatient data. Therefore, additional research is needed to measure the risks, benefits, and efficacy of mood stabilizers in aggressive youth in an array of settings (e.g., outpatient and emergency care).

Mood stabilizers are associated with a variety of adverse side effects. Common side effects of lithium include enuresis, fatigue, ataxia, increased thirst, nausea, vomiting, urinary frequency, and weight gain (Bassarath 2003; Malone et al. 2000). Moreover, frequent blood draws for dose monitoring are needed; thus, lithium may be less suitable for the treatment of aggressive symptoms in children (Malone et al. 2000). Side effects associated with divalproex include gastrointestinal upset and sleepiness (Steiner et al. 2003). Carbamazepine may carry the greatest risk for adverse side effects among mood stabilizers and has been linked to disruption in hepatic, hematological, and metabolic functioning (Cummings and Miller 2004) (see Table 3–7).

Other Agents

Alpha$_2$-Adrenergic Agonists

Clonidine

There is some evidence to support the use of α_2-adrenergic agonists in the treatment of aggressive symptoms and/or DBDs among children and adolescents. Specifically, clonidine has demonstrated efficacy in the treatment of aggression in youth through a meta-analysis of 11 double-blind, controlled, randomized studies (Connor et al. 1999). More recently, Hazell and Stuart (2003) reported gains in a 6-week randomized double-blind, placebo-controlled trial of a combined clonidine + stimulant treatment. Specifically, conduct problems were improved in youth with ADHD and comorbid ODD or CD. Further research on clonidine in the treatment of aggression and DBDs is needed (for dosage information, see Table 3–4).

Guanfacine

Guanfacine has demonstrated efficacy in the treatment of aggressive symptoms in an 8-week RCT involving 34 youth, 7–15 years old, with ADHD and a tic disorder (Scahill et al. 2001). Thus, it appears that guanfacine may be beneficial in the treatment of aggressive symptoms in youth with comorbid psychiatric disorders; however, further research is needed to provide conclusive support in the use of this agent in the treatment of DBDs in youth (see Table 3–4 for dosage information).

Benefits of Alpha$_2$-Adrenergic Agonists

Overall, α_2-adrenergic agonists have been shown to produce medium effect sizes ranging from 0.4 to 1.1 (see Table 3–5) (Pappadopulos et al. 2006). Interestingly, α_2 agonists may reduce the side effects associated with stimulant treatments. Therefore, this agent may be most useful when combined with stimulants in the treatment of aggressive symptoms (see Table 3–6 for detailed efficacy assessment of this class). Additional research is needed to compare the efficacy of α_2 agonists with that of other psychotropic agents in the treatment of aggressive symptoms in youth with behavior disorders.

Risks of Alpha2-Adrenergic Agonists

Alpha$_2$-adrenergic agonists are associated with several adverse side effects, including drowsiness and dizziness (Cantwell et al. 1997). These agents may also be associated with serious adverse risks. Specifically, Cantwell et al. (1997) reported harmful and potentially life-threatening side effects in several children who were treated with clonidine. One child in the study died as a result of an exercise-related syncope, which may have been related to the clonidine treatment. Caution should be executed in administering α_2 agonists to youth with symptoms of aggression and/or DBDs (see Table 3–7 for additional details on the potential adverse effects associated with α_2 agonists).

Beta-Blockers

Current literature on the efficacy of beta-blockers in the treatment of aggression in youth is sparse. In a 1999 review of beta-blockers, Connor et al. found that over 80% of children and adults who used beta-blockers to manage symptoms of aggression demonstrated treatment gains. Specifically, an open-label study found that nadolol, in particular, may be useful in the treatment of aggression and comorbid ADHD in developmentally delayed youth (Connor et al. 1997) (see Table 3–4 for dosage information).

Risks of Beta-Blockers

To date, no RCTs of use of beta-blockers in the treatment of youth have been conducted. Therefore, firm conclusions about the efficacy of these agents cannot be drawn (see Table 3–6). Some of the adverse effects associated with beta-blockers include sedation, mild hypotension, lowered heart rate, bronchoconstriction, hypoglycemia (in patients with diabetes), dizziness, sleep disruption, and potential growth-hormone regulation disturbances (see Table 3–7) (Riddle et al. 1999). Further research on the benefits and risks associated with using beta-blockers to treat youth with aggressive symptoms is needed.

Safety Issues

Monitoring

Antipsychotics

Height and weight should be thoroughly monitored throughout the course of treatment using antipsychotic agents. If weight gain is identified in a child or adolescent who is taking these agents, the physician should implement a diet and exercise plan. Vital signs, with particular attention to cardiac function, should also be routinely assessed in a youth who is taking atypical antipsychotics (Schur et al. 2003). If cardiac symptoms emerge, the physician should consider consulting with a cardiology specialist.

For both typical and atypical antipsychotics, the physician should carefully monitor the youth for EPS such as akathisia, akinesia, tremor, dystonia, and emergent tardive dyskinesia (Connor et al. 2001; McConville and Sorter 2004). Furthermore, the youth should be routinely screened for abnormalities in liver function and lipid production, particularly in the presence of weight gain. Monitoring glucose metabolism is important, given that certain agents may be linked to juvenile diabetes (Clark and Burge 2003). Furthermore, prolactin levels should also be monitored in the case of endocrine symptoms (Wudarsky et al. 1999). Patients should be monitored for rare but life-threatening side effects, including neuroleptic malignant syndrome, seizures, and heat stroke.

Stimulants

Children and adolescents who are taking stimulants should be routinely monitored for adverse symptoms, including insomnia, reduced appetite, stomachache, headache, and dizziness ("A 14-Month Randomized Clinical Trial of Treatment Strategies" 1999; Lisska and Rivkees 2003). Of note, stimulant use has been linked to long-term adverse effects, including height and weight suppression; therefore, it is important that vital signs, height and weight, and abnormalities in metabolic function be thoroughly monitored throughout the course of treatment. Although concerns have been raised about the possibility of cardiac side effects, such effects remain unproven, and electrocardiography or other cardiac monitoring procedures are not indicated in otherwise healthy youth treated for aggression or DBDs. However, if the stimulant is being taken cocurrently with another psychopharmacological agent, such as clonidine, cardiac monitoring is recommended (Fenichel and Lipicky 1994).

Mood Stabilizers

Certain mood-stabilizing agents, such as lithium, require frequent blood draws for dose monitoring and therefore may be less suitable in the treatment of aggressive symptoms and/or behavioral disorders in youth (Bassarath 2003; Malone et al. 2000). In addition, common side effects associated with mood stabilizers include enuresis, fatigue, ataxia, increased thirst, nausea, vomiting, and urinary frequency. Therefore, careful monitoring of these symptoms is required. Moreover, since weight gain is associated with use of mood stabilizers, height and weight should also be monitored during the treatment course. Importantly, it should also be noted that carbamazepine has been linked to serious adverse effects, including hepatotoxic, hematological, and metabolic reactions. Thus, a comprehensive assessment of these systems is important (Cummings and Miller 2004).

Alpha$_2$-Adrenergic Agonists

Careful consideration should be made regarding whether or not to prescribe α_2 agonists to youth with symptoms of aggression. Concerns on the safety of α_2 agonists have been raised because of reports of harmful and potentially life-threatening side effects in several children treated with clonidine (Cantwell et al. 1997). Moreover, clonidine can produce drowsiness and dizziness; thus, patients should be routinely monitored for these symptoms (Hazell and Stuart 2003).

Beta-Blockers

Careful attention should be given to the potential side effects most commonly associated with use of beta-blockers in youth, including sedation, mild hypotension, lowered heart rate, bronchoconstriction, hypoglycemia (in patients with diabetes), dizziness, and sleep disruption (Hazell and Stuart 2003). As with antipsychotics, stimulants, and mood stabilizers, vital signs, height, and weight should be thoroughly monitored throughout the treatment process.

Preventing Adverse Effects

Conservative dosing procedures may prevent the possible occurrence of adverse effects in youth who are taking psychopharmacological agents. The general rule of thumb is to "start low, go slow, and taper slowly" (Pappadopulos et al. 2003). Moreover, potential side effects should be monitored on a systematic basis with rating scales or structured assessment methods (Pappadopulos et al. 2003).

To prevent adverse effects, the physician should avoid prescribing multiple agents whenever possible. In addition, the physician should evaluate and adjust the treatment regimen in youth who do not experience a decrease in aggressive symptoms. Finally, the physician should consider tapering the agent if the youth demonstrates a good response. If the treatment response is maintained during the tapering of a medication, the physician may consider discontinuing the agent.

Interventions to Address Adverse Effects of Psychotropic Agents

Side effects of pharmacological interventions range in severity from life threatening, irreversible, acutely distressing, to those effects that are merely uncomfortable. To more easily distinguish between the potential adverse effects associated with varying psychotropic agents, Table 3–7 separates the potential side effects of each agent into two categories, common and uncommon but serious.

As a general rule of thumb, if the side effect is considered serious, the physician should generally discontinue the use of the agent. Once the serious adverse event is resolved, the physician may consider starting a different psychopharmacological intervention. When appropriate to do so, the physician should consult with specialists (e.g., emergency internal medicine, hematologists, pediatrics) in the care management of youth experiencing serious adverse side effects.

Practical Management Strategies

Treatment Guidelines

Clearly, any conclusions that can be drawn from this review on the pharmacotherapy of aggression are limited by the current scope of the literature. For example, RCTs evaluating the efficacy of atypical medications are a rarity in the current literature. Therefore, until the results of additional RCTs become available, a combination of evidence-based treatment recommendations and expert consensus guidelines may be a useful guide to the use of psychopharmacological agents in the treatment of youth with aggression.

The American Academy of Child and Adolescent Psychiatry has developed several practice parameters geared toward specific mental health issues in children that are based on expert consensus and review of the scientific literature. Several relevant parameters address the assessment and treatment of symptoms of aggression in youth with CD (Steiner 1997), autism (Volkmar et al. 1999), and mental retardation (Szymanski and King 1999). Overall, these parameters stress the importance of using standardized screening instruments and empirically supported multimodal interventions.

Currently, practice parameters are under development with regard to the use of atypical antipsychotics in the treatment of oppositional defiance disorder, CD, aggression, and an array of other psychiatric symptoms and disorders in youth (Findling et al., in press). The focus on the use of atypical agents in the treatment of aggression and/or DBDs in youth is particularly important because aggression is the most common target symptom for which atypicals are prescribed (Cooper et al. 2004; DelBello and Grcevich 2004; Pappadopulos et al. 2003; Simeon et al. 2002; Stigler et al. 2001; Turgay 2005).

Overall, these practice parameters for atypical antipsychotics cite the importance of considering both the age of the study population and the specific diagnosis evaluated in determining whether research findings are applicable to the treatment of child psychiatric disorders in clinical cases (Findling et al., in press). Recommendations for screening, assessment, drug titration, dosage, and other management issues are also addressed (for more details, see Findling et al., in press). Of particular importance in the consideration of aggression typologies, these parameters also note that while atypical antipsychotics have been most rigorously tested as a treatment for impulsive aggression in youth with DBDs, the effectiveness of atypicals in treating other aspects of DBDs has not been as clearly demonstrated. Thus, further research is needed to assess the treatment efficacy of antipsychotics and other psychotropic agents in the treatment of a multitude of aggressive subtypes.

In addition, specific clinical guidelines have been developed for the treatment of aggression and DBDs in youth (Pappadopulos et al. 2003). The Treatment Recommendations for the Use of Antipsychotics for Aggressive Youth (TRAAY) (Jensen et al. 2004) were created using a combination of evidence-

and consensus-based methodologies. Moreover, recommendations were developed from three primary sources of information: current scientific evidence; the expressed needs for guidelines as reported by physicians in focus groups; and consensus of clinical and research experts. Although these guidelines focus primarily on the use of atypical antipsychotics, the use of other classes and agents is addressed. Fourteen treatment recommendations on the use of atypical antipsychotics for aggression in youth with comorbid psychiatric conditions were developed. Each recommendation corresponds to one of the phases of care, evaluation, treatment, stabilization, and maintenance.

The TRAAY guidelines can be briefly summarized as follows: Physicians should conduct an initial diagnostic evaluation (preferably using a standardized assessment tool) before using a pharmacological or psychosocial treatment to manage aggressive symptoms. Typically, a physician should begin with an evidence-based psychosocial intervention as a first-line method of treatment in aggressive youth. If the youth does not make gains in psychotherapy after an adequate time period, the clinician may then consider psychopharmacological treatment, tailoring the agent choice to the primary disorder of the child. If the youth fails to make treatment gains with the agent best suited for the youth's primary disorder, the physician should then consider tapering or switching the agent. Regardless of psychopharmacological approach, the physician should strive to use a conservative dosing strategy. During the course of treatment, the physician should routinely and systematically assess the youth for potential adverse effects. Even for some cases in which adverse effects develop, it is important to ensure an adequate trial of the agent before modifying the treatment plan. Furthermore, the physician should consider tapering and discontinuing medications in youth who show a reduction in aggressive symptoms for a period of 6 months or more (for additional information about the TRAAY guidelines, see Pappadopulos et al. 2003).

Role of Nonmedication Interventions

Whether or not a psychopharmacological intervention is ultimately used, psychoeducation is a critical component of the successful treatment of aggressive disorders in youth. Psychoeducation enables the youth and family to understand and identify aggressive behaviors. Moreover, it also educates the youth and family members about plausible treatment options, including psychopharmacological treatments and behavioral interventions.

As noted in the TRAAY guidelines, empirically supported behavioral interventions should typically constitute the first-line treatment approach in aggressive youth (Pappadopulos et al. 2003). Evidence-based psychosocial interventions for aggression in youth include cognitive-behavioral therapy for aggressive disorders and parent management training (PMT). These evidence-based treatments work to increase positive time spent between youth and family members, help set rules and consequences, and provide training on problem solving and social skills. It should be noted that moderate-to-severe aggressive symptoms in youth typically require a combination of psychoeducation, cognitive and behavioral management strategies, and pharmacological agents.

Conclusions

Additional RCTs are needed to assess the short-term and long-term efficacy, safety, and tolerability of the psychotropic agents used to manage symptoms of aggression and DBDs in youth. More RCTs are also needed to establish the comparative efficacy of the varying psychotropic agents in the treatment of aggression and/or behavioral disorders in youth.

Future RCTs should routinely publish effect size values in order to enhance the clinical interpretation of research findings. Thus far, it appears that the largest effects for the treatment of aggression in youth have been demonstrated with methylphenidate for youth with ADHD and comorbid disruptive behavior problems (mean effect size=0.90) and with risperidone for youth with CD and subaverage intelligence (mean effect size=0.90) (Pappadopulos et al. 2006); however, additional RCTs are needed to test these agents in the management of aggressive youth with nonprimary diagnoses of ADHD and aggressive youth with normal intelligence, respectively.

Additional research is necessary to systematically assess and treat symptoms of proactive and reactive aggression in youth. Because these two forms of aggression may have different etiologic pathways, they may respond differently to different forms of treatment. Thus far, there is some, albeit limited, evidence to suggest that certain psychopharmacological agents may be best suited to manage impulsive aggression in youth; but additional research is needed. Moreover, the development of a standardized measure of aggression subtypes would assist in the goal of understanding and successfully treating the subtypes of aggression.

Although the pharmacological study of aggression and the DBDs is challenged by the severity and chronicity of these conditions, there is some hope that several of our current treatments are among the most effective, in terms of effect sizes, in all of pediatric psychopharmacology. New ways of understanding and assessing aggression, and perhaps the DBDs as well, should be readily available more generally. Overall, although we appear to be making progress in the treatment of severe aggression in youth, this burgeoning area of study and interest bears careful watch in the coming decades.

Clinical Pearls

- Carefully consider using and following currently available evidence- and consensus-based guidelines. Algorithms "provide the framework for facilitating thinking about clinical problems" (Margolis 1983). Available evidence suggests that patients whose doctors generally follow practice guidelines get better outcomes (Emslie et al. 2004; Pliszka et al. 2003; Rush et al. 1995, 1999).

- Remember that less is more (Pappadopulos et al. 2003). Always try to use fewer rather than more medications. Do not add a medication if changing the dose of the current medication is likely to achieve comparable benefit. And do not assume that smaller doses of two or more medications are preferable to higher, appropriate doses of a single medication.

- Don't quit too soon. Do not assume a given medication doesn't work until you have tested it throughout the dose range. As a general rule, in the absence of side effects and lack of response, continue to cautiously raise the dose until you see treatment effects or side effects.

- Start low, go slow, and taper slowly (Pappadopulos et al. 2003).

- Address compliance and adherence issues. Even under optimal circumstances, youth are taking less medication than you are prescribing, even when they assure you they are "taking it as directed." But there are often reasons for less than perfect compliance and adherence—for example, simple forgetting, unexpressed fears about side effects or "addiction," real side effects, cultural factors and

beliefs, child resistance, differing viewpoints between parents—
that can be verbalized and talked through. Often parents are em-
barrassed to admit they have misgivings about the medication or
that they forgot to administer it. They do not want to seem either
like bad parents or mistrustful of your judgment.

- Help children and adolescents to take active roles and responsi-
  bility for controlling and redirecting their behaviors. A kid is not
  simply a receptor or neurotransmitter problem. If the child likes the
  doctor and thinks the doctor likes him or her, considerable progress can be made in using this relationship not just to enhance
  compliance/adherence, but, perhaps more importantly, to influence the child to monitor and *take charge* of his or her behavior
  problems.

- Encourage parents to put optimal parenting and milieu strategies
  into place when managing aggression and DBDs. Parents are not
  automated medication dispensers. Available evidence suggests that
  even in the most challenging cases—those in which comorbid complexity and family stressors are present—benefit is derived from
  careful family support and frequent follow-up (Owens et al. 2003).

- You can't do it alone, so don't pretend you can, and don't even try.
  From the outset, particularly in difficult cases, indicate to parents
  and youth that treating DBDs and aggression with medication can
  be helpful but is rarely sufficient. Tell them that just as with diabetes or severe allergies, changes in family lifestyle are needed; you
  and the family have to work as partners to address situations that
  escalate the child's aggression or DBD symptoms. If you are close
  to even a medium-size city, encourage or require parents to attend
  parent support groups with an organization such as National
  Alliance on Mental Illness (NAMI) (www.nami.org), Children and
  Adults With Attention-Deficit/Hyperactivity Disorder (CHADD)
  (www.chadd.org), Depression and Bipolar Support Alliance
  (DBSA) (www.dbsalliance.org), Federation of Families for Children's Mental Health, (www.ffcmh.org), Mental Health America
  (formerly National Mental Health Association) (www.nmha.org,
  www.mentalhealthamerica.net), and others.

- If you cannot provide evidence-based psychotherapeutic support, get a partner who can. Such support is a must. A range of psychosocial interventions have been developed for treating aggression and related conduct problems, including parent management training (Brestan and Eyberg 1998; Burke et al. 2002; Kazdin et al. 1989, 1992), Parent-Child Interaction Therapy (PCIT) (Schuhmann et al. 1998), some school- and community-based programs (Farmer et al. 2004), and some individual cognitive-behavioral treatments, including anger management training and problem-solving skills training (Brestan and Eyberg 1998; Lochman and Curry 1986; Lochman and Lampron 1988).

References

Aman MG, Teehan CJ, White AJ, et al: Haloperidol treatment with chronically medicated residents: dose effects on clinical behavior and reinforcement contingencies. Am J Ment Retard 93:452–460, 1989

Aman MG, Marks RE, Turbott SH, et al: Clinical effects of methylphenidate and thioridazine in intellectually subaverage children. J Am Acad Child Adolesc Psychiatry 30:246–256, 1991

Aman MG, De Smedt G, Derivan A, et al: Double-blind, placebo-controlled study of risperidone for the treatment of disruptive behaviors in children with subaverage intelligence. Am J Psychiatry 159:1337–1346, 2002

Aman MG, Binder C, Turgay A: Risperidone effects in the presence/absence of psychostimulant medicine in children with ADHD, other disruptive behavior disorders, and subaverage IQ. J Child Adolesc Psychopharmacol 14:243–254, 2004

American Psychiatric Association: Diagnostic and Statistical Manual of Mental Disorders, 4th Edition, Text Revision. Washington, DC, American Psychiatric Association, 2000

Bambauer KZ, Connor DF: Characteristics of aggression in clinically referred children. CNS Spectr 10:709–718, 2005

Bassarath L: Medication strategies in childhood aggression: a review. Can J Psychiatry 48:367–373, 2003

Brestan EV, Eyberg SM: Effective psychosocial treatments of conduct-disordered children and adolescents: 29 years, 82 studies, and 5,272 kids. J Clin Child Psychol 27:180–189, 1998

Brown K, Atkins MS, Osborne ML, et al: A revised teacher rating scale for reactive and proactive aggression. J Abnorm Child Psychol 24:473–480, 1996

Buitelaar JK, van der Gaag RJ, Cohen-Kettenis P, et al: A randomized controlled trial of risperidone in the treatment of aggression in hospitalized adolescents with subaverage cognitive abilities. J Clin Psychiatry 62:239–248, 2001

Bukstein OG, Kolko DJ: Effects of methylphenidate on aggressive urban children with attention deficit hyperactivity disorder. J Clin Child Psychol 27:340–351, 1998

Burke JD, Loeber R, Birmaher B: Oppositional defiant disorder and conduct disorder: a review of the past 10 years, part II. J Am Acad Child Adolesc Psychiatry 41:1275–1293, 2002

Campbell M, Small AM, Green WH, et al: Behavioral efficacy of haloperidol and lithium carbonate: A comparison in hospitalized aggressive children with conduct disorder. Arch Gen Psychiatry 41:650–656, 1984

Campbell M, Adams PB, Small AM, et al: Lithium in hospitalized aggressive children with conduct disorder: A double-blind and placebo-controlled study. J Am Acad Child Adolesc Psychiatry 34:445–453, 1995

Campbell M, Rapoport JL, Simpson GM: Antipsychotics in children and adolescents. J Am Acad Child Adolesc Psychiatry 38:537–545, 1999

Cantwell DP, Swanson J, Connor DF: Case study: adverse response to clonidine. J Am Acad Child Adolesc Psychiatry 36:539–544, 1997

Carlson GA, Rapport MD, Pataki CS, et al: Lithium in hospitalized children at 4 and 8 weeks: mood, behavior and cognitive effects. J Child Psychol Psychiatry 33:411–425, 1992

Center for the Advancement of Children's Mental Health, Office of Mental Health: 10 Tips: Navigating Child and Adolescent Inpatient and Residential Services in New York State. New York, New York State Office of Mental Health, manuscript in preparation

Chalasani L, Kant R, Chengappa KN: Clozapine impact on clinical outcomes and aggression in severely ill adolescents with childhood-onset schizophrenia. Can J Psychiatry 46:965–968, 2001

Clark C, Burge MR: Diabetes mellitus associated with atypical anti-psychotic medications. Diabetes Technol Ther 5:669–683, 2003

Connor DF, Ozbayrak KR, Benjamin S, et al: A pilot study of nadolol for overt aggression in developmentally delayed individuals. J Am Acad Child Adolesc Psychiatry 36:826–834, 1997

Connor DF, Fletcher KE, Swanson, JM: A meta-analysis of clonidine for symptoms of attention-deficit hyperactivity disorder. J Am Acad Child Adolesc Psychiatry 38:1551–1559, 1999

Connor DF, Fletcher KE, Wood JS: Neuroleptic-related dyskinesias in children and adolescents. J Clin Psychiatry 62:967–974, 2001

Connor DF, Glatt SJ, Lopez ID, et al: Psychopharmacology and aggression, I: a meta-analysis of stimulant effects on overt/covert aggression-related behaviors in ADHD. J Am Acad Child Adolesc Psychiatry 41:253–261, 2002

Connor DF, Steingard RJ, Cunningham JA, et al: Proactive and reactive aggression in referred children and adolescents. Am J Orthopsychiatry 74:129–136, 2004

Cooper WO, Hickson GB, Fuchs C, et al: New users of antipsychotic medications among children enrolled in TennCare. Arch Pediatr Adolesc Med 158:753–759, 2004

Croonenberghs J, Fegert JM, Findling RL et al: Risperidone in children with disruptive behavior disorders and subaverage intelligence: a 1-year, open-label study of 504 patients. J Am Acad Child Adolesc Psychiatry 44:969–970, 2005

Cueva JE, Overall JE, Small AM, et al: Carbamazepine in aggressive children with conduct disorder: a double-blind and placebo-controlled study. J Am Acad Child Adolesc Psychiatry 35:480–490, 1996

Cummings MR, Miller BD: Pharmacologic management of behavioral instability in medically ill pediatric patients. Curr Opin Pediatr 16:516–522, 2004

DelBello M, Grcevich S: Phenomenology and epidemiology of childhood psychiatric disorders that may necessitate treatment with atypical antipsychotics. J Clin Psychiatry 65:12–19, 2004

Dodge K: The structure and function of reactive and proactive aggression, in The Development and Treatment of Childhood Aggression. Edited by Pepler DJ, Rubin KH. Hillsdale, NJ, Erlbaum, 1991, pp 201–208

Dodge K, Coie JD: Social-information processing factors in reactive and proactive aggression in children's peer groups. J Pers Soc Psychol 52:1146–1158, 1987

Donovan SJ, Susser ES, Nunes EV, et al: Divalproex treatment of disruptive adolescents: a report of 10 cases. J Clin Psychiatry 58:12–15, 1997

Donovan SJ, Stewart JW, Nunes EV, et al: Divalproex treatment for youth with explosive temper and mood lability: a double-blind, placebo-controlled crossover design. Am J Psychiatry 157:818–820, 2000

Donovan SJ, Nunes EV, Stewart JW, et al: Outer-directed irritability: a distinct mood syndrome in explosive youth with a disruptive behavior disorder? J Clin Psychiatry 64:698–701, 2003

dosReis S, Barnett S, Love RC: A guide for managing acute aggressive behavior of youths in residential and inpatient treatment facilities. Psychiatr Serv 54:1357–1363, 2003

Emslie GJ, Hughes CW, Crismon ML, et al: A feasibility study of the childhood depression medication algorithm: the Texas Children's Medication Algorithm Project (CMAP). J Am Acad Child Adolesc Psychiatry 43:519–527, 2004

Evans RW, Clay TH, Gualtieri CT: Carbamazepine in pediatric psychiatry. J Am Acad Child Adolesc Psychiatry 26:2–8, 1987

Farmer EM, Dorsey S, Mustillo SA: Intensive home and community interventions. Child Adolesc Psychiatr Clin N Am 13:857–884, 2004

Fenichel RR, Lipicky RJ: Combination products as first-line pharmacotherapy. Arch Intern Med 154:1429–1430, 1994

Findling RL, McNamara NK, Branicky LA, et al: A double-blind pilot study of risperidone in the treatment of conduct disorder. J Am Acad Child Adolesc Psychiatry 39:509–516, 2000

Findling RL, Drury SS, Jensen PS, et al: Practice parameter for the use of atypical antipsychotic medications in children and adolescents. J Am Acad Child Adolesc Psychiatry, (in press)

A 14-month randomized clinical trial of treatment strategies for attention-deficit/hyperactivity disorder. The MTA Cooperative Group. Multimodal Treatment Study of Children With ADHD. Arch Gen Psychiatry 56:1073–1086, 1999

Galanter CA, Carlson GA, Jensen PS, et al: Response to methylphenidate in children with attention deficit hyperactivity disorder and manic symptoms in the multimodal treatment study of children with attention deficit hyperactivity disorder titration trial. J Child Adolesc Psychopharmacol 13:123–136, 2004

Gillberg C, Hellgren L: Mental disturbances in adolescents: a knowledge review. Nord Med 101:49–53, 1986

Gittelman-Klein R, Klein DF, Katz S, et al: Comparative effects of methylphenidate and thioridazine in hyperkinetic children, I: clinical results. Arch Gen Psychiatry 33:1217–1231, 1976

Hazell PL, Stuart JE: A randomized controlled trial of clonidine added to psychostimulant medication for hyperactive and aggressive children. J Am Acad Child Adolesc Psychiatry 42:886–894, 2003

Hollander E, Dolgoff-Kaspar R, Cartwright C, et al: An open trial of divalproex sodium in autism spectrum disorders. J Clin Psychiatry 62:530–534, 2001

Horrigan JP, Barnhill, LJ, Courvoisie, HE: Olanzapine in PDD. J Am Acad Child Adolesc Psychiatry 36:1666–1667, 1997

Hunkeler EM, Fireman B, Lee J, et al: Trends in use of antidepressants, lithium, and anticonvulsants in Kaiser Permanente–insured youths, 1994–2003. J Child Adolesc Psychopharmacol 15:26–37, 2005

Jensen PS, Kettle L, Roper MT, et al. Are stimulants overprescribed? Treatment of ADHD in four U.S. communities. J Am Acad Child Adolesc Psychiatry 38:797–804, 1999

Jensen PS, Hinshaw SP, Kraemer HC, et al: ADHD comorbidity findings from the MTA study: comparing comorbid subgroups. J Am Acad Child Adolesc Psychiatry 40:147–158, 2001

Jensen PS, MacIntyre JC, Pappadopulos EA (eds): Treatment Recommendations for the Use of Antipsychotic Medications for Aggressive Youth (TRAAT): Pocket Reference Guide. for Clinicians in Child and Adolescent Psychiatry. New York, New York State Office of Mental Health and Center for the Advancement of Children's Mental Health at Columbia University, Department of Child and Adolescent Psychiatry, 2004

Jensen PS, Youngstrom EA, Steiner H, et al: Consensus report on impulsive aggression as a symptom across diagnostic categories in child psychiatry: implications for medication studies. J Am Acad Child Adolesc Psychiatry 46:309–322, 2007

Jobson KO, Potter WZ: International psychopharmacology algorithm project report. Psychopharmacol Bull 31:457–459, 491–500, 1995

Kafantaris V, Campbell M, Padron-Gayol MV, et al: Carbamazepine in hospitalized aggressive conduct disorder children: an open pilot study. Psychopharmacol Bull 28:193–199, 1992

Kazdin AE: Child, parent and family dysfunction as predictors of outcome in cognitive-behavioral treatment of antisocial children. Behav Res Ther 33:271–281, 1995

Kazdin AE, Bass D, Siegel T, et al: Cognitive-behavioral therapy and relationship therapy in the treatment of children referred for antisocial behavior. J Consult Clin Psychol 57:522–535, 1989

Kazdin AE, Siegel TC, Bass D: Cognitive problem-solving skills training and parent management training in the treatment of antisocial behavior in children. J Consult Clin Psychol 60:733–747, 1992

Klein RG, Abikoff H, Klass E, et al: Clinical efficacy of methylphenidate in conduct disorder with and without attention deficit hyperactivity disorder. Arch Gen Psychiatry 54:1073–1080, 1997

Kranzler H, Roofeh D, Gerbino-Rosen G, et al: Clozapine: its impact on aggressive behavior among children and adolescents with schizophrenia: clinical trial. J Am Acad Child Adolesc Psychiatry 44:55–63, 2005

Lahey BB, Loeber R, Quay HC, et al: Validity of DSM-IV subtypes of conduct disorder based on age of onset. J Am Acad Child Adolesc Psychiatry 37:435–442, 1998

Lisska MC, Rivkees SA: Daily methylphenidate use slows the growth of children: a community based study. J Pediatr Endocrinol Metab 16:711–718, 2003

Lochman JE, Curry JF: Effects of social problem-solving training and self-instruction training with aggressive boys. J Clin Child Psychol 15:159–164, 1986

Lochman JE, Lampron LB: Cognitive-behavioral interventions for aggressive boys: seven months follow-up effects. J Child Adolesc Psychotherapy 5:15–23, 1988

Loeber R, Keenen K, Lahey BB, et al: Evidence for developmentally based diagnoses of oppositional defiant disorder and conduct disorder. J Abnorm Child Psychol 21:377–410, 1993

Loeber R, Burke JD, Lahey BB: What are adolescent antecedents to antisocial personality disorder? Crim Behav Ment Health 12:24–36, 2002

Loeber R, Green SM, Lahey BB: Risk factors for antisocial personality, in Primary Prevention of Adult Antisocial Personality. Edited by Coid J, Farrington DP. Cambridge, England, Cambridge University Press, 2003

Malone RP, Delaney MA, Luebbert JF, et al: A double-blind placebo-controlled study of lithium in hospitalized aggressive children and adolescents with conduct disorder. Arch Gen Psychiatry 57:649–654, 2000

Mannuzza S, Klein RG, Bessler A, et al: Adult outcome of hyperactive boys: educational achievement, occupational rank, and psychiatric status. Arch Gen Psychiatry 50:565–576, 1993

Mannuzza S, Klein RG, Bessler A, et al: Adult psychiatric status of hyperactive boys grown up. Am J Psychiatry 155:493–498, 1998

Margolis CZ: Uses of clinical algorithms. JAMA 249:627–632, 1983

Martin A, Scahill L, Charney DS, et al (eds): Pediatric Psychopharmacology: Principles and Practice. Oxford, England, Oxford University Press, 2003

McConville BJ, Sorter MT: Treatment challenges and safety considerations for antipsychotic use in children and adolescents with psychoses. J Clin Psychiatry 65:20–29, 2004

McCracken JT, McGough J, Shah B: Risperidone in children with autism and serious behavioral problems. N Engl J Med 347:314–321, 2002

MTA Cooperative Group: National Institute of Mental Health Multimodal Treatment Study of ADHD follow-up: 24 month outcomes of treatment strategies for attention deficit/hyperactivity disorder. Pediatrics 113:754–761, 2004

Olfson M, Blanco C, Liu L, et al: National trends in the outpatient treatment of children and adolescents with antipsychotic drugs. Arch Gen Psychiatry 63:679–685, 2006

Owens EB, Hinshaw SP, Kraemer HC: Which treatment for whom for ADHD? Moderators of treatment response in the MTA. J Consult Clin Psychol 71:540–552, 2003

Pappadopulos E, Macintyre JC, Crismon ML, et al: Treatment Recommendations for the Use of Antipsychotics for Aggressive Youth (TRAAY), Part II. J Am Acad Child Adolesc Psychiatry 42:145–161, 2003

Pappadopulos E, Tate Guelzow B, Wong C, et al: A review of the growing evidence base for pediatric psychopharmacology. Child Adolesc Psychiatr Clin N Am 13:817–855, 2004

Pappadopulos EA, Woolston S, Chait A, et al: Pharmacotherapy of aggression in children and adolescents: efficacy and effect size. Journal of the Canadian Academy of Child and Adolescent Psychiatry 15:27–39, 2006

Pliszka SR, Lopez M, Crismon ML, et al: A feasibility study of the Children's Medication Algorithm Project (CMAP) algorithm for the treatment of ADHD. J Am Acad Child Adolesc Psychiatry 42:279–287, 2003

Potenza MN, Holmes JP, Kanes SJ, et al: Olanzapine treatment of children, adolescents, and adults with pervasive developmental disorders: an open-label pilot study. J Clin Psychopharmacol 19:37–44, 1999

Rabinowitz J, Avnon M, Rosenberg V: Effect of clozapine on physical and verbal aggression. Schizophr Res 22:249–255, 1996

Research Units on Pediatric Psychopharmacology Autism Network: Risperidone treatment of autistic disorder: longer-term benefits and blinded discontinuation after 6 months. Am J Psychiatry 162:1361–1369, 2005

Reyes M, Buitelaar J, Toren P, et al: A randomized, double-blind, placebo-controlled study of risperidone maintenance treatment in children and adolescents with disruptive behavior disorders. Am J Psychiatry 163:402–410, 2006a

Reyes M, Croonenberghs J, Augustyns I, et al: Long-term use of risperidone in children with disruptive behavior disorders and subaverage intelligence: efficacy, safety, and tolerability. J Child Adolesc Psychopharmacol 16:260–272, 2006b

Riddle MA, Berstein GA, Cook EH, et al: Anxiolytics, adrenergic agents, and naltrexone. J Am Acad Child Adolesc Psychiatry 38:546–556, 1999

Rush AJ, Kupfer DJ: Strategies and Tactics in the Treatment of Depression, Vol 1, 2nd Edition. Washington, DC, American Psychiatric Press, 1995

Rush AJ, Rago WV, Crismon ML, et al: Medication treatment for the severely and persistently mentally ill: the Texas Medication Algorithm Project. J Clin Psychiatry 60:284–291, 1999

Saxena K, Howe M, Simeonova D, et al: Divalproex sodium reduces overall aggression in youth at high risk for bipolar disorder. J Child Adolesc Psychopharmacol 16:252–259, 2006

Scahill L, Chappell PB, Kim YS, et al: A placebo-controlled study of guanfacine in the treatment of children with tic disorders and attention deficit hyperactivity disorder. Am J Psychiatry 158:1067–1074, 2001

Schuhmann EM, Foote RC, Eyberg SM, et al: Efficacy of Parent-Child Interaction Therapy: interim report of a randomized trial with short-term maintenance. J Clin Child Psychol 27:34–45, 1998

Schur SB, Sikich L, Findling RL, et al: Treatment Recommendations for the Use of Antipsychotics for Aggressive Youth (TRAAY), part I: a review. J Am Acad Child Adolesc Psychiatry 42:132–144, 2003

Sikich L, Hamer RM, Bashford RA, et al: A pilot study of risperidone, olanzapine, and haloperidol in psychotic youth: a double-blind, randomized, 8-week trial. Neuropsychopharmacology 29:133–145, 2004

Simeon J, Milin R, Walker S: A retrospective chart review of risperidone use in treatment-resistant children and adolescents with psychiatric disorders. Prog Neuropsychopharmacol Biol Psychiatry 26:267–275, 2002

Snyder R, Turgay A, Aman M, et al: Effects of risperidone on conduct and disruptive behavior disorders in children with subaverage IQs. J Am Acad Child Adolesc Psychiatry 41:1026–1036, 2002

Steiner H: Practice parameters for the assessment and treatment of children and adolescents with conduct disorder. American Academy of Child and Adolescent Psychiatry. J Am Acad Child Adolesc Psychiatry 36(suppl):122S–139S, 1997

Steiner H: Divalproex sodium for the treatment of conduct disorder: a randomized clinical trial. J Clin Psychiatry 64:1183–1191, 2003

Steiner H, Saxena K, Chang K: Psychopharmacologic strategies for the treatment of aggression in juveniles. CNS Spectr 8:298–308, 2003

Stephens RJ, Bassel C, Sandor P: Olanzapine in the treatment of aggression and tics in children with Tourette's syndrome: a pilot study. J Child Adolesc Psychopharmacol 14:255–266, 2004

Stigler KA, Potenza MN, McDougle CJ: Tolerability profile of atypical antipsychotics in children and adolescents Paediatr Drugs 3:927–942, 2001

Stigler KA, Potenza MN, Posey DJ, et al: Weight gain associated with atypical antipsychotic use in children and adolescents: prevalence, clinical relevance, and management. Paediatr Drugs 6:33–44, 2004

Swanson JM, Kraemer HC, Hinshaw SP, et al: Clinical relevance of the primary findings of the MTA: success rates based on severity of ADHD and ODD symptoms at the end of treatment. J Am Acad Child Adolesc Psychiatry 40:168–179, 2001

Szymanski L, King BH: Practice parameters for the assessment and treatment of children, adolescents, and adults with mental retardation and comorbid mental disorders. American Academy of Child and Adolescent Psychiatry Working Group on Quality Issues. J Am Acad Child Adolesc Psychiatry 38(suppl):5S–31S, 1999

Troost PW, Lahuis BE, Steenhuis MP, et al: Long-term effects of risperidone in children with autism spectrum disorders: a placebo discontinuation study. J Am Acad Child Adolesc Psychiatry 44:1137–1144, 2005

Turgay A: Treatment of comorbidity in conduct disorder with attention-deficit hyperactivity disorder (ADHD). Essent Psychopharmacol 6:277–290, 2005

Turgay A, Binder C, Snyder R, et al: Long-term safety and efficacy of risperidone for the treatment of disruptive behavior disorders in children with subaverage IQs. Pediatrics 110:e34, 2002

U.S. Food and Drug Administration: Antidepressant use in children, adolescents, and adults. Rockville, MD, U.S. Food and Drug Administration, 2005. Available at: http://www.fda.gov/cder/drug/antidepressants/default.htm. Accessed November 18, 2005

U.S. Food and Drug Administration: Drug Safety and Risk Management Advisory Committee (DSaRM), Vol 1. Rockville, MD, U.S. Department of Health and Human Services, Food and Drug Administration, Center for Drug Evaluation and Research, 2006. Available at: http://www.fda.gov/ohrms/dockets/ac/06/transcripts/2006-4202t1.pdf. Accessed July 18, 2006

Vitaro F, Gendreau PL, Tremblay RE, et al: Reactive and proactive aggression differentially predict later conduct problems. J Child Psychol Psychiatry 39:377–385, 1998

Vitiello B, Stoff DM: Subtypes of aggression and their relevance to child psychiatry. J Am Acad Child Adolesc Psychiatry 36:307–315, 1997

Vitiello B, Behar D, Hunt J, et al: Subtyping aggression in children and adolescents. J Neuropsychiatry Clin Neurosci 2:189–192, 1990

Volavka J, Citrome L: Atypical antipsychotics in the treatment of the persistently aggressive psychotic patient: methodological concerns. Schizophr Res 35:23–33, 1999

Volkmar F, Cook EH Jr, Pomeroy J, et al: Practice parameters for the assessment and treatment of children, adolescents, and adults with autism and other pervasive developmental disorders. American Academy of Child and Adolescent Psychiatry Working Group on Quality Issues. J Am Acad Child Adolesc Psychiatry 38(suppl):32S–54S, 1999

Weiner B (ed): Physician's Desk Reference Generics, 2nd Edition. Montvale, NJ, Medical Economics, 1996

Werry JS: Severe conduct disorder: some key issues. Can J Psychiatry 42:577–583, 1997

Wudarsky M, Nicolson R, Hamburger SD, et al: Elevated prolactin in pediatric patients on typical and atypical antipsychotics. J Child Adolesc Psychopharmacol 9:239–245, 1999

4

Anxiety Disorders

Moira A. Rynn, M.D
Jennifer Regan, B.A.

Anxiety disorders begin in childhood and often evolve into adulthood, resulting in lifelong impairment in multiple areas, such as achievement in school, work, relationships, and health. Anxiety disorders are insidious in nature, leading a person to limp along in life, often without relief, because identification and treatment of these disorders are lacking. This results in a waxing and waning course of illness. This lack of acknowledgment and, consequently, treatment is partly due to the fact that the symptoms of anxiety are an expected part of a normal life. Some health care providers seem to have a bias, believing that suffering from an anxiety disorder is not as serious as suffering from other psychiatric disorders, such as major depression.

The sense of anxiety disorders being less serious than other disorders is reflected in the diagnostic definitions given in the revisions of the *Diagnostic and Statistical Manual of Mental Disorders* (DSM). Initially, anxiety disorders were all classified, in DSM-I (American Psychiatric Association 1952), as *psychoneurotic disorders* (reactions) and, in DSM-II (American Psychiatric Association 1968), as neuroses. It was not until DSM-III (American Psychiatric Association 1980) that anxiety disorders started to take shape with delineated criteria for children, including the addition of separation anxiety disorder. In DSM-IV and DSM-IV-TR (American Psychiatric Association 1994, 2000), most childhood anxiety disorders are subsumed under the adult definitions for generalized anxiety disorder (GAD), obsessive-compulsive disorder (OCD), posttraumatic stress disorder (PTSD), social anxiety disorder, and panic disorder (Rickels and Rynn 2001). For example, children who in the past may have been diagnosed with overanxious disorder in childhood would now receive the diagnosis of GAD on the basis of contemporary psychiatric nosology.

Epidemiology

Anxiety disorders, such as overanxious disorder, GAD, and social anxiety disorder, are among the most common diagnoses reported in childhood and adolescent epidemiological studies (Feehan et al. 1994; Lewinsohn et al. 1993; McGee et al. 1990). In community epidemiological studies, the prevalence rates for overanxious disorder have ranged from 2.9% to 4.6%, and rates for separation anxiety disorder have ranged from 2.4% to 4.1% (Anderson et al. 1987; Bowen et al. 1990; Costello 1989). In a general pediatric clinical sample, 8.9% of children met criteria for any anxiety disorder (Costello et al. 1988).

In addition, social avoidance that interferes with functioning and is manifested in worries, isolation, hypersensitivity, sadness, and self-consciousness has been reported in 10%–20% of school-age children (Orvaschel and Weissman 1986; Werry 1986). Prevalence rates for internalizing disorders are also greater in clinical samples, with 14% of patients being diagnosed with an anxiety disorder (Keller et al. 1992).

For specific anxiety disorders, the reported prevalence rates are variable (for review, see Costello et al. 2005): GAD and overanxious disorder are the most common, and separation anxiety disorder is the second most common. The prevalence of OCD and panic disorder approaches 1% in population studies. However, these reported rates vary depending on whether the level of functional impairment is included in the definition. A child with some impaired functioning may not exhibit every symptom to satisfy the full diagnostic criteria and, unfortunately, may not be recommended to receive treatment.

Course and Outcome

Children with anxiety disorders often suffer from low self-esteem and experience social isolation, which fosters inadequate social skills (Strauss 1988). These children also report higher rates of physical symptoms, such as headaches, stomachaches, and irritable bowel syndrome (Livingston et al. 1988). These symptoms can then increase visits to the pediatrician, leading to an increase in family medical costs. Furthermore, there is concern that the presence of anxiety disorders early in childhood provides the pathway for developing subsequent mood and substance abuse disorders (Weissman et al. 1999). Pine and Grun (1998) reported that children with a history of long-term anxiety disorders exhibit increased rates of other psychiatric disorders, psychiatric hospitalization, and suicide attempts as adults.

Anxiety disorders and symptoms are not simply transitory but persist over time (Beidel et al. 1996; Cantwell and Baker 1989; Keller et al. 1992). Dadds et al. (1997) performed a school-based prevention study in which untreated anxious children were identified by self-report and/or teachers' ratings as having features of an anxiety disorder but not meeting the full diagnosis. Results revealed that 54% of those children developed a full anxiety disorder over the remaining 6 months of the study. Children with GAD/overanxious disorder have also been found to be at a higher risk for concurrent additional anxiety disorder (Last et al. 1987a). A prospective 3- to 4-year follow-up study by Last et al. (1996) showed that children with anxiety disorders, though free from their initial anxiety diagnosis at follow-up, were more likely than control subjects to develop new psychiatric disorders, usually a different anxiety disorder, over the time course.

There also appears to be an association between childhood disorders and the presence of adult anxiety disorders. A large number of adults who are given an anxiety diagnosis report childhood histories of separation anxiety or overanxious disorders (Aronson and Logue 1987; Last et al. 1987b, 1987c). One of the few prospective studies that have assessed anxious children's adjustment to early adulthood found that anxious children, especially those with comorbid depression, were less likely than control subjects with no history of psychiatric illness to be living independently, working, or in school (Last et al. 1997). In an outpatient setting, approximately 30% of children with an anxiety disorder have comorbid depression (for review, see Brady and Kendall 1992).

In addition, there is some evidence that as many as 41% of children or adolescents who suffer from major depression had or have an anxiety disorder that preceded the depression (Brady and Kendall 1992; Kovacs et al. 1989). The presence of an anxiety disorder was found to predict a worse prognosis for the depression and, at times, had an effect on the length of or recovery from the depressive episode. Furthermore, after treatment of and recovery from depression, the anxiety disorder usually persisted (Kovacs et al. 1989). Early treatment intervention for anxiety disorders may prevent and alter the course of developing depression and other psychiatric disorders, leading to an improved opportunity for a successful adulthood.

Rationale and Justification for Psychopharmacological Treatment

In recent years, there have been major developments in the treatment of pediatric anxiety disorders with medications. There is strong evidenced-based medicine to suggest that antidepressants, particularly selective serotonin reuptake inhibitors (SSRIs), are safe and efficacious for treating these disorders, as will be reviewed in this chapter. In addition to medication treatment, there is an extensive literature supporting the use of cognitive-behavioral therapy (CBT) for the treatment of pediatric anxiety disorders. The American Academy of Child and Adolescent Psychiatry (2007) anxiety practice parameters recommend that psychosocial treatments, such as CBT, be considered in the treatment of anxious children. Unfortunately, one of the challenges often faced by clinicians recommending CBT is the limited availability of this treatment in many communities. This may lead a clinician to instead initiate medication treatment.

Another issue concerning the use of medications is a consideration of the risk-benefit profile. As of this writing, the safety data from completed randomized clinical trials (RCTs) demonstrate that the adverse-effects profiles of SSRIs in children resemble those of adults and that, overall, these medications are safe and well tolerated. However, the U.S. Food and Drug Administration (FDA) has required a black box warning on various classes of antidepressants because of concern for a potentially increased risk of suicidal ideation and/or behaviors for children taking these medications. In contrast to the pediatric depression RCTs, the majority of pediatric anxiety studies did not show evidence of increased suicidal thinking or behaviors for children taking medications compared with placebo. An alternative option is combined treatment of CBT with medication. An emerging literature, reviewed later in this chapter, suggests combination treatment may provide some advantages.

Medications for Pediatric Anxiety Disorders: Review of Treatment Studies

Selective Serotonin Reuptake Inhibitors

To date, the most widely researched pharmacological treatments for pediatric anxiety disorders are selective serotonin reuptake inhibitors (Table 4–1). The class of SSRIs includes fluvoxamine (Luvox), sertraline (Zoloft), fluoxetine (Prozac), citalopram (Celexa), and paroxetine (Paxil), among others. Although SSRIs are characterized as antidepressants, they are unique in that they specifically inhibit the reuptake of the neurotransmitter serotonin, therefore resulting in increased amounts of serotonin in the synapses of the brain. Decreased serotonin levels are attributed to various disorders, including depression (Roy et al. 1989) and anxiety disorders (Nutt and Lawson 1992; Pigott 1996; Tancer 1993). Extensive empirical literature supports the efficacy of SSRIs in treating adult anxiety disorders (Katzelnick et al. 1995; Liebowitz et al. 2002; Pohl et al. 1998; Pollack et al. 2001).

Efficacy of Acute Treatment

Although the literature assessing the efficacy of SSRIs for pediatric anxiety disorders is not quite as extensive as the adult literature, clinical use in children has grown in recent years. The use of SSRIs and other, newer antidepressants in the U.S. population under 18 years of age increased significantly from 0.8% in 1997 to 1.6% in 2002 ($P < 0.001$; Vitiello et al. 2006). As a result of this frequency of use, the evidence presented in the current literature, and the relatively minimal side effects, SSRIs are presently considered the first-line pharmacotherapy choice for childhood anxiety disorders. Although there have been numerous promising open-label studies (Birmaher et al. 1994; Compton et al. 2001), the RCTs discussed here are those that demonstrate the most compelling evidence for the acute treatment of SSRIs.

Fluoxetine (Prozac).   To date, there have been numerous well-designed fluoxetine studies that test use in pediatric anxiety disorders. Black and Uhde

Table 4–1.   Medications for pediatric anxiety disorders

Drug	Total daily dose	Dosing schedule	Main indications	Side effects
ANTIDEPRESSANTS				
Tricyclic antidepressants				
Tertiary amines				
Clomipramine	2.0–5.0 mg/kg	qd or bid	OCD School refusal	Anticholinergic effects such as dizziness, drowsiness, and dry mouth
Imipramine	2.0–5.0 mg/kg	qd or bid	GAD Panic disorder	Requires electrocardiographic monitoring
Secondary amines				
Desipramine	2.0–5.0 mg/kg	qd or bid	OCD	Potential for cardiac toxicity
Selective serotonin reuptake inhibitors				Gastrointestinal side effects, weight gain and loss, sweating, dry mouth, headaches, irritability, insomnia, fatigue, hypersomnia, restlessness, increased hyperactivity, tremor, increased risk for self-injury and self-injurious behaviors, mania, withdrawal effects, sexual side effects
Citalopram	20–40 mg	qd (A.M.)	Social phobia	
Fluoxetine	10–60 mg	qd (A.M.)	OCD, GAD, SAD, SOC	
Fluvoxamine	50–300 mg	qd (A.M.)	OCD, GAD, SAD, SOC	
Paroxetine	10–40 mg	Once daily (A.M.)	SAD, SOC	
Sertraline	25–200 mg	Once daily (A.M.)	Panic disorder	

Table 4–1. Medications for pediatric anxiety disorders (*continued*)

Drug	Total daily dose	Dosing schedule	Main indications	Side effects
ANTIDEPRESSANTS (*continued*)				
Serotonin-norepinephrine reuptake inhibitors				
Venlafaxine XR	37.5–225 mg	qd	GAD, SAD, SOC	Gastrointestinal side effects, headache, weight loss, fatigue, insomnia, irritability, hypersomnia
				Monitor blood pressure
BENZODIAZEPINES				
Long-acting				
Clonazepam[a]	0.25–2 mg	qd, bid, tid	GAD, panic disorder	Sedation, drowsiness, decreased alertness, disinhibition, taper
Short-to-intermediate acting				
Alprazolam[a]	0.25–4 mg	PRN, qd, bid, tid	GAD, panic disorder	Sedation, drowsiness, decreased alertness, disinhibition, taper
Lorazepam[a]	0.25–6 mg	PRN, qd, bid, tid	GAD, panic disorder	Sedation, drowsiness, decreased alertness, disinhibition, taper
NONBENZODIAZEPINES				
Buspirone	0.2–0.6 mg/kg	bid or tid	OCD, GAD, SOC	Lightheadedness, dizziness, nausea, sedation

Note. GAD=generalized anxiety disorder; OCD=obsessive-compulsive disorder; SAD=separation anxiety disorder; SOC=social anxiety disorder. bid=twice daily; qd=once daily; tid=thrice daily.
[a]Adjunct treatment.

(1994) conducted a double-blind, placebo-controlled trial to examine the efficacy of fluoxetine in treating children (ages 5–16) with the primary diagnosis of elective mutism. Sixteen children were given a placebo run-in for 2 weeks (Phase 1). The nonresponders were then randomly assigned to receive either placebo ($n=9$) or fluoxetine ($n=6$; mean maximum dose$=21.4$ mg/day, range$=$ 12–27 mg/day) for another 12 weeks (Phase 2).

By the end of the trial, although the subjects in the fluoxetine group showed great improvement over time on all parent, patient, and clinician ratings, an analysis of variance (ANOVA) indicated few significant results. The fluoxetine group, compared with the placebo group, showed significantly greater improvement in one symptom—namely, mutism—as reflected by change in ratings on two of the nine parent scales, the mutism CGI scale ($P<0.0003$) and global CGI ($P<0.04$), and on one teacher rating, the Conners Anxiety Scale ($P<0.02$). The proportion of subjects rated as treatment responders based on the parent's rating of mutism change ($P<0.03$) and global change ($P<0.03$) was also significantly greater in the fluoxetine group. Side effects were minimal and did not differ significantly between treatment groups.

Several reasons may account for the lack of significant results in this study. The sample size was relatively small, and the length of the trial may not have been long enough to show the effects of fluoxetine, given that treatment response did not increase markedly until weeks 8–12. In addition, the investigators note that timing may have affected treatment response. Clinical response in an earlier case report (Black and Uhde 1992), in which treatment began before the start of the school year, was more striking than in this study, which was carried out in the last half of the school year, when children with elective mutism may have already known what to expect from their teachers and peers and were less motivated to improve.

In a later, double-blind, placebo-controlled trial, Geller et al. (2001) studied response to fluoxetine in children and adolescents diagnosed with OCD ($N=103$; ages 7–17). Subjects were randomly assigned to receive fluoxetine ($n=71$, mean total daily dose $=24.6$ mg) or placebo ($n=32$) for 13 weeks; the fluoxetine was initiated at 10 mg/day for the first 2 weeks, and the dosage was then increased to 20 mg/day. If subjects were unresponsive after 4 weeks of treatment, as indicated by no change or worsening on the Clinical Global Impression Severity of Illness subscale (CGI-S), the medication could be titrated to 40 mg/day and again to 60 mg/day at week 7.

In an intent-to-treat analysis, Geller et al. (2001) found that subjects randomly assigned to receive fluoxetine showed a greater reduction of OCD severity on the primary efficacy measure, the total Children's Yale-Brown Obsessive Compulsive Scale (CY-BOCS) score ($P=0.026$), with the reduction tending toward significance at week 5 ($P=0.086$) and reaching significance thereafter ($P<0.05$). Almost half (49%) of the subjects in the fluoxetine group were considered responders (with response defined as 40% or greater reduction of symptoms on the CY-BOCS) compared with 25% in the placebo group (Mantel-Haenszel exact $P=0.030$). In addition, significantly more subjects in the fluoxetine group than in the placebo group were rated as *much improved* or *very much improved* on the Clinical Global Impression Improvement (CGI-I) scale (55% vs. 18.8% placebo, $P<0.001$). Patient and parent improvement ratings also reflected this trend ($P<0.001$). Fluoxetine was well tolerated in this trial, with no adverse effects occurring significantly more often in the fluoxetine group than in the placebo group.

Although the results of this study do support the efficacy of fluoxetine in treating children and adolescents with OCD, there are some notable limitations in these findings. The investigators point out that the week in which treatment differences became significant occurred slightly later in this trial than in similar trials using different SSRIs. Also, the study design did not allow for a comparison of efficacy between fixed doses of fluoxetine, so it is difficult to determine whether the higher dosage caused treatment effects or whether subjects would have improved at a later point in the study while taking a lower dose. Results are supported by a similar crossover trial (Riddle et al. 1992).

More recently, Birmaher et al. (2003) completed a fluoxetine treatment study involving children and adolescents diagnosed with separation anxiety disorder, social phobia, and/or GAD. Seventy-four individuals (ages 7–17) were randomly assigned to receive placebo ($n=37$) or fluoxetine ($n=37$; maximum dose = 20 mg/day) for a period of 12 weeks. Two psychiatric research nurses and a child psychiatrist, who were also involved in treatment, assessed subjects weekly using the CGI-I.

Using intent-to-treat analysis, the investigators found that at treatment end, the fluoxetine group showed significantly more improvement on the CGI-I, the primary outcome variable (61% vs. 35% placebo, $\chi^2=4.93$). A survival analysis also showed that subjects in the fluoxetine group were more likely to achieve a high response on the CGI-I (Mantel-Cox χ^2 = 6.55), with a trend of more response by week 4 ($P=0.08$) and significance at week 9 ($P<0.05$). Results from a multivariate analysis of variance (MANOVA) on the combined outcomes indicated that fluoxetine showed greater treatment efficacy ($P=0.003$) and a greater reduction of anxiety symptoms than placebo. Fluoxetine-treated subjects diagnosed with social phobia seemed to have the best outcome, with significantly higher scores on the CGI-I ($\chi^2 =$ 12.13) and the Children's Global Assessment Scale (CGAS) ($\chi^2 = 6.01$) than those on placebo. Side effects in this study were minimal for the most part but included occasional headaches, drowsiness, abdominal pain, nausea, and agitation.

Even though the results of this study are encouraging, the investigators noted that by the end of the trial, approximately half of the subjects remained symptomatic. In consideration of this high percentage, they suggested that some subjects may have required a higher dosage or may have fared better with a different SSRI or concurrent psychotherapy. Also, there are some limitations to the study, given that the same nurses who assessed response to treatment also monitored side effects, possibly indicating a bias. Despite these issues, this study provides promising evidence for using fluoxetine to treat pediatric anxiety disorders.

Sertraline (Zoloft).   RCTs using sertraline as treatment have focused on pediatric populations diagnosed with OCD and GAD. In a double-blind, placebo-controlled trial, March et al. (1998) tested the efficacy of sertraline for children ($n=107$, ages 6–12) and adolescents ($n=80$, ages 13–17) with OCD. Following a 1-week, single-blind, placebo trial, subjects were randomly assigned to receive placebo ($n=95$) or sertraline ($n=92$) for 12 weeks. Sertraline was dosed according to age, with the dosage starting at 25 mg/day for children and 50 mg/day for adolescents and then titrated upward (in a forced design) 50 mg/week to a maximum of 200 mg/day or the best-tolerated dosage (mean total daily dose = 167 mg).

Efficacy analyses revealed that by the end of week 2, subjects treated with sertraline showed significantly greater improvement on the primary outcome variable, the CY-BOCS ($P=0.005$) and the National Institute of Mental Health (NIMH) Global Obsessive-Compulsive Scale (NIMH-GOCS, $P=0.002$) compared with subjects taking placebo. Analysis of responder status, defined as both a greater than 25% reduction of symptoms on the CY-BOCS and *much improved* or *very much improved* status on the CGI-I, also indicated significant results. On the CY-BOCS, 53% of sertraline-treated subjects were considered responders compared with 37% of the placebo group ($P=0.03$). Results were similar on the NIMH-GOCS (42% vs. 26%, $P=0.02$). Side effects in this trial were generally mild to moderate, with sertraline-treated subjects reporting significantly more incidences of insomnia, nausea, agitation, and tremor ($P<0.05$).

The results of March et al. (1998) seem to indicate that sertraline is efficacious in treating children and adolescents with OCD in the short term. It is difficult to comment, however, on dosage and side effects because this trial employed a forced titration, which may have contributed to treatment effects and increased adverse effects. As with other studies, some subjects continued to exhibit symptoms at the end of the trial, which may indicate the need for concurrent psychotherapy. Thus, the investigators advised clinicians to use a more gradual titration schedule and additional therapy to increase the chance of clinical normalization.

Rynn et al. (2001) subsequently conducted a double-blind, placebo-controlled trial assessing the efficacy of a lower daily dose of sertraline in children and adolescents diagnosed with GAD ($N=22$, ages 5–17). Subjects were randomly assigned to receive 9 weeks of placebo or sertraline treatment, 25 mg/day for the first week and 50 mg/day for the subsequent weeks. As subjects tolerated 50 mg/day well, no dosage adjustments were necessary throughout the trial. Assessments were administered weekly and included the Hamilton Anxiety Scale Total, Psychic Factor, and Somatic Factor scores, and CGI scores as primary outcome variables.

An analysis of covariance (ANCOVA) on the primary outcome variables revealed that significant treatment differences were apparent by week 4 and continued until the end of the study. At the end of week 9, subjects receiving sertraline were rated as endorsing fewer symptoms on all Hamilton Anxiety Scale scores (Total F=15.3, $P<0.001$; Psychic Factor F=22.6, $P<0.001$; Somatic Factor F=8.9, $P<0.01$), measuring less severity on the CGI-S (F=30.5, $P<0.001$), and showing greater improvement on the CGI-I (F=14.9, $P<0.001$) than subjects taking placebo.

Similar results were found for secondary assessment measures, including the Hamilton Rating Scale for Depression (F=18.55, $P<0.001$). At treatment endpoint, 90% of sertraline-treated subjects were considered improved based on CGI-I scores (1 or 2), as opposed to 10% of subjects taking placebo ($P<0.001$, Fisher exact test). Yet, only 18% of the subjects in the improved sertraline group were rated as markedly improved, which represents a small remission rate. An additional factorial ANCOVA adjusting for the baseline score on the Hamilton Anxiety Scale revealed a high main treatment effect (F = 11.0, $P<0.005$) favoring sertraline, but no main depression-severity effect and no depression-by-treatment interaction effect, indicating that the anxiolytic effects of sertraline in this trial were independent of its antidepressant effects. Side effects did not differ significantly between the sertraline and placebo groups.

Despite its smaller sample size, this trial suggests that 50 mg/day of sertraline may be an effective, safe dosage for short-term use in young patients diagnosed with GAD, reducing both psychic and somatic symptoms of anxiety with mild side effects. However, placebo response was smaller than indicated in other trials. The investigators noted that the children in the trial had been experiencing symptoms of GAD for years and argued that this may have made them less amenable to placebo response. In addition, the small percentage of those sertraline-treated subjects rated as markedly improved indicates that many of the sertraline-treated subjects still exhibited some symptoms at the end of the trial. Future studies using large sample sizes should more clearly assess dosage requirements and relapse.

Fluvoxamine (Luvox).   In a multisite, randomized, placebo-controlled study, Riddle et al. (2001) examined the effects of fluvoxamine in pediatric OCD. Following a 1- to 2-week, single-blind screening period, eligible subjects ($N=120$, ages 8–17) were randomly assigned to receive placebo ($n=63$) or fluvoxamine ($n=57$) for 10 weeks. During this time, the dosage of fluvoxamine was titrated up 25 mg every 3-4 days to a maximum of 200 mg/day unless severe adverse effects were experienced, in which case the dosage was lowered (but remained above 100 mg/day).

Using an intent-to-treat analysis, the investigators found that fluvoxamine was significantly more effective than placebo in ameliorating OCD symptoms on all measures. A two-way ANOVA on the primary efficacy variable, the CY-BOCS total score, revealed significant treatment effects at weeks 1, 2, 3, 4, 6, and 10. At the end of the study, 42% of subjects taking fluvoxamine were defined as treatment responders, having had a 25% reduction of symptoms on the CY-BOCS since baseline, compared with 25% of subjects taking placebo ($P=0.065$, Cochran-Mantel-Haenszel test).

Similar results were found regarding secondary efficacy variables such as the NIMH-GOCS, the CGI-Clinician, CGI-Parent, and CGI-Subject score ($P<0.05$). The NIMH-GOCS score was also significant at week 8, and the CGI scores were significantly lower in the fluvoxamine group at every follow-up visit. Responder analysis on the CGI-Clinician also revealed that significantly more fluvoxamine-treated subjects had a meaningful response to treatment ("much" or "very much" improved) at the end of 10 weeks (29.8% vs. 17.5% placebo, $P=0.078$, Cochran-Mantel-Haenszel test). Adverse effects that were significantly more prevalent in the fluvoxamine group included asthenia (fatigue, loss of energy, or weakness) and insomnia.

Riddle et al. (2001) demonstrated that fluvoxamine is both fast acting and effective as a short-term pediatric OCD treatment. Treatment differences were significant at an early point in the study and continued throughout the trial, reaching a maximum at the end of 3 weeks. However, it is difficult to comment on effective dosage levels because the study design employed a dose-finding titration phase and, thus, did not allow for dose to be a dependent variable. Another limitation of the study is that most subjects did not have comorbid diagnoses—a sample that is less typical of the OCD population, in which psychiatric comorbidity is high.

In another large-scale study, the Research Units on Pediatric Psychopharmacology (RUPP) Anxiety Study Group ("Fluvoxamine for the Treatment of Anxiety Disorders in Children and Adolescents" 2001) assessed the efficacy of fluvoxamine treatment in children and adolescents ($N=128$, ages 6–17) who met the criteria for social phobia, separation anxiety disorder, or GAD. Children and their families first received 3 weeks of open treatment in supportive, psychoeducational therapy. If the children did not respond to these interventions, they were then randomly assigned to also receive fluvoxamine ($n=63$) or placebo ($n=65$) for 8 weeks. Unless adverse events occurred, the dosage of fluvoxamine was titrated upward 50 mg/week to a maximum of 300 mg/day for adolescents and 250 mg/day for children (age 12 years and younger).

From an intent-to-treat analysis, the investigators found that fluvoxamine-treated subjects had a greater reduction of anxiety symptoms and higher rates of clinical response than did subjects in the placebo group. Treatment differences on one primary outcome variable, the Pediatric Anxiety Rating Scale (PARS), reached significance by week 3 and increased through week 6. By the end of the study, the fluvoxamine group had significantly lower PARS scores, indicating mild symptoms of anxiety ($P<0.001$).

The second outcome variable, the CGI-I score, which defines meaningful clinical response to treatment as scores of 3 (improved), 2 (much improved), or 1 (free of symptoms), revealed that at study endpoint, significantly more fluvoxamine-treated participants received scores of <4 (76% vs. 29% placebo, $P<0.001$). Treatment effects on both measures are considered large in comparison with similar trials. Side effects were generally mild, although fluvoxamine-treated subjects reported significantly more abdominal discomfort ($P=0.02$) and showed a trend for increased motor activity ($P=0.06$). Rates of treatment dropout due to adverse events were also low for a large clinical trial, with only 8% of subjects in the fluvoxamine group discontinuing treatment.

The RUPP study does support the short-term use of fluvoxamine in treating children and adolescents with social phobia, GAD, and separation anxiety disorder ("Fluvoxamine for the Treatment of Anxiety Disorders in Children and Adolescents" 2001). However, trials with longer treatment duration are necessary to establish efficacy and safety of long-term use. Although adverse effects were reported to be mild, the investigators noted that long-term animal studies warrant some concern as to the effects of SSRIs on developmental plasticity in serotonergic neurons.

Following the acute trial, the RUPP group investigated possible moderators and mediators of pharmacological treatment in children and adolescents with anxiety disorders (Walkup et al. 2003). Even though no significant moderators were found, analyses revealed that subjects presenting with social phobia ($P<0.05$) and a greater severity of baseline illness ($P<0.001$) were less likely to improve, regardless of treatment group. The RUPP group also identified the clinician's guess as to a subject's treatment, after having been blind to his or her randomized treatment arm during the acute phase ($P<0.001$), and showed that compliance with treatment tended to improve response ($P=0.05$).

Paroxetine (Paxil).   In a large-scale, placebo-controlled, multicenter trial, Wagner et al. (2004) evaluated the effects of paroxetine in children and adolescents diagnosed with social anxiety disorder (N=319, ages 8–17). Subjects were randomly assigned to receive either paroxetine (N=163, mean dosage= 24.8 mg/day) or placebo (N=156) for a 16-week trial, while their families were provided with psychoeducation in the form of a pamphlet. The primary outcome variable was the CGI-I, with score at week 16 acting as the last observation carried forward.

Analyzing the intent-to-treat population, Wagner et al. (2004) found that at week 16, 77.6% of paroxetine-treated subjects were defined as treatment responders, having a score of *improved* or *much improved* on the CGI-I, compared with 38.3% of subjects taking placebo (P<0.001). This trend appeared even within the first 4 weeks of treatment. A post hoc analysis also revealed that the odds of a subject being considered in remission at the end of the study, measured by a score of 1 or 2 on the CGI-I, were significantly higher in the paroxetine group than in the placebo group (47.8% vs. 14.9% remission status, P<0.001). Adverse effects were rated from mild to moderate in severity, with insomnia (P=0.02), decreased appetite (P=0.11), and vomiting (P=0.07) considered treatment-emergent.

Because paroxetine treatment exhibited a greater response rate than placebo and treatment differences reached significance on all five secondary outcome variables, Wagner et al. (2004) supported the use of paroxetine in treating pediatric social anxiety disorder. This outcome is even more encouraging, given that more than 50% of subjects had a baseline rating from *markedly ill* to among the *most extremely ill* on the CGI-S. Another interesting finding is that the children and adolescents in this study (77.6%) demonstrated a greater response to treatment than socially anxious adults treated with paroxetine (55%; Stein et al. 1998), indicating that social anxiety disorder may be less amenable to treatment in adulthood.

Although this study was much larger in scale than similar studies conducted on SSRIs, it nevertheless contained some limitations. The investigators noted that, given the chronicity of social anxiety disorder, the duration of treatment was short. They also acknowledged that commonly occurring comorbid disorders such as major depression were identified as exclusions and that, therefore, their findings cannot be generalized to a broader population. Finally, some clinicians administered both treatment and assessment measures and, thus, may have exhibited a bias toward active medication. These limitations aside, the strong preliminary data of Wagner et al. (2004) provide evidence of the efficacy of paroxetine in socially anxious children. Similar findings were presented in another large-scale, multisite trial (Geller et al. 2004).

Meta-analytic data.   Currently, there are no meta-analyses of trials using SSRIs on a short-term basis to treat pure pediatric anxiety disorders. However, a meta-analysis of pediatric OCD trials conducted by Geller et al. (2003) reveals some interesting findings regarding the use of antidepressants. Although the investigators found a highly significant pooled effect for each SSRI and clomipramine against placebo ($P < 0.001$), there were no significant pooled mean differences between one SSRI and another, indicating that no one SSRI was more efficacious than another in treating pediatric OCD. There was, however, a significant pooled mean difference favoring clomipramine over the SSRIs ($P = 0.002$, χ^2 test), indicating that clomipramine was more effective in reducing OCD symptoms across studies.

Although this analysis showed clomipramine as superior to the SSRIs, Geller et al. (2003) did not recommend using clomipramine as a first-line pharmacological agent because of its side-effect profile and association with cardiac toxicity. In less severe cases, the investigators suggest that SSRIs should be the first-choice medication, specifying that the choice of individual SSRI should be based more on adverse-effects profiles and pharmacokinetic properties such as half-life, than on efficacy. Although this meta-analysis reviewed data from published RCTs, some caution should be used in applying these recommendations to clinical practice. Because the RCTs involving children and adolescents diagnosed with OCD use multiple exclusion criteria, evidence from them is based on a population with less comorbidity than may be present in a clinical sample.

Risks of Selective Serotonin Reuptake Inhibitors

Currently, the FDA has approved only the following SSRIs for the treatment of pediatric OCD: fluoxetine, sertraline, and fluvoxamine. The consensus is that, in most cases, the benefits of SSRIs outweigh their risks. Yet, the use of psychopharmaceuticals, including SSRIs, for child and adolescent disorders is not without risk. SSRI-related side effects include nausea, diarrhea, gastrointestinal distress, headaches, lack of energy, sweating, dry mouth, restlessness, initial insomnia, sleepiness, increased hyperactivity, and tremor. These problems are usually short-lived, dose-related, and tend to resolve with time.

However, there is the possibility of discontinuation symptoms with some SSRIs, such as paroxetine, which has increasingly been associated with a withdrawal syndrome upon discontinuation (Leonard et al. 1997). Withdrawal symptoms do not generally occur with fluoxetine because of its long half-life, and they are of less concern with sertraline because of the presence of its one weak metabolite. Some trials (Geller et al. 2001; Riddle et al. 2001) also reported cases of subjects who showed abnormal vitals signs, an unsurprising finding, given that medication has been associated with changes in weight and decreases in blood pressure. As with any medication, there is always a risk of allergic reaction.

In addition to these issues, the FDA issued an advisory to physicians that the use of certain classes of antidepressants may lead to suicidal thinking/ attempts in youths. This warning highlights the need for close observation for signs of worsening symptoms and the emergence of suicidality in children treated with these medications. Of note, four paroxetine-treated subjects in the Wagner et al. (2004) trial expressed suicidal ideation or threatened suicide and one exhibited self-harm behavior, whereas no such subjects taking placebo exhibited such behavior. None of the cases were considered serious, involved evidence of a suicide attempt, or were attributed to the study medication by the investigator.

Efficacy of Long-Term Treatment and Maintenance

Benefits. Following their acute trial described in the previous section, the RUPP group conducted a 6-month, open-label extension study (Walkup et al. 2002) to examine the effects of continuing fluvoxamine treatment or treatment with a second SSRI in remaining subjects. The study design was such that active treatment responders from the acute trial continued with fluvoxamine treatment (Group I, $n=35$), active nonresponders switched to fluoxetine treatment (Group II, $n=14$), and placebo nonresponders began fluvoxamine treatment (Group III, $n=48$), with dosage schedules that varied according to treatment group. Subjects were provided with new treating-clinicians, who then continued to administer supportive psychotherapy.

This study was not a double-blind, placebo-controlled trial and therefore data analyses are suggestive and pertain more to clinical functioning. Using the CGI-I as a primary outcome measure, the investigators found that 94% of subjects who continued taking open-label fluvoxamine (mean final dosage=

131 mg/day) were considered responders, with scores of ≤3 after 24 weeks, and maintained their remissions. After 24 weeks, 71% of subjects who were administered fluoxetine (mean final dosage=24 mg/day) met the criteria for response. This result indicates that fluvoxamine nonresponders did show some response to a second SSRI, although only clinician ratings were significant. Finally, 56% of placebo nonresponders initiated on open-label fluvoxamine (135 mg/day) were considered responders at week 24, which is considered a therapeutic response. Side effects were mild and generally transient. The dropout rate was high only in Group III, with seven subjects withdrawing because of somatic complaints or adverse behavioral effects.

Data from this extension study suggest that relapse rates for anxious children maintained on SSRI treatment are low and extended SSRI treatment is generally safe. However, because this study was not a double-blind trial and time was not a controlled factor, there may have been some expectancy effects, and some benefit may have been attributed to medication that could have occurred naturally over time. Future research employing a double-blind design to study long-term SSRI treatment is recommended.

In addition to the RUPP extension study, data from long-term OCD trials can provide some indication of the efficacy and safety of maintenance treatment with SSRIs. Following a 12-week double-blind study (March et al. 1998), Cook et al. (2001) conducted a 52-week sertraline extension trial for subjects who completed the acute phase. Subjects ($N=137$, ages 6–18) began by taking sertraline at a dosage of 25 or 50 mg/day, depending on age (25 mg/day for ages 6–12, 50 mg/day for ages 13–18), and the dosage was then titrated to and maintained at the level at which they exhibited satisfactory clinical response (not to exceed 200 mg/day). Dosages could be decreased by 25 mg at any time to minimize adverse effects.

Data analysis was performed according to age (children: $n=72$, mean dosage = 108 mg/day; adolescents: $n=65$, mean dosage=132 mg/day). Response rates, with response defined as a greater than 25% decrease in the baseline CY-BOCS score and a CGI-I score of 1 or 2 at trial endpoint, were 67% for the combined age groups, 72% for children, and 61% for adolescents. Significant improvements over treatment were evident on all outcome measures ($P<0.05$). By the end of the study, 85% of active treatment responders who completed the full 52 weeks maintained responder status as compared with 43% of nonresponders. Side effects were common, with an incidence of 77%

among all subjects, and included headache, insomnia, nausea, diarrhea, somnolence, abdominal pain, hyperkinesias, nervousness, dyspepsia, and vomiting.

Although these results are also only suggestive, they do seem to provide support for long-term sertraline treatment in OCD youths. The most striking feature of the analyses is that of those subjects who did not respond to sertraline in the acute phase, 43% were considered responders by the end of the extension trial. However, since time was also not a controlled factor in this study, benefit cannot be definitively attributed to the study medication. The study had other limitations, including an absence of blinding, use of a priori criteria to assess relapse, and the uncontrolled-for allowance of concurrent psychotherapy. Finally, although side effects generally improved as treatment continued, the percentage of subjects withdrawing because of adverse events (12%) seems somewhat high in comparison with other trials. Future research should be directed toward more long-term, controlled trials using SSRI treatment in the young OCD population.

A smaller trial assessing the long-term effects of citalopram concurrent with CBT on adolescents with OCD (Thomsen et al. 2001) revealed similar results. After a 10-week, open-label trial (N=23) of citalopram (maximum dosage= 40 mg/day, Thomsen 1997), subjects given citalopram (N=30, ages 13–18) continued in an open trial (mean dosage=46.5 mg/day, range=20–80 mg/day) for a 6-month to 2-year period. Although 28 subjects continued taking citalopram for a year, only 14 completed the 2-year study. Primary outcome measures included the Yale-Brown Obsessive Compulsive Scale (Y-BOCS) (for subjects ≥15 years old) and the CY-BOCS (for subjects <15 years old).

Analyzing data from baseline to the 2-year endpoint, investigators found that the decrease in Y-BOCS/CY-BOCS scores was statistically significant for each time period (baseline–10 weeks, 10 weeks–6 months, 6 months–1 year, and baseline–2 years, $P=0.000$) except for the time from the 1-year endpoint to the 2-year endpoint. This finding indicates that subjects maintaining citalopram treatment for 4.5 months following the acute trial continued to exhibit a reduction of symptoms on the Y-BOCS/CY-BOCS, with an even greater reduction in the next 6 months, and that symptom reduction did not continue in the second year of treatment. Side effects, similar to those reported in other SSRI trials, were generally mild and decreased with continued treatment. Only sexual dysfunction and sedation, causing two subjects to drop out of the trial, were reported as persistent.

Even though the study by Thomsen et al. (2001) provides support for the use of citalopram as long-term treatment for adolescents diagnosed with OCD, the results should be considered cautiously. This is yet another uncontrolled trial in which subjects also received concurrent CBT. Moreover, despite the encouraging levels of symptom reduction after 1 year of treatment, 20% of subjects were still exhibiting clinical OCD at that time. This finding could be partly attributed to the fact that OCD severity at baseline was higher in the extension trial than in the first study. Finally, the treatment sample was small in comparison with other trials.

In addition to these trials, review articles provide guidance on long-term SSRI use in children and adolescents. In his review of acute-anxiety trials and adult and animal studies, Pine (2002) argued that children who have shown satisfactory response to SSRI treatment should be given a medication-free trial instead of maintaining long-term treatment, and should be promptly returned to medication if they show a relapse. Although he noted that side effects in acute SSRI trials were generally low, subjects in these trials often continued to exhibit symptoms at the end of the study, indicating a lack of remission large enough to consider other treatment options.

On the other hand, evidence from longitudinal data suggests that mood and anxiety disorders evident in childhood carry a significant risk for mood and anxiety disorders later in life. If left untreated, these disorders may have considerable harmful effects on development, with possible long-term implications. Pine stated that this finding must be weighed against potential risks in using long-term SSRI medication. Evidence from animal studies also provides an interesting dilemma. Although serotonin plays a role in neural plasticity, and long-term SSRI use may adversely affect cellular processes that involve serotonin, stress in early life can also greatly impact brain development. Thus, Pine put forth the recommendation that another treatment be selected following successful SSRI treatment to minimize risks and still maximize benefit.

There is still much that is unknown about the benefits and safety of long-term SSRI use. Although case reports and extension trials give us some indication that there is a continued benefit, there is no clear suggested duration of treatment. Pine's (2002) recommendations are noteworthy, but longitudinal studies are necessary to understand the effects of continued use of SSRIs.

Risks.   Side effects reported in long-term studies were similar to those reported in acute trials, which included gastrointestinal disturbance, headache, and insomnia. These effects were often mild in nature and decreased with continued treatment. Overall, adverse effects did not typically lead to study withdrawal and most trials had relatively low dropout rates. However, there were reports of hyperkinesia (Cook et al. 2001) severe enough to warrant study withdrawal, in addition to persistent complaints of sexual dysfunction and sedation (Thomsen et al. 2001) in some long-term studies. There have also been reports (Weintrob et al. 2002) documenting a decrease in growth rate among children treated with various SSRIs for a period ranging from 6 months to 5 years (dosage = 20–100 mg/day).

Serotonin-Norepinephrine Reuptake Inhibitors

Pharmacological treatments tend to focus on several neurotransmitter systems believed to form the biological foundation of anxiety disorders, such as serotonin and γ-aminobutyric acid (GABA). Another class of medications under investigation that shows promise in the treatment of pediatric anxiety disorders comprise the selective serotonin-norepinephrine reuptake inhibitors (SNRIs), which target both serotonergic and noradrenergic systems. The SNRI venlafaxine extended-release (XR) has been shown to be effective in adult GAD at total daily doses between 75 and 225 mg in several large, double-blind, placebo-controlled trials (Davidson et al. 1999; Gelenberg et al. 2000; Rickels et al. 2000). As has been the case with SSRI use, children with anxiety disorders appear to respond to venlafaxine XR in the same manner as adults (Rynn et al. 2004).

Duloxetine, another SNRI, is also considered effective for adult major depression and possibly for adult GAD (Rynn et al. 2007). At this time, there do not appear to be any reports about the use of this compound for the treatment of pediatric anxiety disorders.

Efficacy of Acute Treatment

Benefits.   Rynn et al. (2004) presented an abstract at the American Psychiatric Association's annual meeting on the results of a pooled analysis of two combined multisite, 8-week studies examining the efficacy and safety of venlafaxine XR ($n = 154$) compared with placebo ($n = 159$) in the treatment of childhood GAD ($P < 0.001$). Subjects (ages 6–17) met the criteria for GAD in DSM-IV and the Columbia-KIDDIE Schedule for Affective Disorders and Schizophrenia GAD Subsection C (C-KIDDIE-SADS GAD), with symptoms present for at least 6 months. Exclusions included concurrent psychiatric disorders, such as major depressive disorder, social anxiety disorder, and separation anxiety disorder. Dosing for venlafaxine extended-release began with 37.5 mg/day, and the total daily dose was increased on the basis of body weight (children ≥ 50 kg, maximum dose=225 mg; 25–39 kg, dose range= 37.5–112.5 mg; 40–49 kg, minimum dose=75 mg, maximum dose=150 mg).The main outcome measure for both studies was the end-of-study change in total score of the C-KIDDIE-SADS GAD.

Analysis of the two studies revealed that one showed statistically significant improvement favoring venlafaxine extended-release on both primary ($P<$ 0.001) and secondary (all $P<0.01$) outcome measures. The other study showed significant improvement for venlafaxine extended-release in some secondary outcome measures, but not in the primary measure ($P=0.06$). Pooled analysis indicated a greater mean decrease on the primary outcome for venlafaxine extended-release versus placebo (−17.4 vs. −12.7; $P<0.001$). Response rates, with response defined as a CGI-I score <3, were also significantly greater for venlafaxine extended-release (69% vs. 48%; $P=0.004$).

Tourian et al. (2004) found similar results when comparing venlafaxine extended-release ($n=137$) and placebo ($n=148$) in children and adolescents (ages 8–17) with a primary diagnosis of social anxiety disorder ($P<0.001$) over 16 weeks. The semi-structured Anxiety Disorders Interview Schedule for DSM-IV (Silverman and Albano 1996) confirmed the social anxiety disorder diagnosis. Subjects with scores of ≥50 on the Social Anxiety Scale (SAS), a CGI-S score of ≥4, and no concurrent psychiatric disorder were eligible. Dosing was calculated by weight, exactly as in the aforementioned study by Rynn et al. (2004). Results showed that baseline-to-endpoint improvement in total SAS scores was significantly higher for the venlafaxine extended-release group compared with the placebo group (22.5 vs.14.9 points, adjusted change; $P<0.001$).

Risks.   In the Rynn et al. (2004) study, the incidence of asthenia, pain, anorexia, and somnolence in subjects treated with venlafaxine extended-release was twice that (≥5%) of the placebo group. Only the development of anorexia differed significantly between treatment groups (13% vs. 3%); also two medication-treated subjects displayed suicidal ideation and behavior, leading to their removal from the study. In addition, there were statistically significant mean increases from baseline cholesterol serum levels for those children treated with venlafaxine extended-release. There were statistically significant mean changes from baseline in subjects' vital signs, with a difference in pulse rate of approximately 4 beats/minute and a difference in blood pressure (supine diastolic and systolic) of approximately 2 mm Hg for those children treated with venlafaxine extended-release. The venlafaxine extended-release–treated group had a height increase from baseline of 0.3 cm ($P<0.05$), compared with 1.0 cm ($P<0.001$) in children receiving placebo (difference between groups: $P=0.041$).

In Tourian et al.'s (2004) study, the most common adverse effects among venlafaxine extended-release–treated patients were flu, anorexia, asthenia, weight loss, nausea, and pharyngitis. Three adolescents in the medication group also displayed suicidal ideation, as opposed to none in the placebo arm. As found in the GAD study, the venlafaxine extended-release–treated patients experienced significant mean weight loss compared with placebo ($P<0.001$), and in several cases the weight loss was considered clinically significant ($n=8$).

Efficacy of Long-Term Treatment and Maintenance

Two adult venlafaxine XR studies (Allgulander et al. 2001; Gelenberg et al. 2000) were conducted to assess response to 6 months of treatment with venlafaxine XR compared with placebo. Results indicated no tolerance to the efficacy of venlafaxine XR over the 6-month treatment period. Although neither study was designed to assess relapse rates after treatment discontinuation as a function of long-term treatment, both suggest that patients with GAD can benefit from at least 6 months of continuous treatment. Presently, there are no pediatric anxiety studies that evaluate the long-term use of this class of compound, and the risks are unknown.

Benzodiazepines

Benzodiazepines have been used as effective anxiolytics and sedatives in adults since they first appeared in clinical practice in the early 1960s, before their mechanism of action was understood. It was not until almost two decades later that researchers discovered specific benzodiazepine receptors on the neurons of the brain and began to understand how benzodiazepines produce their varying effects. Following this discovery, they postured that benzodiazepines function by activating GABA, an inhibitory neurotransmitter, which slows the response of neural activity in the brain and produces an overall sedating effect.

Although the exact chemical process by which benzodiazepines produce anxiolytic effects has yet to be determined, the effect of benzodiazepines is strongly linked to the relationship between benzodiazepines and the GABA-ergic system. Bernstein and Shaw (1993) hypothesized that because abnormalities in norepinephrine and GABA levels in the brain are thought to underlie anxiety disorders, correcting these levels with agents such as benzodiazepines should lead to a reduction of anxiety symptoms. Future research in the field should indicate the precise mechanism.

Benzodiazepines vary widely in terms of what are considered to be their effective daily dose and half-life, which represents how fast the drug is metabolized by the body. Although, according to the cited literature, some benzodiazepines, such as clonazepam, can be effective in adults at a total daily dose of 0.5–3.0 mg, others, such as lorazepam, are effective at a dosage of 1–6 mg/day (Witek et al. 2005). Clonazepam also has a much longer half-life than lorazepam (18–50 hours compared with 10–20 hours), indicating that clonazepam remains in the body for a longer period of time. This means that clonazepam is long-acting and while it may be useful in relieving long-term anxiety, it may also lengthen the incidence for side effects.

Justification for using benzodiazepines in clinical practice for treatment of anxious children is provided by adult studies on GAD and panic disorder. In a large, multisite, placebo-controlled study, Ballenger et al. (1988) examined the effects of alprazolam on adults diagnosed with panic disorder ($N=481$) in an 8-week trial. Dosages were kept on a flexible schedule, reaching a maximum of 10 mg/day (mean dosage=5.7 mg/day). Side effects were judged to be minimal.

By the end of the trial, Ballenger et al. (1988) found encouraging results. According to the end point analysis, subjects in the alprazolam group were judged to have significantly higher physician and patient global improvement scores ($P<0.0001$) and fewer phobic ($P<0.0001$) and anxiety ($P<0.0001$) symptoms on the Overall Phobia Rating Scale and clinician-rated Hamilton Anxiety Scale, respectively, and they reported significantly fewer panic attacks. Similar results are supported by other RCTs using benzodiazepines to treat adults with panic disorder (Dunner et al. 1986; Pollack et al. 1986).

Benzodiazepines have also been effective in treating adults with GAD. Rickels et al. (1983) found that anxious adults ($N=151$) randomly assigned to receive alprazolam ($n=54$) or diazepam ($n=45$) greatly improved when compared with those on placebo ($n=52$) over a 4-week trial. Although more patients dropped out of the placebo group, ANCOVAs showed that subjects in the medication groups had significantly more improvement on patient and physician ratings as early as 1 week into the study (mean dose: alprazolam = 1.2 mg, diazepam = 20 mg). Significance was also apparent on many of the ratings scales at endpoint analysis, indicating that effects were maintained throughout the trial.

In another interesting double-blind study, Goddard et al. (2001) showed that the addition of benzodiazepines to SSRI treatment in adults diagnosed with panic disorder improved treatment response. Subjects ($N=50$) all received 12 weeks of open-label sertraline (target dosage = 100 mg/day) and were then randomly assigned to receive clonazepam ($n=24$, target dosage = 1.5 mg/day) or placebo ($n=26$) as an additional treatment for 4 weeks, followed by 3 weeks of tapered doses. Primary efficacy was gauged by the clinician, by total scores on the Panic Disorder Severity Scale (PDSS), and by the patient's weekly reports of panic attack frequency. Responder status was determined by a decrease of $\geq 50\%$ from baseline PDSS score.

Although only 68% of subjects completed the trial, an intent-to-treat analysis revealed that there was a greater proportion of responders in the sertraline/clonazepam group than in the sertraline/placebo group at the end of week 1 (41% vs. 4%, $P=0.003$). By the end of week 3, the percentages improved and 63% of subjects in the sertraline + clonazepam group were considered responders compared with 8% of the sertraline + placebo group ($P=0.05$). These between-treatment differences did not continue to be significant throughout the trial, and, on the basis of dropout rates and side-effect profiles, the medications were generally well tolerated.

Closely modeled on clinical practice, the study by Goddard et al. (2001) appears to endorse the efficacy of the coadministration of sertraline and clonazepam for adults with panic disorder. The benefit of concurrent use of a benzodiazepine and an SSRI was large enough after 3 weeks of treatment to warrant future adult research, which may, in turn, justify trials in pediatric samples.

Efficacy of Acute Treatment

Benefits.   Unlike in the substantial literature available on treatment with SSRIs, there are relatively few published, structured investigations assessing the efficacy of benzodiazepines in pediatric anxiety disorders. Whereas a number of open-label trials (Kraft et al. 1965; Pfefferbaum et al. 1987; Simeon and Ferguson 1987) and case reports (Biederman 1987) suggest significant decreases in participants' anxiety levels following treatment with benzodiazepines, RCTs have not supported these findings.

In one of the earliest RCTs measuring the efficacy of benzodiazepines in children with anxiety disorders, Bernstein et al. (1990) examined the effect of alprazolam and imipramine on young school refusers. Encouraged by the positive results of an open-label trial, in which 67% patients randomly assigned to receive alprazolam (N=9) showed marked or moderate improvement and 55% returned to school, they created a double-blind crossover study. Participants were randomly assigned to receive alprazolam, imipramine, or placebo for 8 weeks, and then the medication was tapered for 1–2 weeks and discontinued.

Performing ANOVAs, the investigators discovered that the treatments did show statistically significant differences at week 8 on the Anxiety Rating for Children (ARC) measure. The ANOVA also indicated that on this measure, participants (n=7) randomly assigned to receive alprazolam (maximum dosage = 3 mg/day) showed the most improvement. However, these results failed to reach significance once the baseline scores were factored in as covariates in ANCOVA.

Although the promise of Bernstein et al.'s (1990) results disappears once ANCOVAs are performed on the data, this study supports further research. The Bernstein et al. (1990) study could have benefited from a larger sample size and administration of a higher dosage of alprazolam, given that the investigators indicated the dose was *conservative*. It is also difficult to assess the improvement of the children solely on the basis of the medication, considering that participants were additionally entered into a school reentry program and had weekly individual sessions of psychotherapy. Furthermore, 42% of the subjects in this trial had pure depressive disorders and 42% had comorbid anxiety and depressive disorders, indicating that these results may not truly reflect the effects of alprazolam on children with pure anxiety disorder.

Simeon et al. (1992) conducted an RCT following the results of their open study (Simeon and Ferguson 1987). As in the Bernstein et al. (1990) trial, the follow-up, placebo-controlled, double-blind study failed to corroborate these earlier findings. Subjects ($N=30$) were children meeting DSM-III criteria for anxiety and avoidance. The children were given placebo for 1 week, randomly assigned to receive alprazolam or placebo for 4 weeks (mean maximum dose = 1.57 mg; range = 0.5–3.5 mg), and then the medication was tapered for 2 additional weeks and replaced with a placebo substitute and placebo, respectively.

Although their evaluations, administered after the double-blind trial (day 28), seemed to indicate improvement among children who were administered alprazolam, Simeon et al. (1992) found that differences in clinical global ratings were not statistically significant. Mean improvement on the CGI for the overanxious children ($N=13$) treated with alprazolam was only slightly higher than the rating given for children taking placebo (2.69 vs. 2.85), with similar results for avoidant children (2.5 vs. 3.00). Investigators also found that the overanxious group treated with alprazolam showed a slight relapse (2.90) following the tapering phases (day 42), whereas the placebo group improved (2.42). The avoidant group treated with alprazolam also showed a slight relapse (3.00), whereas the placebo group remained the same (3.00).

Using a cognitive memory search task and electroencephalogram measurements, Simeon et al. (1992) also reported that subjects treated with placebo showed a slight decrease in cognitive efficiency, but subjects treated with alprazolam indicated increased beta power in both hemispheres at day 28 ($P<0.04$). Upon further examination, they discovered that, at baseline, mean beta power in both hemispheres was negatively related to the slope in the memory search task ($r=-0.43–0.47$, $P<0.03$), indicating that low beta power is associated with less efficiency in a memory search task. Based on this relationship, Simeon et al. anticipated that alprazolam, given at the same dosage as in their trial, should not interfere with a child's academic performance.

Although the results of the Simeon et al. (1992) study did not reach significance, they justify undertaking a study with a larger sample size, a longer duration double-blind trial, and a higher dosing schedule. The findings also encourage future studies to discriminate among diagnostic groups, given that clinical effects showed a greater potential for improvement in the avoidant group.

Following the Simeon et al. (1992) trial, Graae et al. (1994) performed a double-blind, crossover pilot study involving children with similar anxiety diagnoses ($N=15$). All but one child were diagnosed with separation anxiety disorder according to the DSM-III criteria, and all but two presented with comorbid anxiety disorders. In this study, unlike the Simeon et al. (1992) study, subjects were immediately randomly assigned to receive either clonazepam (maximum dosage = 2 mg/day) or placebo for a 4-week, double-blind trial.

Although at the end of the study half the children no longer met the criteria for an anxiety disorder, treatment-effect comparisons did not reach significant levels. When levels at baseline were compared with those directly following the medication trial, or when treatment was at maximum dosage (week 3), the Brief Psychiatric Rating Scale (BPRS) and the CGI Scale did not indicate significant improvement for subjects administered either clonazepam or placebo. Additionally, there were no significant treatment differences related to the frequency and severity of anxiety symptoms identified by the other measures, the Diagnostic Interview Schedule for Children and the Children's Manifest Anxiety Scale.

Thus, Graae et al. (1994) did not support using clonazepam at the dosing schedule of 2 mg/day in children and adolescents with anxiety disorders. Results might have shown more improvement if the study sample had been increased to a broader population and the trial lengthened. Although the results of this trial are less promising than those of Simeon et al. (1992), they do warrant further investigation into the use of benzodiazepines in child anxiety disorders, especially if the dose is increased and titration is slowed to decrease possible side effects.

Risks.   Side effects for most benzodiazepines were reported as infrequent and mild, although they varied in severity across studies. The most common side effects were dry mouth and drowsiness. Simeon et al. (1992) also reported that sedation and disinhibition, manifested by aggressivity, irritability, and incoordination, were common. In addition, 71% of subjects in the Bernstein et al. (1990) trial presented with abdominal pain, dizziness, and headaches.

Graae et al. (1994), in their study, reported the most severe side effects. The authors pointed out that disinhibition, irritability, and oppositionalism were notable in their sample; in three cases, these side effects were severe enough to cause the subjects to drop out of the study at Phase I. Although for the remaining 12 subjects the mean rate of side effects for clonazepam was not significantly different from placebo at any study point, this rate does not take study dropouts into account. Future investigators would be advised to record side effects at baseline and monitor adverse events closely, using a severity scale.

Benzodiazepines can lead to dependency with chronic use, which is usually defined as longer than 8 weeks of treatment (Nishino et al. 1995). Because of this concern, increased titration should be gradual and the tapering period should be lengthened in all RCTs. Although none of the reviewed studies indicate withdrawal symptoms during the tapering period, it would be wise to monitor children closely during this period and not administer benzodiazepines on a long-term basis.

Overall, the published literature on benzodiazepine use in children and adolescents with anxiety disorders is very limited. Although the review findings indicate that benzodiazepine treatment offers some benefits for anxious children and adolescents, there have not been enough well-designed clinical trials with large sample sizes to clearly evaluate this class of compounds. However, trends in the current research seem promising and warrant further investigation, if the recommended changes are incorporated in future research.

Efficacy of Long-Term Treatment and Maintenance

Because of concern that dependence will develop as a result of long-term treatment with benzodiazepines, many of the published RCTs have been acute studies, and there are no long-term studies that evaluate treatment for anxious children and adolescents. However, there have been numerous long-term studies using benzodiazepines in adults diagnosed with anxiety disorders, especially panic disorder, because the chronic nature of panic disorder tends to require longer treatment duration.

In a large, placebo-controlled study, Schweizer et al. (1993) investigated the treatment effect of long-term alprazolam (mean dosage=5.7 mg/day) or imipramine (mean dosage=175 mg/day) use in adults diagnosed with panic disorder, with or without agoraphobia (N=106, ages 18–65). Following an acute trial, subjects that improved were randomly assigned to receive alprazolam (n=27), imipramine (n=13), or placebo (n=11) for an additional 6 months of maintenance treatment. Monthly assessments included measures of panic attack frequency and severity, generalized anxiety, and phobias.

Results indicated that following maintenance treatment, panic attack frequency declined for all patients except one in the placebo group. At week 32, only 9% of the alprazolam group, 0% of the imipramine group, and 22% of the placebo group still reported experiencing minor symptom attacks. A measure of nonpanic anxiety, the Hamilton Anxiety Scale, and physician global improvement ratings also indicated sustained treatment gains. Subjects receiving maintenance treatment with alprazolam who showed tolerance to adverse events such as sedation, a common side effect for benzodiazepines, declined from 49% incidence during the acute trial to 7% incidence.

In addition, there was no evidence that alprazolam-treated subjects became tolerant to the clinical, anxiolytic effects of the medication, a feature often associated with withdrawal reactions upon discontinuation. The dosage of alprazolam remained stable throughout maintenance, indicating that no subject required a significant dose increase to maintain treatment effects. Therefore, this trial provides preliminary support for the efficacy of alprazolam in sustaining treatment gains in anxious adults and indicates that no tolerance developed over the 8 months of extended treatment.

After this maintenance trial, Rickels et al. (1993) investigated the outcome following drug taper to address withdrawal reactions. During the tapering phase, subjects receiving maintenance alprazolam treatment ($N=27$) received a dose reduction of 1 mg every 3–4 days until the dosage reached 2 mg/day, at which point they were given half-strength pills, with a decrease in dosage of 0.5 mg every 3–4 days. Subjects were assessed primarily using the Physician Withdrawal Checklist and reported relapse of panic attack symptoms.

Results showed that following taper, there were highly significant statistical differences between alprazolam and the other treatments on the Physician Withdrawal Checklist ($P<0.001$) and a strong trend for an increase in the number of panic attacks reported ($P<0.09$). Withdrawal symptoms were experienced almost exclusively by subjects in the alprazolam group, although 67% showed a decrease of worsening symptoms once taper was finished. Still, 33% of alprazolam-treated subjects were unable to discontinue medication, having a taper success rate that was significantly lower than the other two treatment groups ($P<0.02$). Yet, these subjects were also taking a higher mean pre-taper daily dose of alprazolam (6.9 mg) and reported greater symptom severity than the alprazolam-treated subjects reported to have had a successful taper.

Although this study had a high attrition rate from the acute trial to the maintenance phase, with significantly more subjects remaining in the alprazolam group, the results are striking. Alprazolam-treated patients showed significantly more difficulty than imipramine- or placebo-treated subjects in discontinuing medication. In addition, the investigators note that after 1-year follow-up, patients who had originally been treated with imipramine or placebo did just as well on clinical measures as those who had been treated with alprazolam but without exhibiting any of the physical dependence or withdrawal symptoms. This finding indicates that the sustained treatment effects of long-term therapy with benzodiazepines might not be worth the risk, especially in the pediatric population.

Some studies (Fyer et al. 1987; Rynn et al. 2003) have investigated the efficacy of using other medications, such as imipramine and buspirone, to ease benzodiazepine discontinuation with few significant results, although it appears that benzodiazepine discontinuation is more difficult in adults diagnosed with panic disorder than in adults diagnosed with GAD. There has been some indication (Otto et al. 1993), however, of the efficacy of CBT in aiding patients during discontinuation of benzodiazepine treatment. Further research into this treatment option is recommended.

Tricyclic Antidepressants

Tricyclic antidepressants (TCAs), named for their three-ring structure, are known for their mood-elevating effects. For this reason, they have been used as a front-line pharmacological treatment for adults with depression and anxiety since the mid-1960s (Potter et al. 1995). Precursors to the safer SSRIs, TCAs act by binding to presynaptic transporter proteins in the brain and inhibiting the reuptake of norepinephrine and serotonin in the presynaptic terminal. Although all TCAs are equally effective in inhibiting both norepinephrine and serotonin, some are more preferential to one or the other, causing them to be referred to as "noradrenergic" or "serotonergic," respectively (Meyer and Quenzer 2005).

TCAs may be helpful for long-term treatment of anxiety, because inhibition of norepinephrine and serotonin extends the duration of the transmitter action at the synapse and changes both the pre- and postsynaptic receptors. This adaptation over time may increase the potential for clinical improvement, but it also extends the potential for side effects. In terms of half-life, most TCAs remain in the body for approximately 24 hours, allowing for once-a-day dosing (Potter et al. 1995). In adults, TCAs are used for the treatment of major depression, anxiety disorders (GAD, panic disorder, and OCD), and pain syndromes.

Efficacy of Acute Treatment

Benefits. A review of the existing literature on using TCAs to treat child and adolescent anxiety disorders reveals mixed results. Although some RCTs (Bernstein et al. 2000; Gittelman-Klein and Klein 1971) indicated significant treatment differences between TCAs and placebo, a number of studies were unable to replicate and support these findings (Berney et al. 1981; Bernstein et al. 1990; Klein et al. 1992). Additionally, investigators have reported serious side effects in children taking TCAs, suggesting that the risk involved may outweigh the potential benefits.

Most of the published RCTs evaluating the efficacy of TCAs for childhood anxiety focused on school phobia or school refusal, a disorder that involves comorbid depression and anxiety symptoms. Thus, although they are helpful in demonstrating the possible efficacy of TCAs in school refusal, these studies may not accurately portray results in the treatment of pure anxiety disorders. Also, concurrent psychotherapy was administered in many of these trials. It is important to keep these factors in mind, as they may suggest a lack of efficacy for this class of compounds as a monotherapy.

Gittelman-Klein and Klein (1971) performed the first RCT evaluating the effect of TCAs on children with school phobia. In their double-blind, placebo-controlled study, the investigators randomly assigned school-phobic children ($N=35$) to receive either imipramine or placebo (mean dosage=152 mg/day, range=100–200 mg/day) for 6 weeks. Assessments included measures of global improvement on a 7-point scale, school attendance, and psychiatric ratings of symptoms.

At the end of the 6-week trial, the investigators found that imipramine was significantly more effective than placebo in increasing school attendance and indicated greater improvement on all other measures. Of children taking medication, 81% returned to school, as opposed to 47% who were given placebo ($P<0.05$), and reports indicated a significantly greater frequency of improvement in the imipramine group. Five of the six psychiatric ratings used (depression, phobic behavior, willingness to separate from mother, physical complaints, and fear of going to school) also showed significant improvement with imipramine treatment.

Even though this study supports treating school refusal with TCAs, it does not necessarily indicate that TCAs are a first-line choice. On the Lorr Inpatient Multidimensional Psychiatric Scale (IMPS) measuring depression, 35% of the sample received high scores. In addition, both treatment arms were supplemented with weekly school reentry counseling sessions, calling into question whether the improvements were due solely to the medication.

Berney et al. (1981) followed Gittelman-Klein and Klein's (1971) study with a 12-week trial assessing the efficacy of clomipramine in child and adolescent school refusers (N=46). Subjects were randomly selected to receive clomipramine or placebo, prescribed according to age (40 mg/day for ages 9–10, 50 mg/day for ages 11–12, 75 mg/day for ages 13–14). A psychiatrist and another rater carried out assessments using parent, child, and psychiatric global scores on behavior and clinical judgment on four dimensions: depression, neurotic dimension, separation anxiety, and ability to attend school.

Although the investigators discovered that there was a significant shift toward improvement on global scores within both the placebo and the medication groups, they found that this significance disappeared when the groups were compared in an ANCOVA. By the end of the study, more than one-third of the sample still had serious difficulty returning to school. There are several reasons that may account for this result. The dosages in this study were lower than those in the previous study, and the children's severity levels of separation anxiety were much higher (87%). Response could also have been improved by using higher total daily medication dose.

In a double-blind, placebo-controlled study comparing the use of alprazolam and imipramine in treating school-refusing children and adolescents (N=24), Bernstein et al. (1990) found similar effects. An ANOVA showed that subjects randomly assigned to receive imipramine (N=9; mean total daily dose=164.29 mg) for the full 8 weeks showed significantly less improvement on the ARC scale than those in the alprazolam group, but demonstrated significantly more improvement than those given placebo (P=0.03). However, these results were no longer significant after ANCOVAs were performed.

Considering that plasma levels were carefully monitored in this study and dosage level was based on prior studies, it seems unlikely that the imipramine dose was too low. By week 4, halfway through the trial, only one child had a subtherapeutic plasma tricyclic level (102 ng/mL; therapeutic range 125–250 ng/mL), and this was corrected by a dose increase. Other explanations for the lack of significant results may be the small sample size and the high incidence of comorbidity in the subjects, making it hard to use a target dose. Also, all subjects participated in a concurrent school reentry program.

Following this trial, Klein et al. (1992) conducted another RCT comparing imipramine and placebo in children with separation anxiety disorder ($N=$ 20). If subjects did not respond to a 4-week behavioral treatment, they were randomly assigned to receive placebo or imipramine (mean dosage = 153 mg/ day; range = 75–275 mg/day) for a 6-week trial. By the end of the study, results were not significant on any of the ratings, which included parent and child self-reports, teacher and psychiatrist ratings, and global improvement scores. The following electrocardiogram (ECG) changes were found with medication treatment: trend increase in the PR interval ($P < 0.06$), and a significant increase in QRS ($P < 0.01$). However, none of these changes were considered clinically significant.

Although half the subjects in this study improved, these results do not appear to support use of TCAs as a monotherapy for pediatric anxiety disorders. The targeted sample had pure separation anxiety without comorbid depression, not school phobia, yet the medication did not prove to be any more effective than placebo. Also, children in the medication group reported some severe side effects and were still receiving psychotherapy as an adjunctive treatment.

Studies assessing the efficacy of the serotonergic TCA clomipramine in children with OCD also give some insight into the overall efficacy of TCAs for anxiety disorders. Although children diagnosed with OCD are typically thought to have more severe cases than do generally anxious children, the literature provides compelling results. In a 10-week, double-blind, crossover trial ($N = 48$), Leonard et al. (1989) compared two TCAs: clomipramine, which has been shown to be effective in children with OCD, and desipramine, which is less potent in inhibiting serotonin reuptake (Ross and Renyi 1975).

Following a 2-week, single-blind, placebo phase to assess efficacy, subjects were randomly assigned to receive either clomipramine or desipramine for the first 5 weeks (Phase A), and then their medication was switched to the alternate treatment for another 5 weeks (Phase B). Dosages were on a fixed schedule, with a target total daily dose of 3 mg/kg, and were based on weight (mean dosage: clomipramine, 150 mg/day; desipramine, 153 mg/day; range = 50–250 mg/day).

ANCOVA showed that clomipramine, but not desipramine, produced a significant decrease in all obsessive-compulsive ratings (NIMH-GOCS, $P=0.0002$) and depression ratings (Hamilton Rating Scale for Depression, $P=0.006$; NIMH depression scales, $P=0.0001$), as well as an increase in a measure of global functioning ($P=0.001$).

Drug order was also shown to have a significant effect. Of the subjects who switched from clomipramine in Phase A to desipramine in Phase B, 64% showed a sign of relapse, defined as at least a 1-point decline on the NIMH-GOCS by the fifth week of Phase B. This would indicate that desipramine did not produce the same positive clinical effects as clomipramine and could not sustain those effects following clomipramine treatment. Similar effects have been shown with OCD studies using placebo (Flament et al. 1985).

DeVeaugh-Geiss et al. (1992) found similar results in their 8-week, multisite study assessing clomipramine use in children and adolescents with OCD ($N=60$). Following a 2-week placebo washout period, subjects were randomly assigned to receive clomipramine (maximum dosage by body weight: 25–30 kg, 75 mg/day; 31–45 kg, 100 mg/day; 46–60 kg, 150 mg/day; >60 kg, 200 mg/day) or to continue with placebo. At the end of the trial, subjects in the clomipramine group had a 37% mean reduction of symptoms on the Y-BOCS compared with 8% in those receiving placebo, and a 34% mean reduction on the NIMH-GOCS compared with 6% for the placebo group. Both findings were significant using ANCOVA ($P<0.05$). Patients in the clomipramine group also had a 53% mean reduction of symptoms on self-ratings compared with 8% for the placebo group.

Risks. Side effects for TCAs ranged in severity across studies. Gittelman-Klein and Klein (1971) reported that most side effects disappeared without requiring a dose change. The most common were drowsiness, dizziness, dry mouth, and constipation. Similarly, Berney et al. (1981) argued that, although side effects were reported, they were usually not severe. No subject in the Bernstein et al. (1990) study had side effects that rated higher than mild, the most common being headache, dizziness, dry mouth, abdominal pain, and nausea.

Klein et al. (1992) reported the most severe cases, the most frequent being irritability or angry outbursts and dry mouth. Children in the imipramine group experienced considerably more side effects than those in the placebo group ($\chi^2=5.05$, $P<0.03$), with all complaints lasting at least 3 days and two-thirds reported in the moderate-to-severe range. This is troubling, given that the mean daily dose in this trial was similar to that administered by Gittelman-Klein and Klein (1971), although their sample was significantly smaller. Side effects in studies using clomipramine and desipramine to treat obsessive-compulsive children were similar. Leonard et al. (1989) reported dry mouth, tiredness, and dizziness as the most common adverse effects. However, subjects taking clomipramine experienced more tremor and other side effects, such as chest pain, hot flashes, heartburn, rash, and acne.

Beyond these side effects, there have been some case studies reporting sudden unexplained death in children on TCA medications (Biederman 1991; Riddle et al. 1993; Varley and McClellan 1997). In many of the reported cases, the children were being treated with desipramine at varying but therapeutic or even subtherapeutic levels for attention-deficit disorder or attention-deficit/hyperactivity disorder. Monitoring seems to have been inconsistent among the cases but the cause of death was usually linked to adverse cardiac events. Because of the possibility of cardiac toxicity in young children, clinicians are advised to monitor the effects of TCA levels on their subjects very closely and to follow serial ECGs over the course of treatment to ensure that plasma levels are not above the therapeutic threshold.

Overall, there does not yet appear to be enough evidence to support the frequent use of TCAs as a monotherapy for children and adolescents with anxiety disorders, with the exception of OCD. Although some significant improvements are reflected in research, these are accompanied by significant side effects. Also, since the study populations in much of the literature have a high rate of comorbidity, it is unknown whether these medications would prove useful in pure anxiety disorders, with the exception of OCD. It is recommended that use of TCAs in school refusers continue to be supplemented by some form of psychotherapy and that imipramine blood level be monitored closely to minimize potentially severe side effects.

Efficacy of Long-Term Treatment and Maintenance

Although there have not been many long-term studies assessing the efficacy of TCAs in children with pure anxiety disorders, evidence from long-term OCD trials provides some indication of effects. Following their short-term, placebo-controlled trial, DeVeaugh-Geiss et al. (1992) continued with an open-label extension study for 1 year. They found that efficacy was maintained in subjects who elected to participate and completed the whole year ($N=25$). By the end of the year, the mean Y-BOCS score was 9.5, compared with 23 at the beginning of the extension. The investigators reported that clomipramine was still well tolerated.

Leonard et al. (1991) also performed an 8-month trial similar in design to their previous short-term crossover trial. Children and adolescents from the previous trial receiving maintenance clomipramine treatment ($N=26$) entered into the study and continued to receive clomipramine (mean dosage = 143 mg/day) for 3 months. At month 4, subjects were randomly assigned to receive desipramine substitution (mean dosage = 123 mg/day) or to continue with clomipramine for 2 months. For the final 3-month phase, all subjects continued to receive clomipramine treatment.

For those subjects completing the entire trial ($N=20$), results revealed that during the months of the substitution, those randomized to receive desipramine showed greater impairment across ratings than those continuing with clomipramine. These results were only significant, however, on the NIMH-GOCS scale once the investigators controlled for the error rate.

A survival analysis indicated more significant results. Although 9 of the 11 subjects in the clomipramine group (82%) did not relapse during the substitution period, only one of the subjects on desipramine (11%) did not relapse ($P=0.013$). The desipramine group also gained presubstitution clinical status quickly upon continuance with clomipramine, as there were no significant differences in ratings taken before substitution and after a month of clomipramine reinstatement. Plasma levels for both imipramine and desipramine were not significantly different, nor were side effects.

This study would seem to indicate that efficacy was maintained in subjects on long-term TCA treatment, given that few subjects in the clomipramine group relapsed. However, even those subjects receiving clomipramine for the full 8 months still experienced OCD symptoms, which varied in severity over time. Thus, long-term clomipramine treatment for children and adolescents with OCD seems to be effective in decreasing symptoms, but it does not completely eliminate troubling symptoms.

Buspirone

Buspirone, a nonbenzodiazepine anxiolytic, has been shown to be effective in reducing anxiety symptoms without the side effects of benzodiazepines.

Unlike the sedative-hypnotics, buspirone does not enhance the GABAergic system but acts as an agonist at the serotonin 5-HT_{1A} presynaptic receptors and as a partial agonist at the 5-HT_{1A} postsynaptic receptors. This process is meant to reduce both the flow of serotonin away from the presynaptic neuron and serotonergic activity in the central nervous system (CNS) overall. Buspirone is also not accompanied by the sedation, confusion, or withdrawal that can appear in sedative-hypnotic use (Robinson et al. 1990) and does not enhance the effects of CNS depressants, such as alcohol, making it relatively safe.

However, buspirone does seem to have a relatively long onset of effectiveness. Unlike benzodiazepines, which are usually short-acting, buspirone can take weeks to show significant anxiolytic effects. For this reason and because buspirone may not target all symptoms of anxiety equally, some suggest its use as a supplement to other medications or behavioral therapies in treating anxiety disorders. Several studies have shown the efficacy of buspirone in treating adults diagnosed with GAD (Goldberg and Finnerty 1982; Sramek et al. 1996) and OCD (Pigott et al. 1991).

Efficacy of Acute Treatment

Benefits.   Currently, there are no well-designed, controlled trials assessing the efficacy of buspirone in treating pediatric anxiety disorders. Much of the available information stems from case reports, case series, and open-label trials. Although individual case reports (Alessi and Bos 1991; Balon 1994; Kranzler 1988) seem to indicate some usefulness of buspirone in relieving anxiety symptoms, they do not provide evidence of its efficacy.

In a small open-label study, Pfeffer et al. (1997) investigated the treatment effects of buspirone in child psychiatric inpatients exhibiting symptoms of anxiety and moderate aggression ($N=25$, ages 5–12). Subjects who received high scores on the Revised Children's Manifest Anxiety Scale (RCMAS) and the Measure of Aggression, Violence, and Rage in Children (MAVRIC) were eligible to receive buspirone treatment. After being evaluated for 2 weeks (Phase I), these subjects started receiving buspirone, 5 mg/day. The total daily dose was titrated up 5–10 mg every 3 days (maximum dose = 50 mg) for 3 weeks (Phase II), after which the medication was kept at the optimum dosage for a 6-week maintenance period (Phase III). A registered nurse monitored side effects, blood pressure, and pulse often.

Results indicated that by the end of the 9-week trial subjects had a significant reduction of symptoms on the social anxiety factor of the RCMAS ($P<0.04$) but not on the total RCMAS. Clinicians noted that subjects seemed more eager to engage in interpersonal interactions and more willing to initiate activities with others. There was also a significant reduction in overall aggression, as measured by the MAVRIC ($P<0.02$), and in the number of seclusions and daily physical restraints used ($P<0.01$). However, subjects still showed impairment in global functioning at the endpoint of the study as measured by the CGAS. In addition, some children ($N=6$) had to discontinue use of buspirone because of severe side effects, including agitation, increased aggressivity, euphoric symptoms, increased impulsivity, and out-of-control behavior.

Although the results of this study are limited by its open-label design, they do show some efficacy in treating pediatric social phobia with buspirone. The 19 subjects who completed the trial tolerated buspirone (mean dosage=28 mg/day) well, reporting few side effects, other than headache. However, as the investigators noted, it is troubling that almost 25% of the sample had to discontinue treatment due to interfering adverse events. This finding could be accounted for by the high percentage of subjects with comorbid disorders (90%). Despite these limitations, the findings of Pfeffer et al. (1997) suggest that buspirone warrants future investigation as a potentially effective treatment for childhood anxiety disorders.

A later case series (Thomsen and Mikkelson 1999) also seems to indicate support for the addition of buspirone to SSRI treatment in adolescents diagnosed with OCD ($N=6$, ages 15–19). If patients did not show improvement following past SSRI treatment or CBT in combination, they were treated with buspirone (mean dosage=20 mg/day). Although cases varied in severity, the investigators reported that buspirone in combination with continuing SSRI treatment showed a positive reduction effect on obsessive-compulsive symptoms, especially anxiety and distress. In addition, dramatic clinical improvement, as measured by the Y-BOCS, was seen in three of the six cases. Buspirone was well tolerated, inasmuch as no patients reported severe side effects or had to discontinue combined treatment. Although this case series represents a small percentage of the adolescent OCD population, it does provide some indication that buspirone, when combined with SSRI treatment at a dosage of 20 mg/day, can be effective in reducing OCD symptoms.

Safety Issues

Monitoring

Prior to starting any type of medication treatment, it is important to review the family's medical and psychiatric history, as well as laboratory results and medical evaluation the child may have received by his or her primary care physician. In general, it is recommended that when prescribing a medication, the clinician should document the child's baseline weight, height, and vital signs and then monitor them over time during medication management visits. It is important for the clinician, with the consent of parent and child, to consult with the child's primary care physician in order to obtain additional medical information, such as concomitant medication history and last physical examination, and to establish a collaborative treatment relationship. Informed consent/assent should be obtained from the parent and child following a full explanation of the risks and benefits of the selected medication treatment. It is helpful to develop a list of impairing anxiety symptoms with child and parents, with the expectation that the medication will target these symptoms and will lead to improvement over time.

In general there are no laboratory tests required for the clinical use of SSRIs. Of the studies reviewed in this chapter, SSRIs were well tolerated by children and adolescents. And the pediatric side-effect profile is similar to what is seen in adult clinical studies. The main side effects of concern are the following: gastrointestinal discomfort, drowsiness, headaches, insomnia, nervousness, hyperkinesia, and hostility (Waslick 2006). However, there are reports of withdrawal symptoms accompanying the discontinuation of SSRIs. The child may experience the following symptoms: gastric distress, headache, dizziness, irritability, and agitation (Labellarte et al. 1998). Given this possibility, it is recommended that these medications not be abruptly discontinued.

Recent acute-treatment studies showed that children receiving venlafaxine extended-release had statistically significant changes in blood pressure, heart rate, weight, height, and total cholesterol. From these results it is unclear what impact long-term exposure to this medication would have on these clinical parameters. Given this information, clinicians should monitor vital signs, weight, and height and conduct a periodic laboratory assessment of cholesterol with acute and long-term treatment.

The main concern with TCA use in children is the potential for cardiac risk. When this medication is prescribed, the child should be measured for baseline vital signs, including sitting and standing blood pressure with pulse and ECG. Once the clinician has titrated the medication to the therapeutic dose, another ECG should be performed with a serum level of the medication. This process should be repeated with each dose adjustment and with periodic monitoring for long-term use. Another concern with this class of medication is the risk of lethal overdose, which must be considered when prescribing to a child or adolescent.

There are few available data that can be used to completely evaluate the risk-benefit profile of the benzodiazepines. From the findings obtained so far, there appear to be no serious adverse effects; however, some subjects experienced irritability, drowsiness, and disinhibition.

Prevention and Intervention of Adverse Effects

The best prevention and intervention for the management of medication adverse effects is the education of the family and child about what to expect in terms of potential medication side effects and how the clinician plans to manage the adverse effects if they should occur. As part of this education it must be stressed to the family and child that although there may be mild side effects initially, the majority will usually resolve in the first several weeks of treatment.

In addition, it is important for the clinician to document present, baseline physical symptoms and their levels of severity prior to starting medication and review this with the child and family. This symptom target list should be reviewed at each medication visit to assess change in severity or identify the development of a new symptom. Children with anxiety disorders have somatic symptoms that may be confused with side effects of the medication. If the clinician has documented at baseline the presence of somatic symptoms, this will assist in delineating the development of new adverse events or the worsening of previous symptoms.

In general, for all medications the clinician should initiate treatment at a low dose for the first 7 days and increase the dose slowly over subsequent weeks, depending on the child's clinical response and tolerability of the medication. Unfortunately, there is a dearth of information about dosing guidelines for these medications in treating specific anxiety disorders. Once a clinically efficacious dose is achieved, it should be maintained for 8–12 weeks and later re-evaluated to gauge successful treatment of the primary anxiety target symptoms and its tolerability.

Practical Management Strategies

Treatment Approaches, Algorithms, and Guidelines

Several clinical trials have clearly demonstrated that 10- to 16-week cognitive-behavioral treatments (with in vivo exposure) lead to a significant reduction in anxiety symptoms in children (Barrett et al. 1996; Kendall 1994; Kendall et al. 1997). Given this information, it would be reasonable for a clinician to initially recommend treatment with CBT. However, for some families it may be difficult to obtain CBT treatment because of the limited availability of pediatric therapists proficient in CBT in many parts of the country and the lack of reimbursement for psychotherapy even when CBT is available. If CBT is tried initially, it should be noted that that there is a significant percentage of children who remain symptomatic following CBT treatment. Moreover, one type of treatment will not work for all children. And finally, there are some children who will refuse to engage in CBT treatment.

At this time there are no definitive recommendations on when to use medications for children with anxiety disorders. In the next section of this chapter, we review the use of combination treatment (medications plus CBT) for the various anxiety disorders. In general, medication is often considered for treating pediatric anxiety disorders when a trial of some type of psychosocial intervention has failed and/or when anxiety symptoms are considered to be in the moderate-to-severe range, leading to functional impairment, such as poor school performance, school refusal, insomnia, and the development of comorbid diagnoses (such as major depression).

Combination Treatment

Because, as scientific evidence demonstrates, both CBT and medications such as the SSRIs separately provide efficacious treatments, research has been focused on the effects of combining these two treatments at the onset. Studies that indicate some sense of the potential benefits of combined treatment are reviewed below.

Bernstein et al. (2000) investigated the efficacy of imipramine plus CBT in treating school-phobic adolescents ($N=47$) who were diagnosed with co-morbid anxiety and major depressive disorders in an 8-week trial. Following a 1-week placebo washout, subjects were randomly assigned to receive imipramine or placebo in combination with CBT. Medication dosages were gradually titrated every 3–5 days (mean total daily dose = 182.3 mg). At week 3, a nonblinded psychiatrist monitoring blood levels of imipramine recommended a dose increase if the dose was considered subtherapeutic (imipramine plus desipramine < 150 μg/L) and a decrease if it was too high (imipramine plus desipramine > 300 μg/L).

The results of this study indicate that school attendance improved significantly only in the imipramine plus CBT group ($z = 4.36$, $P < 0.001$) and that the imipramine plus CBT group improved at a faster rate than the placebo plus CBT group (3.6% vs. 0.9%; $z = 2.39$, $P = 0.017$), even when compared with baseline. Anxiety and depression symptoms on various measures decreased significantly for both imipramine and placebo groups, with only one measure, the Children's Depression Rating Scale, Revised (CDRS-R), favoring imipramine ($z = 2.08$; $P = 0.037$). Additionally, remission on clinical measures significantly favored imipramine plus CBT only on the school attendance variable ($\chi^2 = 7.38$, $P = 0.007$).

This study seems to support the use of TCAs in combination with CBT in school-refusing adolescents who suffer from a combination of anxiety and depression symptoms. As with many previous studies, there is a comorbidity factor that precludes recommending TCAs for pure anxiety disorders; nevertheless, school attendance did improve significantly. However, the investigators also pointed out that the placebo group was significantly more symptomatic than the imipramine group at baseline. Additionally, it is difficult to determine how large a factor CBT was in this study. Without a medication-only group, we cannot isolate the benefit of the imipramine.

Another interesting study (Neziroglu et al. 2000) investigated the possible additional benefits of treating children and adolescents with OCD ($N=10$, ages 10–17) with a combination treatment of fluvoxamine and behavior therapy, compared with fluvoxamine alone. Subjects were eligible if they had previously failed a trial of behavior therapy lasting at least 10 sessions by not complying either inside or outside of treatment sessions. Following randomization, all subjects received 10 weeks of fluvoxamine (maximum dosage =

200 mg/day) until week 5, when 20 sessions of behavior therapy were initiated with 5 of the subjects.

Results showed that 8 of the 10 total subjects had improved scores on the primary outcome variable, the CY-BOCS, following the initial 10 weeks of fluvoxamine treatment. At week 43, 3 of the 5 subjects in the fluvoxamine plus behavior therapy group had significantly improved scores on the CY-BOCS, and 2 remained stable; 1 of the 5 subjects in the fluvoxamine-only group significantly improved, 2 remained stable, and 2 deteriorated significantly. At week 52, the pattern was similar, with 1 patient in the combination group and 2 more subjects in the fluvoxamine-only group having deteriorated. By 2-year follow-up, subjects in both treatment groups all continued to improve or remain stable, although data on 2 subjects in the fluvoxamine-only group were unavailable.

The study by Neziroglu et al. (2000), although relatively small, supports the use of combination treatments. Although many subjects improved after the initial fluvoxamine treatment, more subjects continued to improve when this treatment was supplemented with behavior therapy. Interestingly, the combination treatment also seemed to make the children more amenable to behavior therapy, given that all subjects had previously failed an adequate behavior therapy trial. The behavior therapy also seemed to help the children make more clinical gains, a finding supported by investigators noting a plateau effect in the fluvoxamine-only group. Although there are several limitations to this study, such as the small sample size and the lack of a placebo control, the findings suggest that combined SSRI and psychotherapy in treating anxious children warrants future investigation.

The Pediatric OCD Treatment Study (POTS) Team (2004) later conducted a multisite, placebo-controlled, double-blind study assessing the efficacy of sertraline, CBT, and their combination for children and adolescents diagnosed with OCD (N=122, ages 7–17). During Phase I, subjects were randomly assigned to receive sertraline (target dosage=200 mg/day), CBT, combination therapy, or placebo for 12 weeks. Results from intent-to-treat random regression analyses revealed that all active treatments were significantly more effective than placebo, based on change in CY-BOCS score (CBT: $P=0.003$; sertraline: $P=0.007$; combo: $P=0.001$), and that combined treatment was superior to CBT alone ($P=0.008$) and sertraline alone ($P=0.006$). The results for the CBT-alone and sertraline-alone groups did not differ significantly from each other.

Furthermore, the rate of clinical remission, defined as a CY-BOCS score of ≤10 in the combined treatment group, differed significantly from that of the sertraline only ($P=0.03$) and placebo groups ($P<0.001$), but not the CBT-only group. As in the efficacy analysis described above, the CBT-only and sertraline-only groups did not differ significantly. In addition, although the CBT-only group differed significantly from the placebo group ($P=0.002$), the sertraline-only group did not. Side effects were common, with subjects reporting decreased appetite, diarrhea, enuresis, motor activity, nausea, and stomachache. Despite these reports, there were no serious adverse events or reports of suicidality.

POTS (Pediatric OCD Treatment Study [POTS] Team 2004) showed that sertraline, CBT, and their combination are effective treatments for children and adolescents diagnosed with OCD. However, because the combination and CBT-only groups showed both a higher reduction of symptoms on the CY-BOCS and a higher rate of clinical remission, the investigators recommended combination treatment or CBT alone as a first-line treatment option. Because inclusion and exclusion criteria were limited in this study, there were high rates of comorbidity in the sample, with 63% of subjects having exhibited a comorbid internalizing disorder and 26% having exhibited a comorbid externalizing disorder. These high rates of comorbidity make the results even more striking, given that this sample resembled a community sample more than comparable trials.

An ongoing NIMH-funded multisite study, entitled Child/Adolescent Anxiety Multimodal Treatment Study, is comparing the treatment outcomes of children (ages 7–17) with primary diagnoses of GAD, separation anxiety disorder, and social anxiety disorder who were randomly assigned to receive either CBT alone, CBT in combination with sertraline, or sertraline versus placebo. This study is similar to POTS, and it will be interesting to see the results, which will surely have an impact on how these particular disorders are treated in the future.

Conclusions

The empirical evidence provides support for the treatment of pediatric anxiety disorders with pharmacological and psychotherapy (specifically CBT) treatments. The data suggest that there are several classes of medications that can be used safely and lead to an efficacious outcome. It appears that the class of SSRIs should be considered first-line when medication treatment is felt to be necessary. In addition, for pediatric OCD there is evidence to support that a combination treatment approach or CBT alone should be considered first. Additional long-term medication studies are warranted to examine both safety and treatment outcomes.

Clinical Pearls

- Prior to initiation of medication treatment, develop with the child and parent a list of target anxiety symptoms to be tracked during treatment to determine response. This approach can assist with determining the titration of the medication.
- To prevent early termination from a medication trial, spend an adequate amount of time educating the child and parent about potential adverse events.
- Carefully assess the child's response to treatment, and titrate the dose that achieves the maximal response.
- Maintaining a dose that is suboptimal will frustrate the child and family, leading to treatment noncompliance and a prematurely failed trial.
- Remember that as the child responds positively to treatment, his or her behavior may change, and this change may be interpreted by the parent as a possible adverse event. For example, an anxious child who is ordinarily compliant may begin to challenge his or her parent.
- Obtain at baseline a record of all physical symptoms the child experiences prior to medication treatment in order to assess adverse events caused by the medication vs. the child's anxiety symptoms.

References

Alessi N, Bos T: Buspirone augmentation of fluoxetine in a depressed child with obsessive-compulsive disorder. Am J Psychiatry 148:1605–1606, 1991

Allgulander C, Hackett D, Salinas E: Venlafaxine extended release (ER) in the treatment of generalized anxiety disorder: twenty-four week placebo-controlled dose-ranging study. Br J Psychiatry 179:15–22, 2001

American Academy of Child and Adolescent Psychiatry: Practice parameters for the assessment and treatment of children and adolescents with anxiety disorders. J Am Acad Child Adolesc Psychiatry 46:267–283, 2007

American Psychiatric Association: Diagnostic and Statistical Manual: Mental Disorders. Washington, DC, American Psychiatric Association, 1952

American Psychiatric Association: Diagnostic and Statistical Manual of Mental Disorders, 2nd Edition. Washington, DC, American Psychiatric Association, 1968

American Psychiatric Association: Diagnostic and Statistical Manual of Mental Disorders, 3rd Edition. Washington, DC, American Psychiatric Association, 1980

American Psychiatric Association: Diagnostic and Statistical Manual of Mental Disorders, 4th Edition. Washington, DC, American Psychiatric Association, 1994

American Psychiatric Association: Diagnostic and Statistical Manual of Mental Disorders, 4th Edition, Text Revision. Washington, DC, American Psychiatric Association, 2000

Anderson JC, Williams S, McGee R, et al: DSM-III disorders in preadolescent children: prevalence in a large sample from the general population. Arch Gen Psychiatry 44:69–76, 1987

Aronson TA, Logue CM: On the longitudinal course of panic disorder: development history and predictors of phobic complications. Compr Psychiatry 28:344–355, 1987

Ballenger JC, Burrows GD, DuPont RL, et al: Alprazolam in panic disorder and agoraphobia: results from a multicenter trial. Arch Gen Psychiatry 45:413–422, 1988

Balon R: Buspirone in the treatment of separation anxiety in an adolescent boy. Can J Psychiatry 39:581–582, 1994

Barrett PM, Dadds MR, Rapee RM: Family treatment of childhood anxiety: a controlled trial. J Consult Clin Psychol 64:333–342, 1996

Beidel DC, Fink CM, Turner SM: Stability of anxious symptomatology in children. J Abnorm Child Psychol 24:257–268, 1996

Berney T, Kolvin I, Bhate SR, et al: School phobia: a therapeutic trial with clomipramine and short-term outcome. Br J Psychiatry 138:110–118, 1981

Bernstein GA, Shaw K: Practice parameters for the assessment and treatment of anxiety disorders. J Am Acad Child Adolesc Psychiatry 32:1089–1098, 1993

Bernstein GA, Garfinkel BD, Borchardt CM: Comparative studies of pharmacotherapy for school refusal. J Am Acad Child Adolesc Psychiatry 29:773–781, 1990

Bernstein GA, Borchadt CM, Perwien AR, et al: Imipramine plus cognitive-behavioral therapy in the treatment of school refusal. J Am Acad Child Adolesc Psychiatry 39:276–283, 2000

Biederman J: Clonazepam in the treatment of prepubertal children with panic-like symptoms. J Clin Psychiatry 48(suppl):38–41, 1987

Biederman J: Sudden death in children treated with a tricyclic antidepressant. J Am Acad Child Adolesc Psychiatry 30:495–497, 1991

Birmaher B, Waterman GS, Ryan N, et al: Fluoxetine for childhood anxiety disorders. J Am Acad Child Adolesc Psychiatry 33:993–999, 1994

Birmaher B, Axelson DA, Monk K, et al: Fluoxetine for the treatment of childhood anxiety disorders. J Am Acad Child Adolesc Psychiatry 42:415–423, 2003

Black B, Uhde TW: Elective mutism as a variant of social phobia. J Am Acad Child Adolesc Psychiatry 31:1090–1094, 1992

Black B, Uhde TW: Treatment of elective mutism with fluoxetine: a double-blind, placebo-controlled study. J Am Acad Child Adolesc Psychiatry 33:1000–1006, 1994

Bowen RC, Offord DR, Boyle MH: The prevalence of overanxious disorder and separation anxiety disorder: results from the Ontario Child Health Study. J Am Acad Child Adolesc Psychiatry 29:753–758, 1990

Brady EU, Kendall PC: Comorbidity of anxiety and depression in children and adolescents. Psychol Bull 111:244–255, 1992

Cantwell DP, Baker L: Stability and natural history of DSM-III childhood diagnoses. J Am Acad Child Adolesc Psychiatry 28:691–700, 1989

Compton SN, Grant PJ, Chrisman AK, et al: Sertraline in children and adolescents with social anxiety disorder: an open trial. J Am Acad Child Adolesc Psychiatry 40:564–571, 2001

Cook EH, Wagner KD, March JS, et al: Long-term sertraline treatment of children and adolescents with obsessive-compulsive disorder. J Am Acad Child Adolesc Psychiatry 40:1175–1181, 2001

Costello EJ: Child psychiatric disorders and their correlates: a primary care pediatric sample. J Am Acad Child Adolesc Psychiatry 28:851–855, 1989

Costello EJ, Costello AJ, Edelbrock C, et al: Psychiatric disorders in pediatric primary care: prevalence and risk factors. Arch Gen Psychiatry 45:1107–1116, 1988

Costello EJ, Egger HL, Angold A: The developmental epidemiology of anxiety disorders: phenomenology, prevalence, and comorbidity. Child Adolesc Psychiatr Clin N Am 14:631–648, vii, 2005

Dadds MR, Spence SH, Holland DE, et al: Prevention and early intervention for anxiety disorders: a controlled trial. J Consult Clin Psychol 65:627–635, 1997

Davidson JRT, DuPont RL, Hedges D, et al: Efficacy, safety, and tolerability of venlafaxine XR extended release and buspirone in outpatients with generalized anxiety disorder. J Clin Psychiatry 60:528–535, 1999

DeVeaugh-Geiss J, Moroz G, Biederman J, et al: Clomipramine hydrochloride in childhood and adolescent obsessive-compulsive disorder: a multicenter trial. J Am Acad Child Adolesc Psychiatry 31:45–49, 1992

Dunner DL, Ishiki D, Avery DH, et al: Effect of alprazolam and diazepam on anxiety and panic attacks in panic disorder: a controlled study. J Clin Psychiatry 47:458–460, 1986

Feehan M, McGee R, Raja R, et al: DSM-III-R disorders in New Zealand 18 year olds. Aust N Z J Psychiatry 28:87–99, 1994

Flament MF, Rapoport JL, Berg CJ, et al: Clomipramine treatment of childhood obsessive-compulsive disorder: a double-blind controlled study. Arch Gen Psychiatry 42:977–983, 1985

Fluvoxamine for the treatment of anxiety disorders in children and adolescents. Research Units on Pediatric Psychopharmacology Anxiety Study Group. N Engl J Med 344:1279–1285, 2001

Fyer AJ, Liebowitz MR, Gorman JM, et al: Discontinuation of alprazolam treatment in panic patients. Am J Psychiatry 144:303–308, 1987

Gelenberg AJ, Lydiard RB, Rudolph RL, et al: Efficacy of venlafaxine extended-release capsules in nondepressed outpatients with generalized anxiety disorder: a 6-month randomized controlled trial. JAMA 283:3082–3088, 2000

Geller DA, Hoog SL, Heiligenstein JH, et al: Fluoxetine treatment for obsessive-compulsive disorder in children and adolescents: a placebo-controlled clinical trial. J Am Acad Child Adolesc Psychiatry 40:773–779, 2001

Geller DA, Biederman J, Stewart SE, et al: Which SSRI? A meta-analysis of pharmacotherapy trials in pediatric obsessive-compulsive disorder. Am J Psychiatry 160:1919–1928, 2003

Geller DA, Wagner KD, Emslie G, et al: Paroxetine treatment in children and adolescents with obsessive-compulsive disorder: a randomized, multicenter, double-blind, placebo-controlled trial. J Am Acad Child Adolesc Psychiatry 43:1387–1396, 2004

Gittelman-Klein R, Klein DF: Controlled imipramine treatment of school phobia. Arch Gen Psychiatry 25:204–207, 1971

Goddard AW, Brouette T, Almai A, et al: Early coadministration of clonazepam with sertraline for panic disorder. Arch Gen Psychiatry 58:681–686, 2001

Goldberg HL, Finnerty R: Comparison of buspirone in two separate studies. J Clin Psychiatry 43:87–91, 1982

Graae F, Milner J, Rizzotto L, et al: Clonazepam in childhood anxiety disorders. J Am Acad Child Adolesc Psychiatry 33:372–376, 1994

Katzelnick DJ, Kobak KA, Greist JH, et al: Sertraline for social phobia: a double-blind, placebo-controlled crossover study. Am J Psychiatry 152:1368–1371, 1995

Keller MB, Lavori PW, Wunder J, et al: Chronic course of anxiety disorders in children and adolescents. J Am Acad Child Adolesc Psychiatry 31:595–599, 1992

Kendall PC: Treating anxiety disorders in children: results of a randomized clinical trial. J Consult Clin Psychol 62:100–110, 1994

Kendall PC, Flannery-Schroeder E, Panichelli-Mindel SM, et al: Therapy for youths with anxiety disorders: a second randomized clinical trial. J Consult Clin Psychol 65:366–380, 1997

Klein RG, Koplewicz HS, Kanner A: Imipramine treatment of children with separation anxiety disorder. J Am Acad Child Adolesc Psychiatry 31:21–28, 1992

Kovacs M, Gatsonis C, Paulauskas SL, et al: Depressive disorders in childhood, IV: a longitudinal study of comorbidity with and risk for anxiety disorders. Arch Gen Psychiatry 46:776–782, 1989

Kraft IA, Ardali C, Duffy JH, et al: A clinical study of chlordiazepoxide used in psychiatric disorders in children. Int J Neuropsychiatry 1:433–437, 1965

Kranzler HR: Use of buspirone in an adolescent with overanxious disorder. J Am Acad Child Adolesc Psychiatry 27:789–790, 1988

Labellarte MJ, Walkup JT, Riddle MA: The new antidepressants: selective serotonin reuptake inhibitors. Pediatr Clin North Am 45:1137–1155, 1998

Last CG, Hersen M, Kazdin AE, et al: Comparison of DSM-III separation anxiety and overanxious disorders: demographic characteristics and patterns of comorbidity. J Am Acad Child Adolesc Psychiatry 26:527–531, 1987a

Last CG, Phillips JE, Statfeld A: Childhood anxiety disorders in mothers and their children. Child Psychiatry Hum Dev 18:103–112, 1987b

Last CG, Strauss CC, Hersen M, et al: Psychiatric illness in the mothers of anxious children. Am J Psychiatry 144:1580–1583, 1987c

Last CG, Perrin S, Hersen M, et al: A prospective study of childhood anxiety disorders. J Am Acad Child Adolesc Psychiatry 35:1502–1510, 1996

Last CG, Hansen C, Franco N: Anxious children in adulthood: a prospective study of adjustment. J Am Acad Child Adolesc Psychiatry 36:645–652, 1997

Leonard HL, Swedo SE, Rapoport JL, et al: Treatment of obsessive-compulsive disorder with clomipramine and desipramine in children and adolescents: a double-blind crossover comparison. Arch Gen Psychiatry 46:1088–1092, 1989

Leonard HL, Swedo SE, Lenane MC, et al: A double-blind desipramine substitution during long-term clomipramine treatment in children and adolescents with obsessive-compulsive disorder. Arch Gen Psychiatry 48:922–927, 1991

Leonard HL, March J, Rickler KC, et al: Pharmacology of the selective serotonin reuptake inhibitors in children and adolescents. J Am Acad Child Adolesc Psychiatry 36:725–736, 1997

Lewinsohn PM, Hops H, Roberts SE, et al: Adolescent psychopathology, I: prevalence and incidence of depression and other DSM-III-R disorders in high school students. J Abnorm Psychol 102:133–144, 1993

Liebowitz MR, Stein MB, Tancer M, et al: A randomized, double-blind, fixed-dose comparison of paroxetine and placebo in the treatment of generalized social anxiety disorder. J Clin Psychiatry 63:66–74, 2002

Livingston R, Taylor JL, Crawford SL: A study of somatic complaints and psychiatric diagnosis in children. J Am Acad Child Adolesc Psychiatry 27:185–187, 1988

March JS, Biederman J, Wolkow R, et al: Sertraline in children and adolescents with obsessive-compulsive disorder. JAMA 280:1752–1756, 1998

McGee R, Feehan M, Williams S, et al: DSM-III disorders in a large sample of adolescents. J Am Acad Child Adolesc Psychiatry 29:611–619, 1990

Meyer JS, Quenzer LQ: Psychopharmacology: Drugs, The Brain, and Behavior. Sunderland, MA, Sinauer Associates, 2005, pp 412–438

Neziroglu F, Yaryura-Tobias JA, Walz J, et al: The effect of fluvoxamine and behavior therapy on children and adolescents with obsessive-compulsive disorder. J Child Adolesc Psychopharmacol 10:295–306, 2000

Nishino S, Mignot E, Dement WC: Sedative-hypnotics, in The American Psychiatric Press Textbook of Psychopharmacology. Edited by Schatzberg AF, Nemeroff CB. Washington, DC, American Psychiatric Press, 1995, pp 405–416

Nutt D, Lawson C: Panic attacks: a neurochemical overview of models and mechanisms. Br J Psychiatry 160:165–178, 1992

Ollendick T, March J (eds): Developmental epidemiology of anxiety disorders, in Phobic and Anxiety Disorders in Children and Adolescents: A Clinician's Guide to Effective Psychosocial and Pharmacological Interventions. New York, Oxford University Press, 2004, pp 62–91

Orvaschel H, Weissman M: Epidemiology of anxiety in children, in Anxiety Disorders of Childhood. Edited by Gittelman R. New York, Guilford, 1986

Otto MW, Pollack MH, Sacks GS, et al: Discontinuation of benzodiazepine treatment: efficacy of cognitive-behavioral therapy for patients with panic disorder. Am J Psychiatry 150:1485–1490, 1993

Pediatric OCD Treatment Study (POTS) Team: Cognitive-behavior therapy, sertraline, and their combination for children and adolescents with obsessive-compulsive disorder: the Pediatric OCD Treatment Study (POTS) randomized controlled trial. JAMA 292:1969–1976, 2004

Pfeffer CR, Jiang H, Domeshek LJ: Buspirone treatment of psychiatrically hospitalized prepubertal children with symptoms of anxiety and moderately severe aggression. J Child Adolesc Psychopharmacol 7:145–155, 1997

Pfefferbaum B, Overall JE, Boren HA, et al: Alprazolam in the treatment of anticipatory and acute situational anxiety in children with cancer. J Am Acad Child Adolesc Psychiatry 26:532–535, 1987

Pigott TA: OCD: where the serotonin selectivity story begins. J Clin Psychiatry 57:11–20, 1996

Pigott TA, L'Heureux F, Hill JL, et al: A double-blind study of adjuvant buspirone hydrochloride in clomipramine-treated patients with obsessive-compulsive disorder. J Clin Psychopharmacol 12:11–18, 1991

Pine DS: Treating children and adolescents with selective serotonin reuptake inhibitors: how long is appropriate? J Child Adolesc Psychopharmacol 12:189–203, 2002

Pine DS, Grun J: Anxiety disorders, in Child Psychopharmacology. Edited by Walsh TB. Review of Psychiatry, Vol 17 (Series Editors, JM Oldham, MB Riba). Washington, DC, American Psychiatric Press, 1998, pp 115–148

Pohl RB, Wolkow RM, Clary CM: Sertraline for social phobia: a double-blind, placebo-controlled crossover study. Am J Psychiatry 155:1189–1195, 1998

Pollack MH, Tesar GE, Rosenbaum JF, et al: Clonazepam in the treatment of panic disorder and agoraphobia: a one-year follow-up. J Clin Psychopharmacol 6:302–304, 1986

Pollack MH, Zaninelli R, Goddard A, et al: Paroxetine in the treatment of generalized anxiety disorder: results of a placebo-controlled, flexible-dosage trial. J Clin Psychiatry 62:350–357, 2001

Potter WZ, Manji HK, Rudorfer MV: Tricyclic and tetracyclics, in The American Psychiatric Press Textbook of Psychopharmacology. Edited by Schatzberg AF, Nemeroff CB. Washington, DC, American Psychiatric Press, 1995, pp 141–160

Rickels K, Rynn MA: What is generalized anxiety disorder? J Clin Psychiatry 62(suppl):4–12, 2001

Rickels K, Csanalosi I, Greisman P, et al: A controlled clinical trial of alprazolam for the treatment of anxiety. Am J Psychiatry 140:82–85, 1983

Rickels K, Schweizer E, Weiss S, et al: Maintenance drug treatment for panic disorder II: short-and long-term outcome after drug taper. Arch Gen Psychiatry 50:61–68, 1993

Rickels K, Pollack MH, Sheehan DV, et al: Efficacy of venlafaxine XR extended-release capsules in nondepressed outpatients with generalized anxiety disorder. Am J Psychiatry 157:968–974, 2000

Riddle MA, Scahill L, King RA, et al: Double-blind, crossover trial of fluoxetine and placebo in children and adolescents with obsessive-compulsive disorder. J Am Acad Child Adolesc Psychiatry 31:1062–1069, 1992

Riddle MA, Geller B, Ryan N: Case study: another sudden death in a child treated with desipramine. J Am Acad Child Adolesc Psychiatry 32:792–797, 1993

Riddle MA, Reeve EA, Yaryura-Tobias JA, et al: Fluvoxamine for children and adolescents with obsessive-compulsive disorder: a randomized, controlled, multicenter trial. J Am Acad Child Adolesc Psychiatry 40:222–229, 2001

Robinson DS, Rickels K, Feighner J, et al: Clinical effects of the 5-HT$_{1A}$ partial agonists in depression: a composite analysis of buspirone in the treatment of depression. J Clin Psychopharmacol 10(suppl):67S–76S, 1990

Ross SB, Renyi AL: Tricyclic antidepressant agents, I: comparison of the inhibition of the uptake of 3-H-noradrenaline and 14-C-5-hydroxytryptamine in slices and crude synaptosome preparations of the midbrain-hypothalamus region of the rat brain. Acta Pharmacol Toxicol (Copenh) 36 (suppl 5):382–394, 1975

Roy A, De Jong J, Linnoila M: Cerebrospinal fluid monoamine metabolites and suicidal behavior in depressed patients. Arch Gen Psychiatry 46:609–612, 1989

Rynn MA, Siqueland L, Rickels K: Placebo-controlled trial of sertraline in the treatment of children with generalized anxiety disorder. Am J Psychiatry 158:2008–2014, 2001

Rynn MA, Garcia-Espana F, Greenblatt DJ, et al: Imipramine and buspirone in patients with panic disorder who are discontinuing long-term benzodiazepine therapy. J Clin Psychopharmacol 23:505–508, 2003

Rynn M, Yeung PP, Riddle MA, et al: Venlafaxine ER as a treatment for GAD in children and adolescents. Presentation at the 157th annual meeting of the American Psychiatric Association, New York, NY, May 1–6, 2004

Rynn MA, Riddle MA, Yeung PP, et al: Efficacy and safety of extended-release venlafaxine in the treatment of generalized anxiety disorder in children and adolescents: two placebo-controlled trials. Am J Psychiatry 164:290–300, 2007

Schweizer E, Rickels K, Weiss S, et al: Maintenance drug treatment of panic disorder I: results of a prospective, placebo-controlled comparison of alprazolam and imipramine. Arch Gen Psychiatry 50:51–60, 1993

Silverman WK, Albano AM: The Anxiety Disorder Interview Schedule for Children for DSM-IV: Child and Parent Versions. Boulder, CO, Graywind, 1996

Simeon JG, Ferguson HB: Alprazolam effects in children with anxiety disorders. Can J Psychiatry 32:570–574, 1987

Simeon JG, Ferguson B, Knott V, et al: Clinical, cognitive, and neurophysiological effects of alprazolam in children and adolescents with overanxious and avoidant disorders. J Am Acad Child Adolesc Psychiatry 31:29–33, 1992

Sramek JJ, Tansman M, Suri A, et al: Efficacy of buspirone in generalized anxiety disorder with coexisting mild depressive symptoms. J Clin Psychiatry 57:287–289, 1996

Stein MB, Liebowitz M, Lydiard RB, et al: Paroxetine treatment of generalized social phobia (social anxiety disorder): a randomized, controlled trial. JAMA 280:708–713, 1998

Strauss CC: Behavioral assessment and treatment of overanxious disorder in children and adolescents. Behav Modif 12:234–251, 1988

Tancer ME: Neurobiology of social phobia. J Clin Psychiatry 54:26–30, 1993

Thomsen PH: Child and adolescent obsessive-compulsive disorder treated with citalopram: findings from an open trial of 23 cases. J Child Adolesc Psychopharmacol 7:157–166, 1997

Thomsen PH, Mikkelson HU: The addition of buspirone to SSRI in the treatment of adolescent obsessive-compulsive disorder: a study of six cases. Eur Child Adolesc Psychiatry 8:143–148, 1999

Thomsen PH, Ebbesen C, Persson C: Long-term experience with citalopram in the treatment of adolescent OCD. J Am Acad Child Adolesc Psychiatry 40:895–902, 2001

Tourian KA, March JS, Mangano R: Venlafaxine extended release in children and adolescents with social anxiety disorder. Presented at the 157th annual meeting of the American Psychiatric Association, New York, NY, May 1–6, 2004

Varley CK, McClellan J: Case study: two additional sudden deaths with tricyclic antidepressants. J Am Acad Child Adolesc Psychiatry 36:390–394, 1997

Vitiello B, Zuvekas SH, Norquist GS: National estimates of antidepressant medication use among U.S. children, 1997–2002. J Am Acad Child Adolesc Psychiatry 45:271–279, 2006

Wagner KD, Berard R, Stein MB, et al: A multicenter, randomized, double-blind, placebo-controlled trial of paroxetine in children and adolescents with social anxiety disorder. Arch Gen Psychiatry 61:1153–1162, 2004

Walkup J, Labellarte M, Riddle MA, et al: Treatment of pediatric anxiety disorders: an open-label extension of the research units on pediatric psychopharmacology anxiety study. Research Units on Pediatric Psychopharmacology Anxiety Study Group. J Child Adolesc Psychopharmacol 12:175–188, 2002

Walkup J, Labellarte M, Riddle MA, et al: Searching for moderators and mediators of pharmacological treatment effects in children and adolescents with anxiety disorders. Research Units on Pediatric Psychopharmacology Anxiety Study Group. J Am Acad Child Adolesc Psychiatry 42:13–21, 2003

Waslick B: Psychopharmacology interventions for pediatric anxiety disorders: a research update. Child Adolesc Psychiatr Clin N Am 15:51–71, 2006

Weintrob N, Cohen D, Klipper-Aurbach Y, et al: Decreased growth during therapy with selective serotonin reuptake inhibitors. Arch Pediatr Adolesc Med 156:696–701, 2002

Weissman MM, Wolk S, Wickramaratne P, et al: Children with prepubertal-onset major depressive disorder and anxiety grown up. Arch Gen Psychiatry 56:794–801, 1999

Werry J: Diagnosis and assessment, in Anxiety Disorders of Childhood. Edited by Gittelman R. New York, Guilford, 1986

Witek MW, Rojas V, Alonso C, et al: Review of benzodiazepine use in children and adolescents. Psychiatr Q 76:283–296, 2005

5

Major Depressive Disorder

Boris Birmaher, M.D.

Pediatric major depressive disorder (MDD) is a familial recurrent illness associated with poor psychosocial and academic outcome, substance abuse, anxiety, psychosocial difficulties, and an increased risk of suicide and suicide attempts, (Birmaher et al. 1996a, 2002; Lewinsohn et al. 1999; Pine et al. 1998; Weissman et al. 1999a, 1999b).

The prevalence of MDD in children and adolescents is approximately 2% and 6%, respectively (Birmaher et al. 1996a). Because pediatric MDD is continuous into adulthood, early identification and prompt treatment at its early stages are critical.

My main aim in this chapter is to review the current pharmacological treatments for children and adolescents with MDD. Although psychotherapy interventions, including cognitive-behavioral therapy (CBT)—either alone (Brent et al. 1997) or in combination with antidepressants (March et al. 2004)—and interpersonal psychotherapy (IPT) (Mufson et al. 2004), have also been found efficacious for the acute treatment of pediatric MDD, particularly for adolescents, they will not be reviewed here.

The current definitions of outcome (Birmaher et al. 2000; Emslie et al. 1997, 2002, 2004) are presented in Table 5–1.

Assessment of Treatment Response

Treatment response has traditionally been determined by the absence of MDD criteria (e.g., no more than one DSM symptom) or, more frequently, by a significant reduction in symptom severity (usually 50%). However, when the latter criterion is used, patients deemed *responders* may still have considerable residual depressive symptomatology. Therefore, an absolute final score on the Beck Depression Inventory of ≤9 (Beck 1967), on the 17-item Hamilton Rating Scale for Depression of ≤7 (M. Hamilton 1960), or on the Children's Depression Rating Scale, Revised of ≤28 (CDRS) (Poznanski et al. 1984), together with persistent improvement in patient's functioning for at least 2 weeks or longer, may better reflect a satisfactory response. Overall improvement has also been measured with the Improvement subscale of the Clinical Global Impression Scale (CGI-I) (Guy 1976), with scores of 1 and 2 indicating very much or much improvement, respectively.

Functional improvement can be measured using several rating scales such as a score of ≥70 in the Global Assessment Scale (American Psychiatric Association 1994) or the Children's Global Assessment Scale (Shaffer et al. 1983).

Treatment Phases

The treatment of MDD is divided into three phases: acute, continuation, and maintenance ("Practice for the Treatment of Patients With Major Depressive Disorder (Revision)" 2000; "Practice Parameters for the Assessment and Treatment of Children and Adolescents With Depressive Disorder" 1998). The *acute phase* for a youth is the first episode of depression, which usually lasts 6–12 weeks. The main goals of treatment are to achieve response and remission of the depressive symptoms. The *continuation phase* usually lasts 4–12 months, during which remission is consolidated to prevent relapses. The *maintenance phase* lasts 1 year or longer, and its main treatment objective is the prevention of depression recurrences. Almost all studies on children and adolescents have evaluated treatments during the acute phase. There are few continuation studies (Clarke et al. 2005; Emslie et al. 2004; Goodyer et al. 2007)

Table 5–1. Definitions of treatment outcome

Response	No symptoms or a significant reduction in depressive symptoms for at least 2 weeks
Remission	A period of at least 2 weeks and less than 2 months with no or very few depressive symptoms
Recovery	Absence of symptoms of major depressive disorder for 2 months or more (e.g., can have no more than 1–2 symptoms to be considered in recovery)
Relapse	A major depressive episode during the period of remission
Recurrence	Emergence of symptoms of major depressive disorder during the period of recovery (a new episode)

and no maintenance treatment studies. Therefore, recommendations regarding continuation and maintenance treatments are extrapolated from the adult literature. However, caution is warranted because youth may respond differently to continuation and maintenance interventions that thus far have only been tested on adults with MDD (Birmaher et al. 1996b).

Treatment of Major Depressive Disorder With Selective Serotonin Reuptake Inhibitors and Other Novel Antidepressants

Psychoeducation and Supportive Therapy

The optimal pharmacological management of child and adolescent MDD should involve educative and supportive psychotherapy. In fact, at least for youth with mild-to-moderate depression, supportive management and education may be sufficient to ameliorate the symptoms of depression (Goodyer et al. 2007; Mufson et al. 2004; Renaud et al. 1998). Education of the patient and family about the disease, nature of treatment, and prognosis is critical to engagement in treatment and enhancement of compliance (Brent et al. 1993).

Psychosocial scars or complications during and after the depression remission (e.g., family conflict, poor self-esteem and social skills, academic difficulties, problems with peers) need to be addressed with psychotherapy (Birmaher et al. 2000; Kovacs and Goldston 1991; Puig-Antich et al. 1985; Rao et al. 1995; Stein et al. 2000; Strober et al. 1993).

Additionally, the parents of depressed youth may also be experiencing depression and other psychiatric disorders (Klein et al. 2001; Weissman et al. 1987), and parental depression may lead to adverse outcomes in the youth (Brent et al. 1998). To treat the child successfully, the clinician should assess parents and refer them for their own treatment.

Acute Phase

Most studies on the acute treatment of youth with MDD have focused on the effects of the tricyclic antidepressants (TCAs), the selective serotonin reuptake inhibitors (SSRIs), and, more recently, the serotonin-norepinephrine reuptake inhibitors (SNRIs). A few open studies have also shown that monoamine oxidase inhibitors (MAOIs) can be used safely with children and adolescents (Ryan et al. 1988b), but noncompliance with dietary requirements may present a significant problem for youth. Other antidepressants, including the heterocyclics (e.g., amoxapine, maprotiline) and bupropion, have been found to be efficacious for the treatment of depressed adults ("Practice Guideline" 2000), but they have not been well studied for the treatment of MDD in children and adolescents. The TCAs have not been found to be better than placebo for the treatment of youth with MDD (Hazell et al. 2006), and they are associated with significant side effects and high risk for lethality in a case of an overdose. Therefore, this chapter mainly describes the use of SSRIs for youth with MDD.

The SSRIs selectively block the presynaptic neuronal reuptake of serotonin, with little or no affinity for the adrenergic, cholinergic, or histaminic receptors (Emslie et al. 1999; Leonard et al. 1997).

Several, but not all, acute (8–12 weeks) randomized, controlled studies have shown significant improvement in depressive symptomatology for children and adolescents with MDD (Bridge et al. 2007; Cheung et al. 2005; Goodyer et al. 2007; Mann et al. 2006).

Using the score of *much* to *very much* improvement (≤2) on the CGI-I as a positive outcome, three randomized controlled trials (RCTs) using fluoxetine and one each with citalopram, sertraline (two studies combined and reported as one study), and paroxetine showed that children and adolescents with MDD responded significantly better to the acute treatment with these antidepressants (50%-60%) than placebo (30%–50%). Of these SSRIs, fluoxetine showed the largest effect sizes, in part because of a low placebo response rate. Despite the significant rates of response, a smaller proportion (30%–40%) achieved full remission (usually defined as a score of ≤28 on the Children's Depression Rating Scale, Revised) (Emslie et al. 1997, 2004; March et al. 2004; Wagner et al. 2004). A possible explanation for the low rate of remission is that optimal pharmacological treatment may involve a higher dose and/or a longer duration of treatment or that the ideal treatment for some may involve a combination of pharmacological and psychosocial interventions as suggested by the Treatment for Adolescents With Depression Study (TADS) (March et al. 2004). However, in this study, despite that, overall, the rate of remission was higher in combination treatment (37% in combination vs. 23% in medication alone), particularly for less severely depressed subjects, the remission rate was not optimal. Moreover, two other studies did not show an advantage to adding CBT to regular SSRI treatment (Clarke et al. 2005; Goodyer et al. 2007).

Several published or unpublished industry-sponsored studies with SSRIs (one each with citalopram and escitalopram, and two with paroxetine) did not find differences between active medication and placebo (Bridge et al. 2007). In these and some of the above-mentioned positive studies, subjects responded to the SSRIs, but the placebo response was also high, suggesting that depressive symptoms in youth may be highly responsive to supportive management, that these studies included subjects with mild depressions, or that there are other methodological issues responsible for the lack of difference between medication and placebo (for a review of the limitations of current pharmacological RCTs, see Cheung et al. 2005).

A novel way to understand the effect of treatment is through the concept of the *number needed to treat* (NNT) in order to observe one response that it is attributable to active treatment and not placebo. Across all the published and unpublished SSRI RCTs, depressed patients treated with SSRIs have a relatively good response rate (50%–70% clinically improved), but the placebo response rate is also high (30%–60%), resulting in an overall NNT of 9 (Bridge et al. 2007; Cheung et al. 2005). It appears that there is not an age effect (Bridge et al. 2007), and the difference between the response to SSRIs and placebo is inversely related to the number of sites involved in the study (Bridge et al. 2007; Cheung et al. 2005). Fluoxetine is the only medication to be approved by the U.S. Food and Drug Administration for the treatment of child and adolescent depression, and it shows a larger difference between

202 Clinical Manual of Child and Adolescent Psychopharmacology

medication and placebo than do other antidepressants, with an overall NNT of 4. It is not clear whether the difference is due to actual differences in the effect of the medication, to other related properties of the medication (long half-life may lessen the impact of poor adherence to treatment), or to better design and performance of the studies involving fluoxetine, which may have had more severely depressed patients.

Few RCTs have evaluated the effects of other classes of antidepressants for the treatment of depressed youth. One unpublished study showed that nefazodone was significantly more effective than placebo for youth with MDD (Cheung et al. 2005; Mann et al. 2006). However, although the generic form of this medication is still available, the manufacturer has withdrawn Serzone from the market because of a rare but serious side effect—liver damage resulting in hepatic failure. A small RCT comparing venlafaxine with placebo showed no differences between these two conditions (Mandoki et al. 1997). Two unpublished industry-sponsored RCTs with venlafaxine and two with mirtazapine were negative (Bridge et al. 2007; Mann et al. 2006). However, a reanalysis of the venlafaxine trials showed significant effects over placebo for adolescents but not for children. There are no reports on the use of duloxetine in youth. Although bupropion is being used clinically for the treatment of youth with MDD, except for an open study on children with MDD and attention-deficit/hyperactivity disorder (ADHD) (Daviss et al. 2001), no RCTs have been conducted for youth with MDD.

Side Effects

Overall, SSRIs and other novel antidepressants have been well tolerated by both children and adolescents, with only a few short-term side effects commonly reported. It appears that the side effects of SSRIs and SNRIs are similar and dose-dependent, and may subside with time (Cheung et al. 2005; Emslie et al. 1999; Leonard et al. 1997; Safer and Zito 2006). The most common side effects include gastrointestinal symptoms, restlessness, diaphoresis, headaches, akathisia, changes in appetite (increase or decrease), sleep changes (e.g., vivid dreams, nightmares, impaired sleep), and impaired sexual functioning. Approximately 3%–8% of children and adolescents taking antidepressants may show increased impulsivity, agitation, irritability, silliness, and *behavioral activation* (Hammad 2004; Martin et al. 2004; Wilens et al. 1998). These symptoms must be differentiated from the mania or hypomania that may appear in children and adolescents with bipolar disorder or those who are predisposed to develop that disorder (Wilens et al. 1998). More rarely, the use of antidepressants has been associated with serotonin syndrome (Boyer and Shannon 2005), as discussed later in this section (see subsection "Interactions With Other Medications"), and with increased suicidal behaviors (see the next subsection), and bruising (Lake et al. 2000). Because of the risk of bruising, patients treated with SSRIs and SNRIs who are going to have surgery should inform their physicians, and they may wish to discontinue treatment during the preoperative period. Venlafaxine and perhaps other SNRIs may elevate blood pressure and cause tachycardia. Mirtazapine, a serotonin and adrenergic receptor blocker, may increase appetite, weight, and somnolence. Trazodone, a serotonin type 2A (5-HT_{2A}) receptor blocker and weak serotonin reuptake inhibitor, and mirtazapine are mainly utilized as adjunctive and transient treatments for insomnia. Trazodone must be used with caution in males because it can induce priapism. As noted earlier, the brand form of nefazodone (Serzone), a 5-HT_{2A} receptor blocker and weak serotonin reuptake inhibitor, was taken off the market because it may induce liver problems. The long-term side effects of antidepressants have not been systematically evaluated.

Suicidal Behaviors

There appears to be a small but statistically significant increase in *spontaneous* reporting of self-harm behavior and suicidal ideation in antidepressants versus placebo. In a recent FDA-sponsored meta-analysis, in collaboration with Columbia University (Hammad et al. 2006), of the *spontaneous* suicide adverse events (SAEs) reported in 24 RCTs (16 MDD, 4 obsessive-compulsive disorder [OCD], 2 generalized anxiety disorder, 1 social anxiety disorder, and 1 ADHD) comparing several antidepressants versus placebo, the overall risk ratio (RR) for *spontaneous* reported SAEs was 1.95 (95% CI: 1.28–2.98). For only MDD studies the overall RR was 1.66 (95% CI: 1.02–2.68). Only TADS showed a significant difference between active treatment and placebo, and among the antidepressants only venlafaxine showed a statistically significant association with suicidality (March et al. 2004). In general, these results translate to 2 emergent or worsened *spontaneous reported* suicidality for every 100 youth treated with one of the antidepressants included in the FDA meta-analysis. There were very few suicide attempts and *no completions*.

In contrast to the analyses of the SAEs, evaluation of the suicidality ascertained through rating scales in 17 studies did not show significant onset or worsening of suicidality (RR≈0.90) (Hammad et al. 2006). It is not clear why the FDA meta-analysis found increased rates of spontaneously reported suicide-related adverse events for subjects taking drug versus placebo but no differences in suicidality on regularly assessed clinical measures. It is possible that in a subgroup of patients treated with antidepressants, particularly those already agitated and/or suicidal, treatment causes a disinhibition that leads to worsening of ideation and/or a greater tendency to make suicidal threats. Because this event usually leads to removal of the subject from the study and a change in treatment, analyses that look at the slope of suicidal ideation will not find an effect. In addition, suicidal ideation as measured on rating scales is highly correlated with the severity of depression, which is more likely to decline in those given drug than in those given placebo.

These results must be viewed in the context of the limitations of the FDA study, which include use of the metric of relative risk (limited to trials with at least one event), inability to generalize the results to populations not included in RCTs, short-term data, failure to include all available RCTs, and multiple comparisons (Hammad et al. 2006). Also, as stated by the FDA (Hammad et al. 2006), the implications and clinical significance regarding the above-noted findings are uncertain, given that, with the increase in usage of SSRIs, there has been a dramatic decline in adolescent suicide (Olfson et al. 2003). Moreover, pharmacoepidemiological studies, which are correlative rather than causal, support a positive relationship between SSRI use and the reduction in the adolescent and young adult suicide rate (Gibbons et al. 2005; Olfson et al. 2003; Valuck et al. 2004). Another study showed increased suicide attempts only immediately *before* the SSRIs were administered (Simon et al. 2006).

A more recent, thorough meta-analysis extended the FDA analyses by including all existing published and unpublished antidepressants studies (13 MDD, 6 OCD, and 6 anxiety) (Bridge et al. 2007). This meta-analysis found comparable *overall* findings when similar statistical methods (RR) were used rather than the methods used in the FDA study (Bridge et al. 2007)—namely, a significant increased RR for *spontaneous reported* suicidality *only* for subjects with MDD. However, in pooled random-effects analyses of risk differences, which make possible an analysis of *all* the existing RCTs, a nonsignificant risk difference (drug minus placebo) was found for MDD (0.8%; 95% CI: −0.2%

to 1.8%) and other disorders. Moreover, the overall *number needed to harm* (NNH) (number of subjects needed to treat in order to observe one adverse event that can be attributed to the active treatment) for MDD was 125 (Bridge et al. 2007). As stated earlier, the overall NNT for antidepressants in pediatric depression is 9. Thus, nearly 14 times more depressed patients will respond favorably to antidepressants than will *spontaneously report* suicidality (although one must keep in mind the limitations of meta-analyses). The benefit-risk ratio was larger for the SSRIs (10) than for non-SSRI antidepressants (5).

In conclusion, it appears that *spontaneously* reported events are more common in antidepressant treatment. Nevertheless, given the greater number of patients who benefit from antidepressant treatment, particularly the SSRIs, than who experience these SAEs, and the decline in overall suicidal ideation on rating scales, the risk-benefit ratio for SSRI use in pediatric depression appears to be favorable, with careful monitoring. Further work is required to determine if the risk-benefit ratio is indeed less favorable for children than for adolescents. Also, it remains to be clarified whether certain factors are related to increased risk for suicidality (Apter et al. 2006; Brent 2004; Hammad et al. 2006; Safer and Zito 2006)—for example, sex; subject's history of suicidality; family history of suicidality; disorder type (it appears that the effects of the disorder type are more obvious in depressed youth); severity of depressive symptoms at intake; dosages; half-life (in terms of efficacy); type of antidepressants administered; treatment duration; poor adherence to treatment; withdrawal side effects (due to noncompliance or short medication half-life); induction of agitation, activation, or hypomania; and/or susceptibility to side effects (e.g., slow metabolizers or variations in genetic polymorphisms).

Pharmacokinetic Studies

In children and adolescents the half-lives of antidepressants such as paroxetine, sertraline, citalopram, and bupropion SR are between 14 and 16 hours (Axelson et al. 2000a, 2000b; Clein and Riddle 1995; Daviss et al. 2005; Findling et al. 1999, 2000, 2006). One study suggested that sertraline at a dosage of 200 mg/day can be prescribed once a day (Alderman et al. 1998). Results of previously mentioned studies suggest that these medications, particularly when prescribed at lower doses, may need to be given twice a day. Otherwise, children and adolescents may experience withdrawal side effects during the evening, and these symptoms can be confused with lack of response or medication side effects. More pharmacokinetic studies conducted on the other antidepressants are necessary, because it appears that youth metabolize these medications faster than adult populations.

Interactions With Other Medications

Careful attention to possible medication interactions is recommended, given that the antidepressants and/or their metabolites are metabolized in different degrees by the hepatic cytochrome P450 (CYP) enzymes. Of the five major CYP enzymes mediating the oxidative drug metabolism, CYP3A3/4 and CYP2D6 are responsible for approximately 50% and 30%, respectively, of known oxidative drug metabolism. Except for citalopram/escitalopram and sertraline, the currently available SSRIs are mainly metabolized by CYP3A3/4 and/or CYP2D6 enzymes. Bupropion is mainly metabolized by the CYP2B6 enzyme, but it also inhibits the enzyme CYP2D6. Venlafaxine is metabolized by the CYP2D6 enzyme. Substantial inhibition of these enzymes converts a normal metabolizer into a slow metabolizer with regard to this specific pathway. Therefore, it is important to be aware of the possibility that toxicity could result if other medications are prescribed that are also metabolized by the CYP system, such as the TCAs, neuroleptics, atypical antipsychotics, antiarrhythmics, antihypertensives, theophylline, atomoxetine, benzodiazepines, carbamazepine, and warfarin. There are several Web sites with up-to-date information regarding the metabolism of SSRIs and other antidepressants by the CYP system and interactions with other medications (e.g., see http://medicine.iupui.edu/flockhart, www.preskorn.com, and www.pdr.net).

Interactions of the antidepressants with other serotonergic medications, in particular MAOIs, may induce serotonin syndrome, which is marked by agitation, confusion, and hyperthermia (Boyer and Shannon 2005). MAOIs should not be given within 5 weeks after stopping fluoxetine, and for at least 2 weeks after stopping other SSRIs, because of the possibility of inducing serotonin syndrome.

Some antidepressants also have a high rate of protein binding, which can lead to increased therapeutic or toxic effects of other protein-bound medications.

Discontinuation

Especially for antidepressants with shorter half-lives (e.g., paroxetine), sudden or rapid cessation may induce withdrawal symptoms that can mimic a relapse or recurrence of a depressive episode (e.g., tiredness, irritability). Furthermore, there is the clinical impression that rapid discontinuation of antidepressants may induce relapses or recurrences of depression. Therefore, if these medications need to be discontinued, they should be tapered progressively.

Summary and Recommendations

Given that 30%–60% of children and adolescents with MDD respond to placebo (Bridge et al. 2007; Cheung et al. 2005; Mann et al. 2006) and/or very brief or supportive psychotherapy treatments (Goodyer et al. 2007; Mufson et al. 2004; Renaud et al. 1998), it is reasonable, in a patient with a mild depression or mild psychosocial impairment, to offer psychoeducation, support, and case management related to possible environmental stressors in the family and school. If the symptoms of mild depression worsen, or if after 4–6 weeks of supportive therapy the child has not responded, more specific forms of psychotherapy or antidepressants are warranted.

In contrast, children and adolescents who present with chronic or recurrent depressions, moderate to severe psychosocial impairment, comorbid disorder, or a high family history of depression initially require more specific types of psychotherapies and/or antidepressants.

Independent of the treatment administered, patient and family will require education about the nature and treatment of depression, support, and management of daily problems. Problems at school, academic issues, school refusal, abuse of drugs, exposure to negative events (e.g., abuse, conflict with parents), and peer issues must be addressed. For example, family discord is associated with slower recovery and greater chance of recurrence (Birmaher et al. 2000; Rueter et al. 1999), and ongoing disappointments have been associated with chronic depression (Goodyer et al. 1998). Therefore, addressing family discord and improving the patient's coping skills are likely to improve outcome in either psychosocial or psychopharmacological treatment. Moreover, a high incidence of parental mental health problems indicates the need for evaluation and appropriate referral of parents and siblings of depressed youth. Finally, a high degree of comorbidity also emphasizes the importance of a multimodal pharmacological and psychosocial treatment approach (Hughes et al. 1999). For example, a child with MDD and ADHD may not respond to an SSRI alone, and may require either combined treatment with a stimulant plus an SSRI, or an alternative medication such as a TCA, bupropion, or venlafaxine (Daviss et al. 2001; Pliszka et al. 2000).

Currently, the antidepressants of choice to treat children and adolescents with MDD are the SSRIs. So far, fluoxetine is the only SSRI that has shown more consistent positive findings, but until additional studies with better methodologies are available, other SSRIs can also be used with caution. Patients should be treated with adequate doses for at least 6 weeks before the clinician declares a lack of response to treatment (treatment of nonresponders is described in the subsection "Treatment-Resistant Depression" later in this chapter).

The dosages of SSRIs in children and adolescents are similar to those used for adult patients (Leonard et al. 1997) (Table 5–2), except that lower initial doses are used to avoid unwanted effects. To avoid side effects and improve adherence to treatment, it is recommended that the medication be started at a low dosage and that the dosage be increased slowly. Also, it is possible that children require lower dosages than adolescents, but this issue has not been well studied. During the acute phase of treatment, patients should be treated with adequate and tolerable doses for at least 4–6 weeks. Clinical response should be assessed at 4–6 week intervals, and dosage can be increased if a complete response has not been obtained. Although it has not been studied in children, if, at the point of assessment, only a partial response has been achieved, the physician may consider strategies described in the subsection "Treatment-Resistant Depression" later in this chapter. At each step, adequate time should be allowed for clinical response, and frequent, early dose adjustment should be avoided.

Given the small but significant association between antidepressants and worsening or emergent spontaneous SAEs, all patients receiving these medications for suicidal and other symptomatology should be carefully monitored, particularly during the first weeks of treatment. The FDA recommended subjects can be seen every week for the first 4 weeks, and thereafter, biweekly. However, it is not always possible to schedule weekly face-to-face appointments. In that case, evaluations should be briefly carried out by phone. But it is important to emphasize that there are no data to suggest that the face-to-face monitoring schedule proposed by the FDA or telephone calls have any impact on the risk of suicide. Monitoring is important for all patients, but it should be more carefully done for patients who have history of suicidal ideation or suicide attempts or show behavior associated with increased risk for suicide (e.g., prior suicidality, impulsivity, substance abuse, history of sexual

Table 5–2. Dosages of antidepressants usually administered to youth with major depressive disorder

Medication group	Medication	Starting dosage (mg/day)	Dosage range (mg/day)
SSRIs	Citalopram	10	20–60
	Escitalopram	10	10–40
	Fluoxetine	10	20–60
	Fluvoxamine	25	50–150
	Paroxetine	10	20–60
	Sertraline	25	50–300
SNRIs	Venlafaxine XR	37.5	75–225
Others	Bupropion SR	100	150–300
	Bupropion XL	150	150–300

Note. SNRI=serotonin-norepinephrine reuptake inhibitor; SR=sustained release; SSRI=selective serotonin reuptake inhibitor; XL and XR=extended release.

abuse) (Gould et al. 1996; Shaffer and Craft 1999); for patients who have become agitated, disinhibited, or irritable while using an antidepressant; and for those with family history of bipolar disorder or suicide.

Treatment of Major Depressive Disorder Subtypes

Bipolar Depression

Many children and adolescents seeking treatment for depression are usually experiencing their first depressive episode. Because the symptoms of unipolar and bipolar depression are similar, it is difficult to decide whether a patient needs only an antidepressant or concomitant treatment with mood stabilizers. Some symptoms and signs of bipolar illness, such as psychosis or psychomotor retardation, or a family history of bipolar disorder may alert the clinician to the risk that the child could develop a manic episode.

There are no studies of youth with bipolar depression (Kowatch et al. 2005). In adults, RCTs have shown positive effects with lamotrigine, lithium carbonate, valproate, and, more recently, the atypical antipsychotics (either alone or in combination with mood stabilizers) ("Practice Guideline for the

Treatment of Patients With Bipolar Disorder" 1994). A recent meta-analysis (Gijsman et al. 2004) showed that SSRIs are beneficial for the treatment of bipolar depression in adults, and, with the exception of the TCAs, these medications did not induce significantly more manic switches than placebo. Moreover, one RCT found that monotherapy with fluoxetine was better than placebo for the management of depressed adult patients with bipolar II disorder and did not induce significant increase in manic switches (Amsterdam et al. 1998). Some studies have also suggested that bupropion is less likely to induce a mania or rapid cycling (Compton and Nemeroff 2000; "Practice Guideline" 1994). It is important to mention that children and adolescents do not always respond to medications in the same way as adults, and youth may be more prone to switch to mania with antidepressants. Therefore, these recommendations must be followed with caution until controlled studies of children and adolescents are available.

Psychotic Depression

There are no controlled studies of psychotic depression in youth. In adults, only 20%–40% respond to antidepressant monotherapy ("Practice Guideline" 2000). Thus, recommended treatment often consists of antidepressants combined with an antipsychotic. The antipsychotics are usually tapered after remission of the depression. The newer antipsychotic medications (e.g., risperidone, olanzapine) may prove useful as monotherapy for psychotic depression. Electroconvulsive therapy (ECT) is particularly effective for the psychotic subtype of depression in adults ("Practice Guideline" 2000) and may be useful for depressed teens as well (Ghaziuddin et al. 2004). Treatment with antidepressants in psychotic depressed children should be conducted with caution, because the presence of psychosis is a marker for possible development of bipolar disorder (Geller et al. 1994; Strober and Carlson 1982).

Seasonal Affective Disorder

Studies in adults have shown that SSRIs and bright-light therapy are beneficial for the treatment of subjects with recurrent seasonal affective disorder (SAD). One small RCT focusing on children and adolescents suggested that bright-light therapy is efficacious for the treatment of SAD (Swedo et al. 1997), but no studies with antidepressants have been conducted.

Treatment-Resistant Depression

As in adults ("Practice Guideline" 2000), approximately 20%–30% of youth with MDD have a partial (moderate response on the CGI-I; presence of significant symptoms of MDD, but the full syndrome is not present) or no response to treatment (Birmaher et al. 2000; Emslie et al. 2004; March et al. 2004). Patients with partial response have a significantly higher rate of relapse during the first 6 months following therapy and have significantly more psychosocial, occupational, and medical problems ("Practice Guideline" 2000). Moreover, among children, chronic depressions do not usually remit spontaneously and are not responsive to placebo ("Practice Guideline" 2000; "Practice Parameters" 1998), indicating the need for aggressive treatment of patients with these conditions.

The first step in the management of patients with treatment-resistant depression is to establish the nonresponse. Several definitions of nonresponse have been used, including the presence of a significant number of depressive symptoms, less that 50% improvement as measured by rating scales (e.g., the Children's Depression Rating Scale, Revised), and no change or worsening in the CGI. Once it has been established that the patient has not responded, it is crucial to try to find out why. The most common reasons for treatment failure are inappropriate diagnoses, inadequate drug dosage or length of drug trial, lack of compliance with treatment, comorbidity with other psychiatric disorders (e.g., dysthymia, anxiety, ADHD, covered substance abuse, personality disorders) or comorbid medical illnesses (e.g., hypothyroidism), presence of bipolar depression, and exposure to chronic or severe life events (e.g., abuse, chronic conflicts) that require different modalities of therapy (Brent et al. 1998; Hughes et al. 1999; "Practice Guideline" 2000).

There are very few pharmacological studies of children and adolescents with treatment-refractory depression. After noncompliance with treatment has been ruled out, the following strategies, based on the adult literature, have been recommended:

1. *Optimize initial treatments.* Although few studies have evaluated the efficacy of this strategy, initial treatment can be maximized by increasing the length of the trial or increasing the dose.

   a. *Extend the initial medication trial.* For patients with at least partial response after receiving a therapeutic dose of antidepressant for 6 weeks, the first and simplest strategy is to extend the treatment for another 2–4 weeks, if the patient's clinical and functional status allows ("Practice Guideline" 2000; Thase and Rush 1997).

b. *Increase the dose.* This strategy can be used for partial responders, but occasionally, increasing the dose in a patient with no response for another 2–3 weeks may help (Heiligenstein et al. 2006; "Practice Guideline" 2000).

2. *Switch strategies.* For patients who do not respond to a specific antidepressant medication or who do not tolerate its side effects, other antidepressants of the same class or different classes (e.g., venlafaxine for a patient treated with an SSRI) can be tried. The few adult studies published so far suggest that, because of the probable heterogeneity in depression mechanisms, it is more efficacious to switch antidepressant classes than to stay within the same class. Also, it has been suggested that severe depressions appear to respond better to antidepressants with both serotonergic and adrenergic properties (e.g., venlafaxine; Poirier and Boyer 1999). MAOIs have been found beneficial for patients who have not responded to other medications ("Practice Guideline" 2000; Thase and Rush 1997). An open study suggested that adolescents with depression who had not responded to TCAs responded to MAOIs (Ryan et al. 1988b). However, it is possible that these adolescents did not respond to TCAs because this group of medications is not efficacious for the treatment of pediatric MDD (Birmaher et al. 1996b).

3. *Augmentation or combination strategies.* The most common augmentation or combination strategies include adding lithium carbonate at therapeutic levels for a period of 4 weeks, or L-triiodothyronine (T_3) (25–50 µg/day), or stimulants, or combining an SSRI with a TCA (Bauer et al. 2000; "Practice Guideline" 2000). In adults, the combination of lithium and antidepressants has yielded response rates of 50%–65% in studies that administered lithium at therapeutic levels for at least 4 weeks (e.g., see "Practice Guideline" 2000; Thase and Rush 1997). The interval before response to the augmentation with lithium has been reported to be from several days to 3 weeks ("Practice Guideline" 2000). After this period, the chance to observe improvement with lithium decreases.

In adolescents with MDD, an open study showed significant improvement of refractory depressive symptoms after augmentation of TCA treatment with lithium (Ryan et al. 1988a). On the other hand, another open-label study did not replicate this finding (Strober et al. 1992).

Case reports have suggested that adding stimulant medications or combining an SSRI and a TCA or bupropion may also be effective ("Practice Guideline" 2000), but these combinations need to be used with caution because of the possibility of interactions (as with, e.g., SSRIs and TCAs). In adolescents and adults, the combination of antidepressants and psychotherapy (CBT, IPT) for patients with severe or treatment-resistant depression has also been found useful (Keller et al. 2000; March et al. 2004).

4. *Electroconvulsive therapy.* ECT is one of the most efficacious treatments for adults with nonresistant (70% response) and resistant MDD (50% response) (Ghaziuddin et al. 2004; "Practice Guideline" 2000). However, because of the invasiveness of this treatment, it remains the treatment of choice only for the most severe, incapacitating forms of resistant depression. No controlled studies have been conducted in adolescents, but anecdotal reports suggest that adolescents with refractory depression may respond to ECT without significant side effects (Ghaziuddin et al. 2004; Rey and Walter 1997). Approximately 60% of adult patients treated successfully with ECT tend to relapse after 6 months ("Practice Guideline" 2000). Therefore, they also have to receive maintenance treatment with antidepressants and sometimes maintenance ECT. However, maintenance ECT has never been reported in adolescents.

5. *Other biological treatments.* Other innovative treatments, such as intravenous clomipramine, transcranial magnetic stimulation (TMS), and, more recently, vagal nerve stimulation (VNS) have been used for the treatment of depressed adults who have not responded to standard treatment. In adolescents, intravenous clomipramine has been shown to be efficacious for patients who have failed to respond to other antidepressant treatment (Sallee et al. 1997). No studies using TMS or VNS have been conducted in depressed youth.

All of these strategies require implementation in a systematic fashion (for reviews, see "Practice Guideline" 2000; "Practice Parameters" 1998; Thase and Rush 1997).

Psychoeducation for the patient and family is also required in order to avoid the development of hopelessness both in the patient and family and in the clinician. Comparing these strategies with other treatments of medical disorders can be useful to help patients and their families understand the medication plan and to improve compliance with and tolerance of treatment. The example of hypertension is appropriate: diuretics may be used alone, or combined with other antihypertensives in different trials, according to response.

Treatment of Comorbid Conditions and Suicidality

Comorbid disorders may influence the onset, maintenance, and recurrence of depression (Birmaher et al. 1996a, 1996b). Therefore, in addition to treating the depressive symptoms, it is of prime importance to treat the comorbid conditions that frequently accompany the depressive disorders (Hughes et al. 1999).

For example, depressed adolescents with comorbid ADHD respond less well to treatment (Emslie et al. 1997; J.D. Hamilton and Bridge 1999). For these patients, it has been suggested that the ADHD be treated first. If, after stabilization of the ADHD the depressive symptoms continue, an SSRI should be added (Hughes et al. 1999; Pliszka 2000); but this strategy has not been validated. An open study using bupropion suggested that this medication can be efficacious to treat both MDD and ADHD (Daviss et al. 2001), although its effect on ADHD is not as impressive as that obtained by treatment with stimulants (Conners et al. 1996).

Treatment of comorbid anxiety, which most often precedes depression, is essential, insofar as it contributes to improvement, and because the anxiety, if left untreated, may predispose to future depressive episodes (Hayward et al. 2000; Kovacs et al. 1989). Fortunately, similar pharmacotherapy and psychotherapy treatments found useful for the treatment of MDD have also been found beneficial for the treatment of youth with anxiety disorders (Birmaher et al. 2003; "Fluvoxamine for Anxiety in Children" 2001; Kendall 1994).

Other comorbid conditions, such as OCD, conduct disorder, eating disorders, and posttraumatic stress disorder, have also been found to affect treatment response; these conditions must be addressed for the successful treatment of depressed youth (Birmaher et al. 1996a; Brent et al. 1998; Goodyer et al. 1997).

Suicidal ideation and behavior are common symptoms accompanying major depression and are more likely to occur in the face of comorbid disruptive disorders, substance abuse, physical or sexual abuse, impulsive behaviors, prior suicide attempts, and family history of suicidal behavior (e.g., Gould et al. 1996). Assessment of suicidality, securing of any lethal agents (e.g., medications, firearms), and development of no-suicide contracts with the patient and family are essential components of the management of the suicidal, depressed patient. Patients who cannot agree to a no-suicide contract may require inpatient hospitalization. Treatment of the underlying depression may be necessary but not sufficient to prevent recurrent attempts. Placebo-controlled medication trials in adults show that greater improvement in depression is associated with medication, but equal rates of attempts and completions are cited in medication plus placebo conditions (Khan et al. 2000). Other contributors to suicidality, such as sexual abuse, drug and alcohol use, ADHD, conduct problems, impulsivity and aggression, personality disorders, and family discord, must be assessed and targeted (Brent et al. 1999).

Continuation Therapy

Naturalistic longitudinal studies have shown that the rate of MDD relapse is very high (Birmaher et al. 2002). An RCT fluoxetine discontinuation study showed that continued treatment with fluoxetine was associated with much lower rate of relapse compared with treatment with placebo (Emslie et al. 2004). Similar results have been reported in adults with MDD ("Practice Guideline" 2000). Thus, until further research results are available, to consolidate the response and prevent relapse of symptoms, *all patients* should be offered continuation treatment for 6–12 months after complete symptoms remission. During this phase, patients should be seen biweekly or monthly depending on the patient's clinical status, functioning, support systems, environmental stressors, motivation for treatment, and the existence of other psychiatric/medical disorders. The patient and his/her family should be taught to recognize early signs of relapse.

During the continuation phase, antidepressants must be maintained at the same dose used to attain remission of acute symptoms, provided that there are no significant side effects or dose-related negative effects on the patient's compliance ("Practice Guideline" 2000). At the end of the continuation phase, if a decision is made to discontinue the antidepressant, the medication should be tapered gradually (e.g., over a period of 6 weeks) in order to avoid withdrawal effects (e.g., sleep disturbance, irritability, or gastrointestinal symptoms) that may lead the clinician to misinterpret the need for continued medication treatment. In addition, clinical practice has suggested that rapid discontinuation of antidepressants may precipitate a relapse/recurrence of depression. It is recommended that treatment discontinuation occur while children and adolescents are on extended vacation, rather than during the school year.

If relapse occurs, it should first be determined whether the patient has been compliant. If the patient has not been compliant, resumption of the antidepressant medication should occur. If the patient has been compliant and had been previously responding to the medication (without significant side effects), the clinician should consider the presence of ongoing stressors (e.g., conflict, abuse), comorbid psychiatric disorders (anxiety disorders, ADHD inattentive or combined, substance abuse, dysthymia, bipolar II disorder, eating disorder), and medical illnesses.

In this case, and depending on the circumstances, an increase in the medication dose, change to other medication, augmentation strategies, or psychotherapy may be indicated. For patients receiving only psychotherapy, the clinician should consider adding medications and/or utilizing new psychotherapeutic strategies.

Maintenance Therapy

After the patient has been asymptomatic for a period of approximately 6–12 months (continuation phase), the clinician has to decide *whether* the patient should receive maintenance therapy, *which* therapy to use, and for *how long*.

The main goal of the maintenance phase is to prevent recurrences. This phase may last from 1 year to much longer and is typically conducted at a visit frequency of every 1–3 months depending on the patient's clinical status, functioning, support systems, environmental stressors, motivation for treatment, and the existence of other psychiatric/medical disorders.

Who Should Receive Maintenance Therapy?

The recommendation for maintenance therapy depends on several factors, such as severity of the initial depressive episode (e.g., suicidality, psychosis, functional impairment), number and severity of prior depressive episodes, chronicity, comorbid disorders, family psychopathology, presence of support, patient and family willingness to adhere to the treatment program, and contraindications to treatment.

Factors associated with increased risk for recurrence in naturalistic studies of depressed children and adolescents may serve as a guide for the clinician in deciding who needs maintenance treatment. These factors include history of prior depressive episodes, female sex, late onset, suicidality, double depression, subsyndromal symptoms, poor functioning, personality disorders, exposure to negative events (e.g., abuse, conflicts), and family history of recurrence (≥ 2 MDD) (Birmaher et al. 1996a, 1996b; Goodyer et al. 1998; Klein et al. 2001; Lewinsohn et al. 1999; Rao et al. 1999; Rueter et al. 1999; Weissman et al. 1999a, 1999b).

There are no maintenance studies on depressed children and adolescents. In depressed adults, patients who have only a single uncomplicated episode of depression, mild episodes, or lengthy intervals between episodes (e.g., 5 years) probably should not start maintenance treatment ("Practice Guideline" 2000). There is also a consensus in adults that patients with three or more depressive episodes (especially if they occur in a short period of time and have deleterious consequences) and chronic depressions should have maintenance treatment.

There is controversy about whether to treat patients with two previous episodes using maintenance treatment. Overall, maintenance treatment has been recommended for adult depressed patients who have had two depressive episodes and who meet one or more of the following criteria (Depression Guideline Panel 1993): 1) a family history of bipolar disorder or recurrent depression; 2) early age at onset of the first depressive episode (before age 20); and 3) both episodes were severe or life threatening and occurred during the past 3 years. Given that depression in youth has similar clinical presentation, sequela, and natural course as in adults, the previously noted guidelines should probably be applied for youth who have experienced two previous major depressive episodes.

Which Treatment Should Be Used?

Practically, unless there is any contraindication (e.g., medication side effects), the treatment that was efficacious in the induction of remission of the acute episode should be used for maintenance therapy. However, patients who are maintained only with medications should be offered psychotherapy to help them cope with the psychosocial scars induced by the depression. Furthermore, many depressed youth live in environments charged with stressful situations, and their parents usually have psychiatric disorders, emphasizing the need for multimodal treatments.

In selecting medication for maintenance therapy, the clinician should consider the side-effect profile and the way the side effects may affect the patient's compliance. For example, dry mouth, weight gain, increased sweating, sexual dysfunction, and polyuria (if patient is taking lithium) may be very troublesome and may induce discontinuation of treatment. In addition, in children and adolescents, the long-term consequences of using antidepressant medications (e.g., chronic inhibition of the serotonin reuptake by the SSRI) are not known.

Other factors, such as a patient's embarrassment with friends, uneasiness about the idea of having his or her mind "controlled by a medication," view of treatment with medications as a sign of "weakness," and uncertainty about the risk of relapse in spite of doing well while taking medications, should all be addressed with both patient and parents.

How Long Should the Maintenance Phase Last?

It is recommended that adult patients with second episodes, who fulfill the criteria for maintenance therapy noted above, should be maintained for several years (up to 5 years in adult studies) with the same dose of antidepressant used to achieve clinical remission during the acute treatment phase. However, patients with three or more episodes and patients with second episodes associated with psychosis, severe impairment, and severe suicidality who proved very difficult to treat should be considered for treatment for longer periods of time or even lifelong treatment ("Practice Parameters" 1998).

TCAs, SSRIs, and lithium have been found to be efficacious for the prevention of depressive recurrences in adults ("Practice Guideline" 2000). However, given the apparent lack of efficacy of TCAs in youth, and the advantages of SSRIs and their efficacy in the acute treatment of MDD, the SSRIs are considered first-line medications in maintenance therapy. Antidepressant medication, unless it is not tolerated, should be continued at the full dose used to exert the initial therapeutic effect.

For most children and adolescents, multimodal therapies are recommended. However, if antidepressant medications are used alone, psychosocial maintenance strategies should be implemented to help the patient's inner and interpersonal conflicts, improve coping and social skills, deal with the psychosocial and personal scars left by the depression, and improve academic and social functioning. The reduction of family stress, promotion of a supportive environment, and effective treatment of parents and siblings with psychiatric disorders may also help diminish the risk for recurrence.

Clinical Pearls

- The treatment of major depressive disorder includes three phases: acute, continuation, and maintenance.
- The goal of treatment is to achieve remission and good psychosocial functioning.
- During all phases of treatment, depressed youth and their families should be offered education and support. Some mildly depressed youth may respond well to short management with education and support.
- Depending on the severity and chronicity of the depression and other factors, treatment during the acute phase should include antidepressants and/or psychotherapy. So far, there is evidence that cognitive-behavioral therapy and interpersonal psychotherapy, and among the antidepressants the SSRIs (and in particular fluoxetine), are efficacious for the treatment of depressed youth. These medications may induce side effects, and 1 in 100 children and adolescents treated with these medications may show onset or worsening of suicidal ideation and, more rarely, suicide attempts.
- After successful acute treatment, all youth should be offered continuation treatment with SSRIs and/or psychotherapy for 6–12 months to prevent relapses.

- After the continuation phase, some depressed youth, especially those with severe depressions or frequent recurrences, should have maintenance treatment with SSRIs and/or psychotherapy for at least 1 year or more to prevent recurrences.

- Treatment of subtypes of depression, including seasonal, psychotic, and bipolar depression, may require special treatments such as light therapy, antipsychotics, and mood stabilizers, respectively.

- Management of comorbid disorders, ongoing conflicts, and family psychopathology is necessary to achieve remission.

- Management of resistant depressions should take into account factors associated with poor response to treatment, such as poor adherence to treatment, misdiagnoses, ongoing negative life events, and presence of comorbid disorders.

References

Alderman J, Wolkow R, Chung M, et al: Sertraline treatment of children and adolescents with obsessive-compulsive disorder or depression: pharmacokinetics, tolerability, and efficacy. J Am Acad Child Adolesc Psychiatry 37:386–394, 1998

American Psychiatric Association: Diagnostic and Statistical Manual of Mental Disorders, 4th Edition. Washington, DC, American Psychiatric Association, 1994

Amsterdam JD, Garcia-Espana F, Fawcett J, et al: Efficacy and safety of fluoxetine in treating bipolar II major depressive episode. J Clin Psychopharmacol 18:435–440, 1998

Apter A, Lipschitz A, Fong R, et al: Evaluation of suicidal thoughts and behaviors in children and adolescents taking paroxetine. J Child Adolesc Psychopharmacol 16:77–90, 2006

Axelson D, Perel, J, Rudolph G, et al: Sertraline pediatric/adolescent PK-PD parameters: dose/plasma level ranging for depression (abstract). Clin Pharmacol Ther 67:169, 2000a

Axelson D, Perel J, Rudolph G, et al: Significant differences in pharmacokinetics/dynamics of citalopram between adolescents and adults: implications for clinical dosing (abstract). Proceedings of the 39th Annual Meeting of the American College of Neuropsychopharmacology, San Juan, Puerto Rico, 2000b

Bauer M, Bschor T, Kunz D, et al: Double-blind, placebo-controlled trial of the use of lithium to augment antidepressant medication in continuation treatment of unipolar major depression. Am J Psychiatry 157:1429–1435, 2000

Beck AT: Depression: Clinical, Experimental and Theoretical Aspects. New York, Harper & Row, 1967

Birmaher B, Ryan ND, Williamson D, et al: Childhood and adolescent depression: a review of the past 10 years, part I. J Am Acad Child Adolesc Psychiatry 35:1427–1439, 1996a

Birmaher B, Ryan ND, Williamson DE, et al: Childhood and adolescent depression: a review of the past 10 years, part II. J Am Acad Child Adolesc Psychiatry 35:1575–1583, 1996b

Birmaher B, Brent DA, Kolko D, et al: Clinical outcome after short-term psychotherapy for adolescents with major depressive disorder. Arch Gen Psychiatry 57:29–36, 2000

Birmaher B, Arbelaez C, Brent D: Course and outcome of child and adolescent major depressive disorder. Child Adolesc Psychiatr Clin N Am 11:619–637, 2002

Birmaher B, Axelson DA, Monk K, et al: Fluoxetine for the treatment of childhood anxiety disorders. J Am Acad Child Adolesc Psychiatry 42:415–423, 2003

Boyer EW, Shannon M: The serotonin syndrome. N Engl J Med 352:1112–1120, 2005

Brent DA: Antidepressants and pediatric depression: the risk of doing nothing. N Engl J Med 351:1598–601, 2004

Brent DA, Poling K, McCain B, et al: A psychoeducational program for families of affectively ill children and adolescents. J Am Acad Child Adolesc Psychiatry 32:770–774, 1993

Brent DA, Holder D, Birmaher B, et al: A clinical psychotherapy trial for adolescent depression comparing cognitive, family, and supportive therapy. Arch Gen Psychiatry 54:877–885, 1997

Brent DA, Kolko D, Birmaher B, et al: Predictors of treatment efficacy in a clinical trial of three psychosocial treatments for adolescent depression. J Am Acad Child Adolesc Psychiatry 37:906–914, 1998

Brent DA, Kolko D, Birmaher, et al: A clinical trial for adolescent depression: predictors of additional treatment in the acute and follow-up phases of the trial. J Am Acad Child Adolesc Psychiatry 38:263–270, 1999

Bridge JA, Iyengar S, Salary CB, et al: Clinical response and risk for reported suicidal ideation and suicide attempts in pediatric antidepressant treatment: a meta-analysis of randomized controlled trials. JAMA 297:1683-1696, 2007

Cheung AH, Emslie GJ, Mayes TL: Review of the efficacy and safety of antidepressants in youth depression. J Child Psychol Psychiatry 46:735–754, 2005

Clarke G, Debar L, Lynch F, et al: A randomized effectiveness trial of brief cognitive-behavioral therapy for depressed adolescents receiving antidepressant medication. J Am Acad Child Adolesc Psychiatry 44:888–898, 2005

Clein PD, Riddle MA: Pharmacokinetics in children and adolescents. Child Adolesc Psychiatr Clin N Am 4:59–75, 1995

Compton MT, Nemeroff CB: The treatment of bipolar depression. J Clin Psychiatry 61:57–67, 2000

Conners CK, Casat CD, Gualtieri CT, et al: Bupropion hydrochloride in attention deficit disorder with hyperactivity. J Am Acad Child Adolesc Psychiatry 35:1314–1321, 1996

Daviss WB, Bentivogli P, Racusin R, et al: Bupropion sustained release in adolescents with comorbid attention deficit hyperactivity. J Am Acad Child Adolesc Psychiatry 40:307–314, 2001

Daviss WB, Perel JM, Rudolph GR, et al: Steady-state pharmacokinetics of bupropion SR in juvenile patients. J Am Acad Child Adolesc Psychiatry 44:349–357, 2005

Depression Guideline Panel: Depression in Primary Care, Vol 2: Treatment of Major Depression (Clinical Practice Guideline No 5). AHCPR Publication No 93-0551. Rockville, MD, U.S. Department of Health and Human Services, Public Health Service, Agency for Health Care Policy and Research, April 1993

Emslie GJ, Rush AJ, Weinberg WA, et al: A double-blind, randomized, placebo-controlled trial of fluoxetine in children and adolescents with depression. Arch Gen Psychiatry 54:1031–1037, 1997

Emslie GJ, Walkup JT, Pliszka SR, et al: Nontricyclic antidepressants: current trends in children and adolescents. J Am Acad Child Adolesc Psychiatry 38:517–528, 1999

Emslie GJ, Heiligenstein JH, Wagner KD, et al: Fluoxetine for acute treatment of depression in children and adolescents: a placebo-controlled, randomized clinical trial. J Am Acad Child Adolesc Psychiatry 41:1205–1215, 2002

Emslie GJ, Heiligenstein JH, Hoog SL, et al: Fluoxetine treatment for prevention of relapse of depression in children and adolescents: a double-blind, placebo-controlled study. J Am Acad Child Adolesc Psychiatry 43:1397–1405, 2004

Findling RL, Reed MD, Myers C, et al: Paroxetine pharmacokinetics in depressed children and adolescents. J Am Acad Child Adolesc Psychiatry 38:952–959, 1999

Findling RL, Preskorn SH, Marcus RN, et al: Nefazodone pharmacokinetics in depressed children and adolescents. J Am Acad Child Adolesc Psychiatry 39:1008–1016, 2000

Findling RL, McNamara NK, Stansbrey RJ, et al: The relevance of pharmacokinetic studies in designing efficacy trials in juvenile major depression. J Child Adolesc Psychopharmacol 16:131–145, 2006

Fluvoxamine for the treatment of anxiety disorders in children and adolescents. Research Unit on Pediatric Psychopharmacology Anxiety Group. N Engl J Med 344:1279–1285, 2001

Geller B, Fox LW, Clark KA: Rate and predictors of prepubertal bipolarity during follow-up of 6- to 12-year-old depressed children. J Am Acad Child Adolesc Psychiatry 33:461–468, 1994

Ghaziuddin N, Kutcher SP, Knapp P, et al; Work Group on Quality Issues; AACAP: Practice parameter for use of electroconvulsive therapy with adolescents. J Am Acad Child Adolesc Psychiatry 43:1521–1539, 2004

Gibbons RD, Hur K, Bhaumik DK, et al: The relationship between antidepressant medication use and rate of suicide. Arch Gen Psychiatry 62:165–172, 2005

Gijsman HJ, Geddes JR, Rendell JM, et al: Antidepressants for bipolar depression: a systematic review of randomized, controlled trials. Am J Psychiatry 161:1537–1547, 2004

Goodyer IM, Herbert J, Secher SM, et al: Short-term outcome of major depression, I: comorbidity and severity at presentation as predictors of persistent disorder. J Am Acad Child Adolesc Psychiatry 36:179–187, 1997

Goodyer IM, Herbert J, Altham PM: Adrenal, steroid secretion and major depression in 8- to 16-year-olds, III: influence of cortisol/DHEA ratio at presentation on subsequent rates of disappointing life events and persistent major depression. Psychol Med 28:265–273, 1998

Goodyer IM, Dubicka B, Wilkinson P, et al: Selective serotonin reuptake inhibitors (SSRIs) and routine specialist care with and without cognitive behaviour therapy in adolescents with major depression: randomised controlled trial. BMJ 335 (7611):142, 2007

Gould MS, Fisher P, Parides M, et al: Psychosocial risk factors of child and adolescent completed suicide. Arch Gen Psychiatry 53:1155–1162, 1996

Guy W: Clinical Global Impressions, in ECDEU Assessment Manual for Psychopharmacology, Revised (NIMH Publ No 76-338). Rockville, MD, National Institute of Mental Health, 1976, pp 218–222

Hamilton JD, Bridge J: Outcome at 6 months of 50 adolescents with major depression treated in a health maintenance organization. J Am Acad Child Adolesc Psychiatry 38:1340–1346, 1999

Hamilton M: A rating scale for depression. J Neurol Neurosurg Psychiatry 23:56–61, 1960

Hammad TA: Review and Evaluation of Clinical Data: Relationship Between Psychotropic Drugs and Pediatric Suicidality. Rockville, MD, U.S. Food and Drug Administration, 2004. Available online at http://www.fda.gov/ohrms/dockets/ac/04/briefing/2004-4065b1-10-TAB08-Hammads-Review.pdf, 2004.

Hammad TA, Laughren T, Racoosin J: Suicidality in pediatric patients treated with antidepressant drugs. Arch Gen Psychiatry 63:332–333, 2006

Hayward C, Killen JD, Kraemer HC, et al: Predictors of panic attacks in adolescents. J Am Acad Child Adolesc Psychiatry 39:207–214, 2000

Hazell P, O'Connell D, Heathcote D, et al: Tricyclic drugs for depression in children and adolescents. Cochrane Database of Systematic Reviews, Issue 2. Art No: CD002317. DOI: 10.1002/14651858.CD002317, 2006

Heiligenstein JH, Hoog SL, Wagner KD, et al: Fluoxetine 40–60 mg versus fluoxetine 20 mg in the treatment of children and adolescents with a less-than-complete response to nine-week treatment with fluoxetine 10–20 mg: a pilot study. J Child Adolesc Psychopharmacol 16:207–217, 2006

Hughes CW, Emslie GJ, Crismon ML, et al: The Texas Childhood Medication Algorithm Project: update from the Texas Consensus Conference Panel on Medication Treatment of Childhood Major Depressive Disorder. J Am Acad Child Adolesc Psychiatry 38:1442–1454, 1999

Keller MB, McCullough JP, Klein DN, et al: A comparison of nefazodone, the cognitive behavioral-analysis system of psychotherapy, and their combination for the treatment of chronic depression. N Engl J Med 342:1462–1470, 2000

Kendall PC: Treating anxiety disorders in children: results of a randomized clinical trial. J Consult Clin Psychol 62:100–110, 1994

Khan A, Warner HA, Brown WA: Symptom reduction and suicide risk in patients treated with placebo in antidepressant clinical trials: an analysis of the Food and Drug Administration database. Arch Gen Psychiatry 57:311–317, 2000

Klein DN, Lewinsohn PM, Seeley JR, et al: A family study of major depressive disorder in a community sample of adolescents. Arch Gen Psychiatry 58:13–20, 2001

Kovacs M, Goldston D: Cognitive and social cognitive development of depressed children and adolescents. J Am Acad Child Adolesc Psychiatry 30:388–392, 1991

Kovacs M, Gatsonis C, Paulauskas SL, et al: Depressive disorders in childhood, IV: a longitudinal study of comorbidity with and risk for anxiety disorders. Arch Gen Psychiatry 46:776–782, 1989

Kowatch RA, Fristad MA, Birmaher B, et al: Treatment guidelines for children and adolescents with bipolar disorder. J Am Acad Child Adoles Psychiatry 44:213–235, 2005

Lake MB, Birmaher B, Wassick S, et al: Bleeding and selective serotonin reuptake inhibitors in childhood and adolescence. J Child Adolesc Psychopharmacol 10:35–38, 2000

Leonard HL, March J, Rickler KC, et al: Pharmacology of the selective serotonin reuptake inhibitors in children and adolescents. J Am Acad Child Adolesc Psychiatry 36:725–736, 1997

Lewinsohn PM, Allen NB, Seeley JR, et al: First onset versus recurrence of depression: differential processes of psychosocial risk. J Abnorm Psychol 108:483–489, 1999

Mandoki MW, Tapia MR, Tapia MA, et al: Venlafaxine in the treatment of children and adolescents with major depression. Psychopharmacol Bull 33:149–154, 1997

Mann JJ, Emslie G, Baldessarini RJ, et al: ACNP Task Force report on SSRIs and suicidal behavior in youth. Neuropsychopharmacology 31:473–492, 2006

March J, Silva S, Petrycki S, et al: Fluoxetine, cognitive-behavioral therapy, and their combination for adolescents with depression: Treatment for Adolescents With Depression Study (TADS) randomized controlled trial. JAMA 292:807–820, 2004

Martin A, Young C, Leckman JF, et al: Age effects on antidepressant-induced manic conversion. Arch Pediatr Adolesc Med 158:773–780, 2004

Mufson L, Dorta KP, Wickramaratne P, et al: A randomized effectiveness trial of interpersonal psychotherapy for depressed adolescents. Arch Gen Psychiatry 61:577–584, 2004

Olfson M, Shaffer D, Marcus SC, et al: Relationship between antidepressant medication treatment and suicide in adolescents. Arch Gen Psychiatry 60:978–982, 2003

Pine DS, Cohen P, Gurley D, et al: The risk for early adulthood anxiety and depressive disorders in adolescents with anxiety and depressive disorders. Arch Gen Psychiatry 55:56–64, 1998

Pliszka S: Patterns of psychiatric comorbidity with attention-deficit hyperactivity disorder. Child Adolesc Psychiatr Clin N Am 9:525–540, 2000

Poirier MF, Boyer P: Venlafaxine and paroxetine in treatment-resistant depression: double blind, randomized comparison. Br J Psychiatry 175:12–16, 1999

Poznanski EO, Freeman LN, Mokros HB: Children's Depression Rating Scale–Revised. Psychopharmacol Bull 21:979–989, 1984

Practice guideline for the treatment of patients with bipolar disorder. American Psychiatric Association. Am J Psychiatry 151 (12, suppl):1–36, 1994

Practice guideline for the treatment of patients with major depressive disorder (revision). American Psychiatric Association. Am J Psychiatry 157 (4, suppl):1–45, 2000

Practice parameters for the assessment and treatment of children and adolescents with depressive disorder. J Am Acad Child Adolesc Psychiatry 37(suppl):63S–83S, 1998

Puig-Antich J, Lukens E, Davies M, et al: Psychosocial functioning in prepubertal depressive disorders, II: interpersonal relationships after sustained recovery from the affective episode. Arch Gen Psychiatry 42:511–517, 1985

Rao U, Dahl RE, Ryan ND, et al: Unipolar depression in adolescents: clinical outcome in adulthood. J Am Acad Child Adolesc Psychiatry 34:566–578, 1995

Rao U, Hammen C, Daley SE: Continuity of depression during the transition to adulthood: a 5-year longitudinal study of young women. J Am Acad Child Adolesc Psychiatry 38:908–915, 1999

Renaud J, Brent D, Baugher MA, et al: Rapid response to psychosocial treatment for adolescent depression: a 2-year follow-up. J Am Acad Child Adolesc Psychiatry 37:1184–1190, 1998

Rey JM, Walter G: Half a century of ECT use in young people. Am J Psychiatry 154:595–602, 1997

Rueter MA, Scaramella L, Wallace LE, et al: First onset of depressive or anxiety disorders predicted by the longitudinal course of internalizing symptoms and parent–adolescent disagreements. Arch Gen Psychiatry 56:726–732, 1999

Ryan N, Meyer V, Dachille S, et al: Lithium antidepressant augmentation in TCA-refractory depression in adolescents. J Am Acad Child Adolesc Psychiatry 27:371–376, 1988a

Ryan N, Puig-Antich J, Rabinovich H, et al: MAOIs in adolescent major depression unresponsive to tricyclic antidepressant. J Am Acad Child Adolesc Psychiatry 27:755–758, 1988b

Safer DJ, Zito JM: Treatment-emergent adverse events from selective serotonin reuptake inhibitors by age group: children versus adolescents. J Child Adolesc Psychopharmacol 16:159–169, 2006

Sallee FR, Vrindavanam NS, Deas-Nesmith D, et al: Pulse intravenous clomipramine for depressed adolescents: a double-blind, controlled trial. Am J Psychiatry 154:668–673, 1997

Shaffer D, Craft L: Methods of adolescent suicide prevention. J Clin Psychiatry 60(suppl):70–74, discussion 75–76, 113–116, 1999

Shaffer D, Gould MS, Brasic J, et al: A Children's Global Assessment Scale (CGAS). Arch Gen Psychiatry 40:1228–1231, 1983

Simon GE, Savarino J, Operskalski B, et al: Suicide risk during antidepressant treatment. Am J Psychiatry 163:41–47, 2006

Stein D, Williamson DE, Birmaher B, et al: Parent–child bonding and family functioning in depressed children and children at high-risk and low risk for future depression. J Am Acad Child Adolesc Psychiatry 39:1220–1226, 2000

Strober M, Carlson G: Bipolar illness in adolescents with major depression: clinical, genetic, and psychopharmacologic predictors in a three-to four-year prospective follow-up investigation. Arch Gen Psychiatry 39:549–555, 1982

Strober M, Freeman R, Rigali J, et al: The pharmacotherapy of depressive illness in adolescence, II: effects of lithium augmentation in nonresponders to imipramine. J Am Acad Child Adolesc Psychiatry 31:16–20, 1992

Strober M, Lampert C, Schmidt S, et al: The course of major depressive disorder in adolescents, I: recovery and risk of manic switching in a follow-up of psychotic and nonpsychotic subtypes. J Am Acad Child Adolesc Psychiatry 32:34–42, 1993

Swedo S, Allen AJ, Glod CA, et al: A controlled trial of light therapy for the treatment of pediatric seasonal affective disorder. J Am Acad Child Adolesc Psychiatry 36:816–821, 1997

Thase ME, Rush AJ: When at first you don't succeed: sequential strategies for antidepressant nonresponders. J Clin Psychiatry 58:23–29, 1997

Valuck RJ, Libby AM, Sills MR, et al: Antidepressant treatment and risk of suicide attempt by adolescents with major depressive disorder: a propensity-adjusted retrospective cohort study. CNS Drugs 18:1119–1132, 2004

Wagner KD, Robb AS, Findling RL, et al: A randomized, placebo-controlled trial of citalopram for the treatment of major depression in children and adolescents. Am J Psychiatry 161:1079–1083, 2004

Weissman MM, Gammon GD, John K, et al: Children of depressed parents: increased psychopathology and early onset of major depression. Arch Gen Psychiatry 44:847–853, 1987

Weissman MM, Wolk S, Goldstein RB, et al: Depressed adolescents grown up. JAMA 281–1707–1713, 1999a

Weissman MM, Wolk S, Wickramaratne PJ, et al: Children with prepubertal-onset major depressive disorder and anxiety grown up. Arch Gen Psychiatry 56:794–801, 1999b

Wilens TE, Wyatt D, Spencer TJ: Disentangling disinhibition. J Am Acad Child Adolesc Psychiatry 37:1225–1227, 1998

6

Bipolar Disorders

Kevin W. Kuich, M.D.
Robert L. Findling, M.D.

Research over the past 10 years has helped better define the phenomenology and course of bipolar disorder in children and adolescents. Pediatric bipolar disorder has been shown to have a chronic course with little interepisode recovery that can lead to substantive psychosocial dysfunction (Biederman et al. 2004; Findling 2001; Geller et al. 2004). For these reasons, effective treatments are needed for youth suffering from bipolar illness. The purpose of this chapter is to present a rational, practical, and commonsense approach to the pharmacotherapeutic management of bipolar disorder in children and adolescents.

When thinking about the pharmacotherapy of pediatric bipolar disorder, one should begin by considering which agent, or agents, might be prescribed. The question of initiating treatment with either monotherapy or combination therapy often depends on symptom presentation and a careful, meticulous review of past medication response. Strong consideration should be given to restarting agents that have been helpful in the past. Similarly, agents that have been problematic or ineffective during prior therapeutic trials should generally be avoided.

Many medications used to treat bipolar illness may be associated with substantial risks, have a narrow therapeutic index, and/or require monitoring of drug levels and other laboratory parameters. For this reason, a careful review with both the patient and caregivers about medication treatment options, as well as a thoughtful consideration of anticipated barriers to medication or monitoring adherence, must be considered. Possible adherence barriers can include medication cost, lack of nearby laboratory facilities, and social factors that may interfere with adherence to the regular administration of medications.

Recently, pharmacotherapy guidelines for treating pediatric bipolar disorder have been published (Kowatch et al. 2005). The authors of these guidelines based their recommendations on the available scientific literature and current clinical practice. The guidelines also provide useful algorithms that may assist in medication selection. Briefly, use of lithium, an anticonvulsant, or an atypical antipsychotic as monotherapy is suggested in the initial treatment of manic or mixed bipolar presentations in outpatients without psychosis. It is recommended that partial response to monotherapy with a given agent may be addressed by adding another drug from a different class of compounds to the preexisting pharmacological regimen. It is also suggested that a rational approach to patients who do not respond at all to a given agent might be to treat the youth with a medication from a different drug class.

In this chapter, we review individual medications that have been studied in the treatment of pediatric bipolar illness and summarize the extant evidence for combination pharmacotherapy.

Lithium

Lithium has been widely used in the acute treatment of mania in adults. In addition, research has demonstrated that lithium also has efficacy as a maintenance therapy for bipolar disorder in adults. There is also evidence that lithium may be helpful in treating the depressed phase of bipolar illness.

At present, lithium is the only medication that is approved by the U.S. Food and Drug Administration (FDA) for use in treating bipolar disorder in teenagers. However, this indication had been given based on the results of adult research. Definitive studies of lithium in the acute and maintenance treatment of pediatric mania have not been performed. However, in 2006, the Collaborative Lithium Trials group began the definitive testing of lithium in juvenile mania under the auspices of a National Institute of Child Health and Human Development contract.

Supporting Studies in Youth

Although much of the published literature on lithium consists of case reports and studies lacking methodological rigor, more recent prospective studies have provided evidence to suggest that lithium is both effective and reasonably well-tolerated in the treatment of pediatric bipolar disorder. In an open-label monotherapy study, Kowatch et al. (2000) described lithium as being effective in the short-term treatment of pediatric mania. In a short-term, double-blind trial, Geller et al. (1998) found lithium helpful in reducing substance abuse and improving global functioning in a dually diagnosed adolescent population. Yet another prospective trial found lithium combined with divalproex was effective and tolerated in treating severe manic symptoms (Findling et al. 2003). Other studies that have found lithium to be useful involved treatment of young patients with both lithium and antipsychotics (Kafantaris 2003; Pavuluri et al. 2004). As for maintenance studies, one 18-month study evaluating the effectiveness of lithium monotherapy in pediatric bipolar disorder found it to be as useful as divalproex monotherapy (Findling et al. 2005).

In summary, although lithium can be a complicated medication to use, there exists good evidence supporting its effectiveness. Definitive efficacy trials must still be performed.

Formulations

Lithium is available in tablets, liquid, and long-acting formulations. Lithium carbonate is perhaps the most widely used formulation and carries the brand name of Eskalith. Generic preparations are also available and come in tablets at strengths of 150 mg, 300 mg, and 600 mg. Lithobid and Eskalith CR, both sustained-release preparations in film-coated dissolving tablets, are available in strengths of 300 mg and 450 mg, respectively. The 450-mg sustained-release tablets are scored. Lithium citrate is an oral solution of lithium with a concentration of 300 mg per teaspoon (8 mEq/5 mL).

Preliminary Evaluation

Prior to initiating any medication regimen, thoughtful consideration should be given to the target symptoms and their severity, anticipated barriers to medication adherence, and the patient's ability to swallow pills. Before lithium treatment is initiated, a careful medical history should be obtained. Particular attention should be paid to reviewing organ systems known to be affected by lithium administration: renal, endocrinological, neurological, and cardiovascular. Given that lithium is known to be a teratogen, increasing the likelihood of Ebstein's anomaly, especially during the first trimester of pregnancy, a pregnancy test should be completed for females of childbearing capacity prior to initiating treatment.

Discussions with females of childbearing potential should also be considered both before and throughout treatment in order to assess whether these patients are sexually active or intend to become pregnant. Baseline laboratories including blood urea nitrogen (BUN)/creatinine, electrolytes, and thyrotropin (thyroid-stimulating hormone; TSH) should be obtained to evaluate for the possibility of any preexisting renal impairment, electrolyte imbalances, or hypothyroidism that may lead the clinician to eschew prescribing lithium to an individual patient. We also recommend that a pretreatment electrocardiogram (ECG) be obtained for each patient in order to rule out any cardiac conduction abnormalities.

Medication Dosing

Lithium has a narrow therapeutic index. For this reason, it is important for the correct dose of lithium to be identified in a given patient in order to maximize therapeutic effectiveness while minimizing untoward side effects. Unfortunately, there are limited data available to guide clinicians about how to initiate lithium dosing in children and teenagers. Weight-based approaches suggest that the initial dosing of lithium can be made based on a milligram-per-kilogram (mg/kg) basis, with lithium doses subsequently titrated based on clinical response and serum level (Weller 1986). Another approach that has been described includes the administration of an initial test dose of lithium and the use of a nomogram. Serum levels are then measured at the 24-hour time point, with daily dosing prescribed according to the nomogram (Cooper et al. 1973; Geller and Fetner 1989). Both methods were compared head-to-head in a small inpatient sample and found to be equally effective (Hagino 1998).

Because the available studies included limited sample sizes, definitive conclusions about how to dose lithium in young people are still lacking. We recommend using a weight-based dosing strategy when starting lithium treatment because of the practical considerations associated with using a test dose and nomogram. Typically, lithium is started at a dosage of 15–20 mg/kg/day taken in divided doses (twice daily or thrice daily). If the dose cannot be divided evenly, an attempt should be made to give the larger dose at night to avoid daytime side effects. We try to avoid single doses greater than 900 mg because we have found that such high single doses are generally not well tolerated. Lithium can be increased by 300 mg every 4–5 days, based on clinical response and serum levels. Serum levels should be taken approximately 12 hours after the last dose and repeated every 4–5 days as the dosage is being adjusted. The therapeutic range for lithium appears to be between 0.6 and 1.4 mEq/L in pediatric patients, similar to what has been reported in adults.

Serum levels at the higher end of this therapeutic range appear to be associated with better symptom amelioration but are associated with greater side effects. When the lithium dose is stable, we recommend that screening laboratories be repeated. Subsequently, lithium levels, TSH, and renal function (BUN/creatinine or creatinine clearance) are evaluated every 3 months, or more frequently if necessary.

Side Effects

Adverse effects are common and involve the central nervous system (CNS) and the renal, dermatological, endocrine, and gastrointestinal (GI) systems (Table 6–1). Although side effects during lithium treatment are common, they generally do not lead to lithium discontinuation. It appears that GI symptoms (stomachache, nausea, vomiting, and diarrhea) are the most common side effects noted. Often, GI side effects can be addressed by recommending that the patient take lithium with food, dividing the doses more frequently throughout the course of the day, or administering lithium in the liquid citrate formulation. It should be noted, though, that persistent nausea, vomiting, and diarrhea (as well as other side effects noted below) may all signal the presence of lithium toxicity. For this reason, careful inquiry and reassessment of serum lithium levels should be considered for patients presenting with these

Table 6–1. Management of common lithium side effects

System	Side effect	Suggested intervention
Gastrointestinal	Nausea, emesis, diarrhea	Reduce dose or split dose Take with food Change to citrate formulation
CNS	Tremor, ataxia, slowed mentation	Reduce or split dose
Renal	Polyuria, changes in renal function	Allow for bathroom breaks Monitor kidney function every 3 months
Dermatological	Acne, rash	Provide education about side effects
Endocrine	Weight gain, thyroid abnormalities	Encourage exercise and healthy habits diet Monitor thyroid function every 3–6 months

concerns. If the lithium level is indeed high, lithium doses may be stopped for 24 hours while the level is rechecked and reinitiation at a lower dose is considered.

Other side effects appear to be less common. CNS side effects that have been reported include tremor, ataxia, and slowed mentation. Tremor is usually mild and can be aided by dose reduction. Although the use of propranolol has been described as a treatment for lithium-related tremor in adults, this management strategy is not one we generally recommend for youth.

Renal side effects include polyuria/polydipsia and possible morphological changes to the kidney after long-term use. Unfortunately, there are insufficient data regarding the long-term renal effects of lithium in the young. Dermatologically, an acne-like rash can be a troubling side effect for adolescents, and education concerning this possibility is suggested. Rash and hair loss have been infrequently described in relation to lithium therapy. Lastly, endocrine side effects can include weight gain and hypothyroidism.

Drug Interactions and Cautions

Lithium is excreted by the kidney. Thus, drug–drug interactions may occur as a result of modification of renal excretion by other agents. Concomitant use of other drugs or substances may either increase or decrease lithium levels. For example, nonsteroidal anti-inflammatory drugs (NSAIDs) can increase lithium levels by reducing renal excretion. Although use of NSAIDs is not necessarily contraindicated for patients prescribed lithium, care should given if NSAIDs are taken during lithium therapy, with particular attention being paid to symptoms of lithium toxicity. Thiazide diuretics, though not commonly used in young people, may substantively increase lithium levels. On the other hand, theophylline and caffeine may decrease lithium levels by enhancing renal excretion. Lastly, sodium chloride can also affect the renal excretion of lithium. Thus, excessive intake of salty snack foods or salt-repleting sports drinks can lower the lithium level. Therefore, discussion about these drug-drug interactions, dietary considerations, and the encouragement of adequate hydration, especially during summer months and during vigorous physical activities, is recommended.

In summary, lithium use in pediatric bipolar disorder is supported by numerous case studies and open-label reports, with limited data available from randomized controlled trials (RCTs). However, lithium is an agent that has a great deal of support in the adult literature for use in bipolar disorder. At present, lithium remains the only mood stabilizer that is FDA-approved for the treatment of pediatric bipolar disorder. Although use of lithium does have substantive burdens in terms of monitoring and its side-effect profile, its potential for significant benefit allows it to remain a first-line agent in treating pediatric bipolar disorder.

Anticonvulsants

Although anticonvulsants appear to be widely used in treating pediatric bipolar disorder, there are no anticonvulsants that are FDA-approved for treating acute mania or as a maintenance therapy for bipolar disorder in children and adolescents. In adults, divalproex sodium, lamotrigine, and Equetro (extended-release carbamazepine) have approved uses for bipolar disorder. Carbamazepine, oxcarbazepine, divalproex sodium, lamotrigine, and topiramate have all been investigated in youths with bipolar illness. Other, newer agents, such as zonisamide, levetiracetam, and tiagabine, have not received rigorous testing to date in children and adolescents with bipolar disorders.

Carbamazepine

Carbamazepine was the first anticonvulsant extensively studied as a potential treatment for bipolar disorder in adults. However, recently, it appears that carbamazepine is generally not commonly used in the treatment of bipolar disorder in the young. This is most likely due to a paucity of clinical trials data in this patient population when compared with lithium or divalproex sodium. Another possible contributing factor is that there are sometimes challenges associated with the administration of carbamazepine that might complicate its use. These challenges include the possibility of drug–drug interactions, concerns regarding aplastic anemia and agranulocytosis, and metabolic auto-induction.

Supporting Studies in Youths

As noted above, there are limited data regarding the use of carbamazepine in pediatric bipolar illness. The data that do exist suggest that carbamazepine may be useful in the treatment of this patient population. In an open-label trial comparing carbamazepine, lithium, and divalproex sodium, 5 of 13 children, ages 6–18 years, with bipolar I or II disorder achieved a 50% reduction in manic symptoms within 6 weeks of initiation of carbamazepine therapy (Kowatch et al. 2003). The reported serum level that led to these results was 7.11 ± 1.79 μg/mL. Nausea and sedation were noted as adverse effects in the carbamazepine-treated subjects. In addition, case studies have suggested that carbamazepine may be useful in treating symptoms of mania in children as young as age 5 years, and in those who might be unresponsive to lithium (Craven 2000; Tuzun 2002; Woolston 1999).

Formulations

Carbamazepine is available in several forms. Generic carbamazepine is available as 100-mg chewable tablets, 200-mg tablets, and an oral solution of 100 mg/5 mL strength. These forms of carbamazepine are generally dosed thrice daily or four times daily. An extended-release formulation of carbamazepine is also available in 100-mg, 200-mg, and 300-mg capsule form (Carbatrol), which allows twice-daily dosing. The contents of a Carbatrol capsule may be sprinkled over food, such as applesauce. This form is similar to the newest extended-release formulation, Equetro, available in sprinkle capsules of strengths of 100 mg, 200 mg, and 300 mg. The tablet version of extended-release carbamazepine, Tegretol-XR, is available in strengths of 100 mg, 200 mg, and 400 mg.

Preliminary Evaluation

A thorough medical history should be obtained before starting carbamazepine. Particular attention should be paid to any history of hepatic dysfunction, hematological abnormalities, cardiac conduction problems, or immunological concerns. Laboratory work should include a complete blood count (CBC) with differential and platelets, electrolytes, BUN/creatinine, transaminases, and a urine pregnancy test, if applicable. Careful discussion regarding the teratogenic potential of carbamazepine should occur with all females of childbearing capacity, both prior to the initiation of treatment and throughout maintenance therapy. Because carbamazepine can auto-induce its metabolism, blood levels should be monitored carefully and dose adjustments made accordingly (Kudriakova et al. 1992). In addition, carbamazepine can significantly affect the metabolism of numerous other medications, so a complete assessment of concomitant medications is recommended.

Medication Dosing

Carbamazepine use in the child and adolescent population has been extensively studied in the pediatric neurology literature, and the following recommendations are based on those studies. In children younger than 6 years, carbamazepine should be initiated at 10–20 mg/kg/day in twice-daily or thrice-daily dosing, and the dosage is titrated at weekly intervals to symptom resolution or dose-limiting side effects. As noted earlier, the carbamazepine oral solution should be administered in a thrice-daily or four-times-daily dosing regimen to minimize any side effects from the higher peak serum levels seen with this formulation. In children ages 6–12 years, carbamazepine may be initiated at 100 mg bid and increased weekly by 100 mg, with the total daily dose not to exceed 1 gram. For individuals older than age 12, the carbamazepine can be initiated at 200 mg twice daily and titrated by 200 mg weekly. Adequate serum levels in individuals over age 12 are generally achieved at dosages similar to those used in adults (800–1,200 mg/day). Of note, in the only published open-label study to compare carbamazepine, lithium, and divalproex sodium in children and adolescents with bipolar disorder, all of the subjects in the carbamazepine arm had carbamazepine initiated at a dosage of 15 mg/kg/day (Kowatch et al. 2000).

We have generally found that initiating carbamazepine at a dosage of approximately 15 mg/kg/day is reasonably well tolerated. The therapeutic serum level range is 4–12 µg/mL, with 7–10 µg/mL being a common maintenance drug level. Since auto-induction may occur during carbamazepine therapy, doses that were initially found to be therapeutic may subsequently be inadequate. For this reason, careful laboratory and symptom monitoring are indicated. We recommend that drug levels, CBC with differential and platelets, and liver enzyme measurements be completed at least every other week during the first 2 months of treatment, then at least every 3 months thereafter.

Side Effects

Common side effects of carbamazepine affect both the GI system and the CNS (Table 6–2). Nausea and sedation are commonly experienced and can often be minimized with gradual titration of treatment and divided dosing. Blurred vision and ataxia can also be noted as well.

Hematological, dermatological, and hepatic side effects seem to be less common. Mild leukopenia and thrombocytopenia may occur in some individuals. Rarely, some patients develop aplastic anemia or agranulocytosis. Transient skin rashes may occur. Stevens-Johnson syndrome may occur very rarely with carbamazepine use as well. Transaminase levels may become mildly elevated with carbamazepine administration. Hyponatremia has been reported, in addition to abnormal renal function, in some individuals. Weight gain does not appear to be a substantive problem with this drug.

Drug Interactions and Cautions

Carbamazepine is metabolized through the cytochrome P450 (CYP) 3A3 and 3A4 systems and so has the potential to interact with many commonly used medications. A partial listing of drugs that can *increase* carbamazepine levels include fluoxetine, fluvoxamine, valproate, tricyclic antidepressants, prednisolone, and macrolide antibiotics (erythromycin). Similarly, use of carbamazepine may *decrease* the blood levels of the following medications: oral contraceptives, benzodiazepines, theophylline, sertraline, and neuroleptics, among other medications. Carbamazepine has been associated with fetal abnormalities when used by pregnant women in the first trimester.

In summary, carbamazepine has limited data on its effectiveness in treating pediatric mania. No randomized, double-blind trials currently exist to support the routine use of carbamazepine. In addition, the numerous risks related to carbamazepine use and its extensive interactions with other concomitant medications suggest it should be considered a second-line or adjunctive agent in treating pediatric bipolar disorder until further studies are performed.

Table 6–2. Management of common carbamazepine side effects

System	Side effect	Suggested intervention
Gastrointestinal	Nausea	Reduce dose or split dose Take with food Change formulation used
CNS	Blurred vision, ataxia, sedation.	Reduce or split dose
Hematological	Leukopenia, thrombocytopenia, agranulocytosis, aplastic anemia	Advise patients to immediately notify clinician if flu symptoms or signs of infection occur Monitor laboratory values regularly Agranulocytosis/aplastic anemia: Immediately discontinue drug and consider medical hospitalization
Hepatic	Elevated transaminases	Monitor laboratory values regularly Educate patient on symptoms of hepatic failure (jaundice, fatigue)
Dermatological	Skin rash	Carefully monitor and consider discontinuation

Divalproex Sodium

Divalproex sodium (Depakote) received FDA approval for treatment of mania in adults in 1994. It appears that valproate, unlike carbamazepine, is commonly prescribed to children and adolescents with bipolar disorder.

Supporting Studies in Youth

Acute treatment of manic, hypomanic, and mixed mania symptoms in children and adolescents has been evaluated in open-label trials of up to 8 weeks in length (Papatheodorou et al. 1995; Scheffer et al. 2005; Wagner et al. 2002). These studies suggest that divalproex may be effective in the treatment of bipolar disorder in the young. Headache, GI complaints, and sedation were commonly observed side effects in these reports.

Two published studies have evaluated the longer-term use of divalproex sodium in pediatric bipolar disorder. In a 6-month, prospective, open-label trial by Pavuluri et al. (2005), treatment with divalproex sodium was started at a dose of 250–500 mg the first night, and the dosage was then adjusted to 15–20 mg/kg/day given in divided doses. Children and adolescents ages 5–18 years achieved a response rate of 73.5% and a remission rate of 52.9% during the study period, while weight gain and transient transaminase elevations were noted. Findling et al. (2005) reported on an 18-month, double-blind, maintenance comparison of lithium and divalproex sodium in youth ages 5–18 years with bipolar disorder. Divalproex was initiated in divided doses and gradually increased to a target dosage of 20 mg/kg/day. In this trial, lithium and divalproex treatment appeared to have similar effectiveness as maintenance treatments. GI complaints, tremor, and headache were commonly reported side effects.

Formulations

Standard valproic acid without enteric coating is available in the form of Depakene in 250-mg capsules and an elixir of 250 mg/5 mL. Enteric-coated valproic acid (divalproex sodium) is available as Depakote in 125-mg, 250-mg, and 500-mg tablets. Depakote Sprinkles are available in 125-mg capsules. The beaded contents of the sprinkle capsules can be put over applesauce for those children having difficulty swallowing pills. Depakote ER is available in 250-mg and 500-mg tablets, and once-daily dosing may be possible with this form.

Preliminary Evaluation

A detailed medical history is recommended prior to initiating treatment with valproate. Particular attention should be paid to any history of hepatic and/or hematological dysfunction. Concomitant medications that are hepatically metabolized should also be reviewed. The teratogenic potential for neural tube defects has been well established with valproate therapy, and urine pregnancy testing and documentation of education regarding this possibility is suggested in females of childbearing potential. Concerns regarding polycystic ovary syndrome (PCOS) have prompted some clinicians to document pretreatment menstrual patterns in order to facilitate the identification of any changes in menses that might occur during valproate therapy. Baseline laboratory work should include a CBC with differential and platelets, as well as an assessment of liver function (e.g., transaminases, bilirubin). Because treatment with divalproex may lead to weight gain, monitoring of weight and height prior to and during valproate treatment is also recommended.

Medication Dosing

Enteric-coated preparations are generally preferred for the treatment of pediatric patients with bipolar illness when compared with generic valproic acid, given that enteric-coated formulations are associated with a reduced risk for GI side effects such as dyspepsia and abdominal pain. For outpatients, we generally recommend initiating divalproex sodium at a dosage of approximately 10–15 mg/kg/day (given in divided doses). Then, based on the results of serum levels and clinical response, dose increases in 250-mg to 500-mg increments may be considered. Serum levels of valproic acid should be obtained shortly after initiation of treatment, during dose titration periods, or when clinically indicated. Adequate serum levels have been reported in the 50–125 μg/mL range, and the total daily dose should not exceed 60 mg/kg. After dose stabilization, liver function tests, CBC with differential and platelets, and serum levels should be obtained at least every 6 months, or when clinical symptoms change.

Side Effects

Side effects reported to be associated with divalproex pharmacotherapy in the pediatric bipolar population have included GI, CNS, hepatic, and hematological events (Table 6–3). Weight gain was noted in 59% of the sample treated by Pavuluri et al. (2005). CNS effects that have been reported include cognitive dulling, headaches, tremor, and somnolence. Although the enteric-coated divalproex sodium preparations can minimize GI symptoms, nausea, stomach pain, diarrhea, and emesis have been reported with these formulations. Rare cases of hepatic failure and potentially fatal pancreatitis have also been observed. Therefore, we routinely advise patients to notify their physician about new-onset symptoms of nausea, lethargy, jaundice, or anorexia. Thrombocytopenia may occur, so monitoring for bleeding or easy bruising is suggested.

The issue surrounding PCOS has received renewed interest in the past several years. PCOS is a syndrome of hyperandrogenism (menstrual irregularities, hirsutism, acne, and alopecia). Small studies have failed to consistently show a relationship between PCOS and valproate use among patients without seizure disorders (H. Joffe et al. 2003; R. T. Joffe et al. 2003). However, more recent work has identified a functional polymorphism, SNP-71G, which may contribute to the creation of excessive testosterone production (Qin 2005).

Table 6–3. Management of divalproex sodium–related side effects

System	Side effect	Suggested intervention
Gastrointestinal	Nausea, emesis, stomach pain, diarrhea	Take with food Switch to Depakote formulation Consider checking serum level for toxicity
CNS	Tremor, headache, sedation, cognitive dulling	Reduce or split dose
Hematological	Leukopenia, thrombocytopenia	Consider hematology consultation Consider medication discontinuation
Hepatic	Elevated transaminases/ pancreatic enzymes	Consider rechecking of laboratory values Consider medication discontinuation
Endocrinological	Menstrual irregularities, hyperandrogenism	Consider referral to an endocrinologist Consider switching mood-stabilizing agents

Furthermore, valproate has been shown to potentiate this gene's expression in ovarian cells (Nelson-DeGrave 2004; Wood 2005). In sum, it appears that valproate treatment may play a role in the potentiation of PCOS in certain patients, so careful monitoring may be indicated until a clearer picture of the association between valproate administration and PCOS is available.

Drug Interactions and Cautions

Like many other psychotropic agents, valproate is metabolized in the liver. Because of the possibility of drug–drug interactions, care should be used when valproate is prescribed with concomitant medications. Commonly used agents that can *increase* valproate levels include erythromycin, fluoxetine, aspirin, and ibuprofen. Similarly, carbamazepine is a medication that may *decrease* valproate levels during concomitant use. In addition, valproate can lead to substantive increases in lamotrigine levels when both agents are used together. This elevation in lamotrigine concentrations may result in serious dermatological reactions. Therefore, dosing of lamotrigine should be modified when prescribed concomitantly with valproate.

Other Anticonvulsants

Evidence for the use of other, newer anticonvulsants in treating pediatric bipolar disorder is sparse. For this reason, we generally do not prescribe these compounds to patients unless other agents with more extensive empirical support do not provide adequate therapeutic benefit.

Lamotrigine has been considered in a case series of adolescents ages 14–18 years taking concomitant medications (Carandang et al. 2003) and in one small open-label study in adolescents with bipolar depression (Chang et al. 2006). The adjunctive use of lamotrigine in the depressed phase of adolescent bipolar disorder was also considered in a five-subject case report (Soutullo et al. 2006). These data provide the basis for a possible role for lamotrigine in young people with bipolar illness.

There are data from one methodologically stringent clinical trial that examined the use of topiramate. In that study, DelBello et al. (2005) conducted a double-blind, placebo-controlled trial of topiramate in children ages 6–17 years with bipolar I disorder. This trial was ended before the entire planned sample was ascertained when it was learned that results of concurrent adult mania studies failed to demonstrate efficacy for the compound. However, in this pediatric trial, there did appear to be a trend toward topiramate indeed having some therapeutic efficacy. However, because this pediatric study had a limited sample size, and therefore reduced statistical power to detect a drug–placebo difference, definitive conclusions about the short-term efficacy of topiramate cannot be made on the basis of the results of this trial.

Similar to what had been suggested in adults (Benedetti et al. 2004; Hummel et al. 2002), in two separate case reports, oxcarbazepine was described as possibly being beneficial in the treatment of pediatric bipolar disorder (Davanzo et al. 2004; Teitelbaum 2001). However, in a large, multi-site, randomized, double-blind, placebo-controlled study in children and adolescents, treatment with oxcarbazepine was found not to be superior to treatment with placebo (Wagner et al. 2006).

It should be noted there have been reports that have considered zonisamide, levetiracetam, and tiagabine in the adult literature. However, these published reports are not placebo controlled and generally lack methodological rigor. At present, we do not prescribe these three agents to youth, given that there are no available data to support their use in the management of pediatric bipolar disorder.

Maintenance Therapy

Most studies of lithium and anticonvulsants in the pediatric bipolar literature have been open label and typically no longer than 8 weeks in duration. However, bipolar illness is a chronic, long-term condition. Although the pediatric neurology literature provides some insights into the long-term safety of several of the anticonvulsants, there are limited data about the long-term effectiveness and use of these medications in children and adolescents with bipolar illness. One 18-month study compared the efficacy of lithium with that of divalproex sodium as maintenance therapy. Results indicated that both drugs were generally well tolerated and showed equal effectiveness in preventing relapse over the 18-month trial period (Findling et al. 2005). Clearly, more studies are needed to address the long-term effectiveness and safety of lithium and anticonvulsants in the pediatric bipolar population.

Atypical Antipsychotics

At present, there are seven atypical antipsychotic agents that are available to clinicians in the United States: aripiprazole, clozapine, olanzapine, paliperidone (the active metabolite of risperidone), quetiapine, risperidone, and ziprasidone. The mood-stabilizing properties of atypical antipsychotic medications have received significant attention in the literature on adult bipolar disorder over the past several years. In the adult literature, it has been established that atypical antipsychotic monotherapy can provide similar benefits to traditional mood-stabilizer monotherapy in acute mania. Researchers in pediatric bipolar illness have also begun to explore the usefulness of atypical antipsychotics as a monotherapy and as an adjunctive therapy in this often difficult-to-treat population.

General Evaluation and Monitoring

Prior to prescribing any atypical antipsychotic medication, care must be taken to obtain an accurate psychiatric, medical, and family history. Particular attention should be paid to a medical history, family history, and physical examination that consider weight/obesity, endocrine and cardiovascular system issues, and neurological status/movement disorders. Similar to all psychotropic medications prescribed to children and adolescents, documentation that the potential for short-term and long-term side effects was reviewed with both the patient and the patient's guardians is strongly encouraged. Besides considerations that pertain to this entire class of drugs, there are specific issues that are particular to some of the individual agents. These drug-specific topics are discussed as each agent is considered individually below.

Before considering specific agents, it should be recalled that one of the key aspects that confers *atypicality* to this class of drugs is their reduced propensity to cause extrapyramidal side effects (EPS) when compared with the older, *typical* antipsychotics. However, neurological side effects such as dystonia, parkinsonism, and tardive dyskinesia have been reported with these agents. The potential for these risks should be reviewed with patients and their guardians. In addition, we recommend that extra care be specifically paid to the assessment of extrapyramidal symptoms prior to and during the course of treatment with this group of drugs. In addition, because tardive dyskinesia is a possibly irreversible side effect, we carefully evaluate and monitor for this possibility. A commonly used instrument that can facilitate this process is the Abnormal Involuntary Movement Scale (AIMS) (National Institute of Mental Health 1985).

Much discussion has occurred in the past several years concerning the potential for metabolic/endocrinological and cardiovascular complications when prescribing atypical antipsychotics. Although the adult literature has data to support the assertion that atypical antipsychotics are effective and reasonably well-tolerated medications for acutely treating symptoms of psychosis and mania, the concerns over developing glucose intolerance, adverse lipid-profile changes, and dramatic weight increases during longer-term treatment with these drugs have been notable. Consensus guidelines (based on adult data) to assist clinicians with suggested monitoring strategies that address these concerns regarding treatment with atypical antipsychotics are available (American Diabetes Association et al. 2004).

Avoiding drug interactions with atypical antipsychotics generally involves avoiding specific concomitant therapies. Because atypical antipsychotic medications can be sedating, combined use with other CNS depressants is cautioned. In addition, medications that affect cardiac conduction by lengthening the QT interval should be avoided as well. Concomitant use of medications affecting hepatic metabolism can reduce (e.g., carbamazepine) or increase (e.g., fluvoxamine, atomoxetine) blood levels of certain atypical antipsychotics.

Aripiprazole

Aripiprazole has recently been determined to be an effective monotherapy treatment in adult bipolar disorder (Keck et al. 2003). Of the atypical antipsychotics, it is unique in that it acts as a partial dopamine agonist.

Supporting Studies

Retrospective chart reviews suggest that aripiprazole may be effective in treating pediatric bipolar disorder. Two chart reviews evaluating aripiprazole use in children and adolescents suggested aripiprazole might be an effective agent in pediatric bipolar illness (Barzman et al. 2004; Biederman et al. 2005a). Methodologically stringent data from efficacy trials or prospective long-term effectiveness studies are currently not available.

Formulations

Aripiprazole is available under the brand name Abilify in both tablet and liquid forms. Tablet strengths include 2 mg, 5 mg, 10 mg, 15 mg, 20 mg, and 30 mg. The liquid preparation is available as a 1 mg/mL elixir. An orally disintegrating tablet formulation is available in strengths of 10 mg and 15 mg. Aripiprazole is also available in an injectable form that has not yet been studied in children.

Medication Dosing

Because methodologically stringent RCTs of aripiprazole are not available, specific dosing strategies have not been clearly established for use of aripiprazole in young people with bipolar illness. With its long half-life, aripiprazole is routinely prescribed in once-daily dosing. On the basis of our clinical experience, we generally recommend initiating aripiprazole at a dose of 2 mg or 5 mg at bedtime and titrating the dose by 2- to 5-mg increments every 5–7 days to maximize salutary effects while minimizing side effects. We do not recommend exceeding the FDA-approved maximum dosage for adults of 30 mg/day.

Side Effects

Common side effects that have been reported with aripiprazole in youth include sedation, motoric activation, and nausea/emesis (Table 6–4). Studies in adults suggest that aripiprazole may have a reduced propensity for inducing weight gain compared with some of the other atypical agents. However, this has yet to be definitively confirmed or refuted. It does appear that clinically

Table 6–4. Management of aripiprazole side effects

System	Side effect	Suggested intervention
Gastrointestinal	Nausea, emesis	Take with food Slower titration Reduce dose
CNS	Headache, sedation, activation, akathisia	Reduce or split dose Change time of daily administration
General	Weight gain	Educate patient about appropriate diet and exercise Consider nutrition consultation Switch to another treatment

significant electrocardiographic changes are not common with aripiprazole. In addition, because of its unique partial dopamine agonism mechanism of action, prolactin levels do not seem to increase during aripiprazole therapy.

Clozapine

Whereas the other atypical antipsychotic agents are considered to be first-line agents, clozapine is generally reserved for patients who fail to respond to other forms of therapy, and appears to be only rarely used in pediatric patients with bipolar illness. This is due to clozapine's associated risk for potentially fatal agranulocytosis. It should also be noted that clozapine can lower the seizure threshold and lead to both electroencephalographic changes as well as overt seizures in youth who are prescribed this drug.

There is some evidence that clozapine may be of benefit to adolescents with treatment-resistant bipolar illness (Masi et al. 2002). Unfortunately, there have been no prospective RCTs of clozapine in youth with bipolar illness.

Olanzapine

Olanzapine was introduced in the United States in 1996. It is approved for use in adults for the treatment of schizophrenia and mania in bipolar disorder. Concerns over weight gain and endocrine abnormalities (diabetes, dyslipidemias) associated with olanzapine therapy have received attention in adults. These issues are of important clinical concern for children and adolescents, who may be at greater risk for antipsychotic-related weight gain.

Supporting Studies

One of the first publications to suggest that olanzapine might be effective in youths was a case series involving 12- to 17-year-old patients with acute mania (Soutullo et al. 1999). Frazier et al. (2001) subsequently conducted an open-label olanzapine monotherapy trial. Over the course of the 8-week study, treatment with olanzapine was effective in reducing symptoms of mania in patients who ranged in age from 5 to 14 years. More recently, Biederman et al. (2005b) described the treatment of 4- to 6-year-old children with bipolar disorder who were administered olanzapine (1.25–10 mg) with risperidone (0.25–2 mg). The authors noted that both medications appeared to be effective.

Of particular note are the results of a double-blind, randomized, placebo-controlled, 3-week trial (Tohen et al. 2005). In that study, patients with mania between the ages of 13 and 17 years were treated with olanzapine ($n=107$) or placebo ($n=54$) at dosages ranging from 2.5 to 20 mg/day. The investigators found that treatment with olanzapine was associated with greater reductions in manic symptoms than treatment with placebo. Patients randomly assigned to receive olanzapine gained more weight (3.7 kg) than did those treated with placebo (0.3 kg).

Formulations

Olanzapine is available as Zyprexa tablets, an intramuscular preparation, and the dissolving formulation Zydis. Tablets are available in strengths of 2.5 mg, 5 mg, 7.5 mg, 10 mg, 15 mg, and 20 mg. Zydis orally disintegrating tablets, which are available in strengths of 5 mg, 10 mg, 15 mg, and 20 mg, may be useful for those children unable to swallow tablets. The injectable form of olanzapine is generally reserved for management of emergencies and potentially dangerous situations.

Preliminary Evaluation

Given that olanzapine therapy may be associated with weight gain and endocrine dysfunction in the adult population, care should be exercised to establish any history of endocrine dysfunction or obesity in both the child/adolescent and his or her biological family prior to therapy. Discussions with patients and their families should include both the short-term risks noted in the previously conducted acute pediatric trials and long-term risks seen in adult studies. Active participation of the patient and family in monitoring side effects is also suggested.

Table 6–5. Management of olanzapine side effects

System	Side effect	Suggested intervention
Endocrine	Glucose intolerance	Monitor fasting glucose and hemoglobin A_{1C} at least annually Consider nutrition consultation
CNS	Headache, sedation	Reduce or split dose Administer dose at bedtime
General	Weight gain	Educate patient about appropriate diet and exercise Consider nutrition consultation Switch to another atypical Consider addition of topiramate

Medication Dosing

No consensus dosing guidelines have been established for the use of olanzapine in pediatric bipolar disorder. In the Biederman et al. (2005b) olanzapine study of children ages 4–6, olanzapine was initiated at 1.25 mg at bedtime, and the dosage was increased weekly to a maximum of 10 mg/day. In the open-label study of Frazier et al. (1999), olanzapine was initiated at 2.5 mg as a single evening dose, and the dosage was increased by that same amount every 3 days, as tolerated. Whether higher starting doses are more or less effective remains an empirical question.

Side Effects

Weight gain has been noted in the published pediatric bipolar trials (Table 6–5). Although sedation is commonly reported with olanzapine use, GI problems appear to be relatively uncommon. Unfortunately, there is a paucity of methodologically stringent long-term studies of olanzapine. Therefore, the magnitude of weight gain associated with long-term olanzapine therapy in the pediatric population has yet to be adequately characterized.

Quetiapine

Quetiapine monotherapy is FDA-approved in adults for the treatment of schizophrenia, acute mania in bipolar disorder, and depressive episodes associated with bipolar disorder. As with all atypical antipsychotic medications that may be prescribed to children, its use remains off-label. Quetiapine was introduced in the U.S. market in 1997.

Supporting Studies

Quetiapine has mainly received attention in the pediatric bipolar literature as an adjunct to the mood stabilizers. In a retrospective chart review, the response rate for youth receiving quetiapine monotherapy to treat a bipolar spectrum illness was 78.6% (Marchand et al. 2004). In one prospective study, 50 patients with mania between the ages of 12 and 18 years were randomly assigned to receive treatment with either quetiapine, at dosages ranging from 400 to 600 mg/day, or divalproex, at dosages necessary to achieve serum levels of 80–120 µg/mL, for up to 4 weeks. The authors found both medications to be equally effective in symptom amelioration of mania and both agents to be reasonably well tolerated (DelBello et al. 2006).

Other studies have evaluated the usefulness of quetiapine as an adjunctive treatment in pediatric bipolar disorder. These clinical trials are considered in the section "Combination Pharmacotherapy" later in this chapter.

Formulations

Quetiapine is branded as Seroquel and is available in strengths of 25 mg, 50 mg, 100 mg, 200 mg, 300 mg, and 400 mg.

Preliminary Evaluation

It should be mentioned that cataract formation was noted in laboratory animals administered quetiapine. Although a relationship between quetiapine use and cataract formation has not been established in humans, in addition to the previously noted evaluations that might be considered prior to beginning atypical antipsychotic therapy, the clinician may consider ophthalmologic examinations for patients prescribed this drug.

Medication Dosing

There are no clear guidelines on pediatric dosing of quetiapine in the treatment of bipolar disorder. In the quetiapine-adjunctive inpatient study by DelBello et al. (2002), quetiapine was initiated at 25 mg bid, and the dosage was titrated to 150 mg tid over the course of 1 week. Our clinical practice has suggested that upward dosage increments of 50–100 mg/day are generally well

Table 6–6. Management of quetiapine side effects

System	Side effect	Suggested intervention
CNS	Sedation, orthostasis	Reduce or split dose to thrice daily, with larger dose at night Caution patient to be careful when getting out of bed or standing up
Visual	Cataracts	Educate patient about possible changes in eyesight Recommend regular ophthalmologic evaluation
General	Weight gain	Educate patient about appropriate diet and exercise Consider nutrition consultation Consider switch to another agent

tolerated in adolescents, and that increases of 25–50 mg/day are reasonably well tolerated in younger patients. Sedation is the dose-limiting side effect that we observe most frequently during dosing increases. As with adults, we generally administer quetiapine in twice-daily doses that are equal in size. Future research is needed in order to characterize the most effective means to achieve optimal dosing levels in children and adolescents.

Side Effects

The adult literature notes sedation and orthostatic hypotension as common adverse effects that occur with quetiapine treatment (Table 6–6). Although weight gain appears to be less than that noted with olanzapine and clozapine treatment, we do observe weight gain with quietiapine in our clinical practice. It appears that the risk of EPS may be relatively modest with quetiapine when compared with the other atypical agents.

Risperidone

Like other atypical antipsychotics, risperidone is FDA-approved in adults as a monotherapy for schizophrenia and acute mania in bipolar disorder. However, it has also been FDA-approved in children ages 5–16 years for treatment of irritability associated with autistic disorder, as covered elsewhere in this text (see Chpater 7, "Autism and Other Pervasive Developmental Disorders").

Supporting Studies

Frazier et al. (1999) in one of the first communications regarding the use of risperidone in pediatric bipolarity, reported that with risperidone at an average dosage of 1.7 mg/day, youth ages 4–17 years demonstrated substantive improvement in symptoms of mania and aggression over the treatment period. Biederman et al. (2005b) compared risperidone with olanzapine monotherapy in preschool children ages 4–6 years with bipolar disorder. At dosages of up to 2 mg/day, risperidone was found to be generally beneficial. In another study from the same research group (Biederman et al. 2005c), patients ages 6–17 years were treated in a prospective 8-week long, open-label study. In this trial of 30 subjects, the authors found that treatment with risperidone at a mean dosage of 1.25 mg/day was associated with symptom amelioration and was reasonably well tolerated.

Formulations

Risperidone (Risperdal) is available in tablet, liquid, disintegrating tablet, and long-acting injectable forms. The tablets are available in strengths of 0.25 mg, 0.5 mg, 1 mg, 2 mg, 3 mg, and 4 mg. The concentration of the liquid formulation is 1 mg/mL. The orally disintegrating form, Risperdal M-Tab, is available in strengths of 0.5 mg, 1 mg, 2 mg, 3 mg, and 4 mg. Neither injectable Risperdal Consta nor long-acting oral paliperidone (Invega) has been studied in the pediatric population.

Preliminary Evaluation

The preliminary assessment that was recommended prior to atypical antipsychotic initiation, as noted earlier, should be considered. It appears that risperidone, compared with other atypical antipsychotics, has a greater propensity to increase prolactin concentrations. Because in our experience prolactin-related side effects are not often problematic, we generally do not monitor prolactin concentrations over time. However, we do recommend a pretreatment prolactin level be obtained for youths prior to risperidone initiation. Thus, if side effects that might be attributable to prolactin develop de novo (e.g., irregular menses/amenorrhea, galactorrhea, breast enlargement), and a prolactin measurement is subsequently obtained, there is a baseline level with which this on-treatment assessment can be compared.

Table 6–7.   Management of risperidone side effects

System	Side effect	Suggested intervention
CNS	Sedation, headache	Reduce the total dose Administer more of the daily dose at night
Endocrine	Glucose intolerance; prolactin elevation	Monitor fasting glucose Monitor for changes in menses, galactorrhea, or gynecomastia
General	Weight gain	Educate patient about appropriate diet and exercise Consider switching to another agent

Medication Dosing

Clear guidelines for the most effective risperidone dosing paradigm in treating pediatric bipolar disorder are unavailable. In our experience, dose-limiting side effects during risperidone titration are sedation and EPS.

For younger children, we generally suggest starting at 0.25 mg/day, with titration every 2–3 days, to a total daily dose that does not exceed 2 mg. This total daily dose is typically administered twice daily in relatively equal amounts. For older children and adolescents (typically weighing more than 40 kg), a similar dosing strategy that employs 0.5-mg dosing increments and a total daily dose that does not exceed 4 mg is what we generally consider.

Side Effects

The most commonly reported side effects seen during risperidone treatment include increased/weight gain, headache, and sedation (Table 6–7). It appears that a more rapid rate of dose titration, as well as higher final total-daily doses, increases the risk of EPS during pediatric risperidone therapy. As noted earlier, the rates of hyperprolactinemia seem higher with risperidone than with other atypicals.

Ziprasidone

Ziprasidone has been marketed in the United States since 2000 and is FDA-approved as monotherapy for schizophrenia and acute mania in adults. It does not appear to cause weight gain in adults. Ziprasidone does have a generally modest effect on intracardiac conduction. The risks associated with this effect in adults appear to be modest (Daniel 2003). Although concerns have been raised (Blair et al. 2005), at present, the effects of ziprasidone on cardiac electrophysiology have not been well characterized in children or adolescents. There is, as of yet, no FDA-approved pediatric indication for ziprasidone.

Supporting Studies

The published literature on the use of ziprasidone in the treatment of pediatric bipolar disorder as of the time of this writing consists of one case series. All subjects described in the report received concomitant medications along with ziprasidone (Barnett 2004) and appeared to have received some benefit at dosages ≤80 mg/day.

Formulations

Ziprasidone is marketed in the United States as Geodon and is available in both capsules and as an intramuscular injection. Capsules are available in strengths of 20 mg, 40 mg, 60 mg, and 80 mg. The injectable form is reserved for acute agitation, and although its use has been described in case reports (Hazaray et al. 2004; Staller 2004), this formulation has not been examined in methodologically stringent research in the pediatric population.

Preliminary Evaluation

The evaluation prior to initiating ziprasidone therapy is similar to that mentioned previously for the other atypical antipsychotic medications. Particular attention should be paid to inquiring about any individual or family history of cardiac conduction problems or symptoms associated with cardiac disease (such as syncope, arrhythmias, or family history of sudden cardiac death). In the absence of adequate data to characterize ziprasidone's effects on intracardiac conduction, we recommend that an ECG be obtained prior to the initiation of ziprasidone, as well as during the course of ziprasidone therapy (see subsection "Side Effects" below).

Medication Dosing

Considering the paucity of published literature, it is not surprising that there are no definitive guidelines about the dosing of ziprasidone in pediatric bipolar patients. Our experience suggests that in teenagers, optimal final doses of ziprasidone are similar to those doses reported to be beneficial to adults. Lower doses appear to be effective in younger children (putatively attributable

Table 6–8.   Management of ziprasidone side effects

System	Side effect	Suggested intervention
CNS	Sedation, akathisia, extrapyramidal side effects	Reduce the daily dose Administer the total daily dose in thrice-daily rather than twice-daily divided doses Administer a larger proportion of the total daily dose at bedtime
Cardiovascular	QTc prolongation, elevated heart rates	Monitor for any syncopal events or dizziness Consider electrocardiographic monitoring at baseline and during upward dose titration Consider electrocardiographic monitoring when optimal dosage achieved, then periodically, or if symptoms change

to their smaller size). On the basis of the available data, it is recommended that ziprasidone be administered twice daily in divided doses. Because ingestion of ziprasidone with food increases this agent's bioavailability, we generally recommend that patients take their ziprasidone consistently with food in order to achieve predictable drug exposure.

Side Effects

Sedation, akathisia, and elevated heart rates have been noted when ziprasidone is prescribed to youth (Barnett 2004) (Table 6–8). Unlike many of the other atypical agents, there does not appear to be substantive weight increases or dyslipidemias associated with ziprasidone therapy in adults. In the absence of definitive information regarding the magnitude of QTc prolongation that may occur in youth, no definitive recommendations about electrocardiographic monitoring in youth treated with ziprasidone can be made. However, in our practice, in addition to a baseline ECG, we generally suggest that an ECG be repeated after every 40–60 mg/day increase in dosage.

It should also be noted that ziprasidone-associated mania has been described (Keating et al. 2005). The mechanism for this action and the frequency of this occurrence in young people remain empirical questions for which further research is needed.

Combination Pharmacotherapy

Much of the recent treatment research into pediatric bipolarity suggests that the use of lithium, mood stabilizers, and atypical antipsychotics may be effective as drug monotherapy in treating this illness. However, there is increasing evidence to suggest that combination pharmacotherapy, consisting of more than one agent, might be appropriate for some patients. These include inpatients, youth with psychosis, and patients who have only a partial response to one class of medications. It appears that most clinicians opt to treat pediatric mania with psychosis with either lithium or divalproex sodium in combination with an atypical antipsychotic.

Combining lithium with divalproex sodium has also demonstrated effectiveness in treating pediatric mania (Findling et al. 2003). However, there are data to suggest that lithium, in combination with other antipsychotics, may also be a rational therapeutic strategy (Kafantaris et al. 2001). Similarly, adjunctive administration of quetiapine with divalproex has been found to be an effective approach in pediatric bipolar illness (DelBello et al. 2002). In addition, risperidone administered concomitantly with either lithium or divalproex sodium has been noted to be an effective combination treatment (Pavuluri et al. 2004).

Despite the fact that combination pharmacotherapy may be a reasonable mood-stabilizing strategy for some patients, this observation should not be used to infer that all patients should be treated with more than one thymoleptic. Unfortunately, at present, identifying which patients will or will not respond to drug monotherapy prior to treatment initiation is not possible. For this reason, with the exception of mania accompanied by psychosis, and mania of the severity requiring inpatient hospitalization, we generally recommend that mood-stabilizer pharmacotherapy for children with bipolar disorder begin with one agent.

There appears to be a significant number of young patients with bipolar illness who are being treated with multiple medications (sometimes in excess of five psychotropic agents) concurrently. Because of the inherent risks of such combinations, this degree of polypharmacy should be avoided, if at all possible. Clinicians should remember that incremental benefits should be seen when a new medication is added to an existing pharmacological regimen that has been partially effective. If improvement is not clearly observed with the addition of a new drug, it is not recommended that more medications simply be added to a youth's pharmacological regimen. Rather, it is recommended that the potential benefit and risk of each agent be assessed and the option of discontinuing one or more of the agents be considered for mood stabilization.

Besides mood states that can be difficult to manage in pediatric bipolarity, it should be recalled that psychiatric comorbidity is the rule, not the exception, in pediatric bipolar disorder. Therefore, the clinician should pay careful attention to discerning whether other psychiatric conditions are present when faced with a young patient with bipolarity. Unfortunately, there are very few data available about how to treat psychiatric comorbidities in pediatric bipolar illness.

The best evidence available pertains to the treatment of comorbid attention-deficit/hyperactivity disorder (ADHD). Scheffer et al. (2005) demonstrated that addition of mixed amphetamine salts was effective in treating ADHD symptoms after mood stabilization with divalproex monotherapy was established. Similarly, it was found that in youths who had achieved a stable mood with lithium and/or divalproex sodium, treatment with stimulants did not lead to an increased risk of relapse when compared with youths who were not treated with a psychostimulant (Findling et al. 2005).

Conclusions

Quite a bit of progress has occurred over the past 10 years in the pharmacological treatment of pediatric bipolar disorder. Clinicians are now better able to both recognize and more effectively treat this condition. Continued research into the phenomenology, longitudinal course, genetics, and therapeutics of this spectrum of illnesses will eventually provide insights into the pathophysiology of pediatric bipolar disorder. Those insights, in turn, should contribute to the development of a broader, evidence-based foundation for pediatric bipolarity's identification and management. As research into those domains continues, and as a better appreciation and understanding of the development and course of the illness develops, it is possible these avenues of research may eventually lead to useful preventive strategies for this chronic, debilitating illness.

Clinical Pearls

The clinical pearls below might be helpful when considering pharmacotherapy for a young person with bipolar illness. Although many of the concepts noted are applicable to the pharmacotherapy of young people in general, the reasons for which these constructs are particularly salient in the medication treatment of this population are also noted.

- Be sure the diagnosis is correct. In many instances, pediatric bipolar disorder is a difficult diorder to diagnose. As many of the treatments for this condition are associated with risks of side effects, it is important to be sure the right patients are receiving the correct interventions.

- Select an evidence-based medication regimen. Many medications are not adequately studied in pediatric populations. However, treatment efficacy and tolerability may differ between adults and youths. For this reason, it is important to consider selecting a medication regimen that is based on scientific data from pediatric populations.

- Use the right dose of medication. Several agents that may be useful in the treatment of pediatric bipolar illness have narrow therapeutic windows, with some medicines requiring therapeutic drug concentration monitoring. In addition, many agents will be less effective if underdosed or may be less safe if prescribed at too high a dose. Thus, it is important to use the right dose of medication.

- Ensure the medication trial continues for an adequate period of time. Some drugs do not provide noteworthy salutary effects until after several weeks of treatment have been provided at an appropriate dose. Thus, in order to confirm or refute a medication's effects in a given patient, in some instances several weeks of treatment are required.

- Be aware of any psychiatric comorbidities. Comorbidities might contribute to what seemingly is "treatment nonresponse." Pediatric bipolar illness is oftentimes associated with other psychiatric illnesses. Thus, even if the pediatric bipolar illness is treated effectively, substantive psychiatric symptomatology might remain. For this reason, it is important to distinguish between residual mood symptomatology from the patient's bipolar illness and untreated psychiatric comorbidity.

- Carefully assess for side effects. The medications used in the treatment of pediatric bipolarity may be associated with substantive risks. Thus, vigilant monitoring for these risks is important in hopes of reducing the likelihood of serious untoward events happening to the patient.

- Remove agents that might be exacerbating the illness. Some medications can worsen the course of illness in some patients. For this reason, it is important to ensure a youngster is not being prescribed a medication that is making matters worse rather than better.

References

American Diabetes Association, American Psychiatric Association, American Association of Clinical Endocrinologists, North American Association for the Study of Obesity: Consensus and development conference on antipsychotic drugs and obesity and diabetes. J Clin Psychiatry 65:267–272, 2004

Barnett MS: Ziprasidone monotherapy in pediatric bipolar disorder. J Child Adolesc Psychopharmacol 14:471–477, 2004

Barzman DH, DelBello MP, Kowatch RA, et al: The effectiveness and tolerability of aripiprazole for pediatric bipolar disorders: a retrospective chart review. J Child Adolesc Psychopharmacol 14:593–600, 2004

Benedetti A, Lattanzi L, Pini S, et al: Oxcarbazepine as add-on treatment in patients with bipolar manic, mixed or depressive episodes. J Affect Disord 79:273–277, 2004

Biederman J, Mick E, Faraone SV, et al: A prospective follow-up study of pediatric bipolar disorder in boys with attention-deficit/hyperactivity disorder. J Affect Disord 82(suppl):S17–S23, 2004

Biederman J, McDonnell MA, Wozniak J, et al: Aripiprazole in the treatment of pediatric bipolar disorder: a systematic chart review. CNS Spectr 10:141–148, 2005a

Biederman J, Mick E, Hammerness P, et al: Open-label, 8-week trial of olanzapine and risperidone for the treatment of bipolar disorder in preschool-age children. Biol Psychiatry 58:589–594, 2005b

Biederman J, Mick E, Wozniak J, et al: An open-label trial of risperidone in children and adolescents with bipolar disorder. J Child Adolesc Psychopharmacol 15:311–317, 2005c

Blair J, Scahill L, State M, et al: Electrocardiographic changes in children and adolescents treated with ziprasidone: a prospective study. J Am Acad Child Adolesc Psychiatry 44:73–79, 2005

Carandang CG, Maxwell DJ, Robbins DR, et al: Lamotrigine in adolescent mood disorders. J Am Acad Child Adolesc Psychiatry 42:750–751, 2003

Chang K, Saxena K, Howe M: An open-label study of lamotrigine adjunct or monotherapy for the treatment of adolescents with bipolar depression. J Am Acad Child Adolesc Psychiatry 45:298–304, 2006

Cooper TB, Bergner PE, Simpson GM: The 24-hour serum lithium level as a prognosticator of dosage requirements. Am J Psychiatry 130:601–602, 1973

Craven C, Murphy M: Carbamazepine treatment of bipolar disorder in an adolescent with cerebral palsy. J Am Acad Child Adolesc Psychiatry 39:680–681, 2000

Daniel DG: Tolerability of ziprasidone: an expanding perspective. J Clin Psychiatry 64(suppl):40–49, 2003

Davanzo P, Nikore V, Yehya N, et al: Oxcarbazepine treatment of juvenile-onset bipolar disorder. J Child Adolesc Psychopharmacol 14:344–345, 2004

DelBello MP, Schwiers ML, Rosenberg HL, et al: A double-blind, randomized, placebo-controlled study of quetiapine as adjunctive treatment for adolescent mania. J Am Acad Child Adolesc Psychiatry 41:1216–1223, 2002

DelBello MP, Findling RL, Kushner S, et al: A pilot controlled trial of topiramate for mania in children and adolescents with bipolar disorder. J Am Acad Child Adolesc Psychiatry 44:539–547, 2005

DelBello MP, Kowatch RA, Adler CM, et al: A double-blind randomized pilot study comparing quetiapine and divalproex for adolescent mania. J Am Acad Child Adolesc Psychiatry 45:305–313, 2006

Findling RL, Gracious BL, McNamara NK, et al: Rapid, continuous cycling and psychiatric comorbidity in pediatric bipolar I disorder. Bipolar Disord 3:202–210, 2001

Findling RL, McNamara NK, Gracious B, et al: Combination lithium and divalproex sodium in pediatric bipolarity. J Am Acad Child Adolesc Psychiatry 42:895–901, 2003

Findling RL, McNamara NK, Youngstrom EA, et al: Double-blind 18-month trial of lithium versus divalproex maintenance treatment in pediatric bipolar disorder. J Am Acad Child Adolesc Psychiatry 44:409–417, 2005

Frazier JA, Meyer MC, Biederman J, et al: Risperidone treatment for juvenile bipolar disorder: a retrospective chart review. J Am Acad Child Adolesc Psychiatry 38:960–965, 1999

Frazier JA, Biederman J, Tohen M, et al: A prospective open-label treatment trial of olanzapine monotherapy in children and adolescents with bipolar disorder. J Child Adolesc Psychopharmacol 11:239–250, 2001

Geller B, Fetner HH: Children's 24-hour serum lithium level after a single dose of predicts initial dose and steady-state plasma levels. J Clin Psychopharmacol 9:155, 1989

Geller B, William M, Zimerman D, et al: Prepubertal and early adolescent bipolarity differentiate from ADHD by manic symptoms, grandiose delusions, ultra-rapid or ultradian cycling. J Affect Disord 51:81–91, 1998

Geller B, Tillman R, Craney JL, et al: Four-year prospective outcome and natural history of mania in children with a prepubertal and early adolescent bipolar phenotype. Arch Gen Psychiatry 61:459–467, 2004

Hagino OR, Weller EB, Weller RA, et al: Comparison of lithium dosage methods for preschool and early school-age children. J Am Acad Child Adolesc Psychiatry 37:60–65, 1998

Hazaray E, Ehret J, Posey DJ, et al: Intramuscular ziprasidone for acute agitation in adolescents. J Child Adolesc Psychopharmacol 14:464–470, 2004

Hummel B, Walden J, Stamper R, et al: Acute antimanic efficacy and safety of oxcarbazepine in an open-label trial with an on-off-on design. Bipolar Disord 4:412–417, 2002

Joffe H, Hall JE, Cohen LS, et al: A putative relationship between valproic acid and polycystic ovarian syndrome: implications for treatment of women with seizure and bipolar disorders. Harv Rev Psychiatry 11:99–108, 2003

Joffe RT, Brasch JS, MacQueen GM: Psychiatric aspects of endocrine disorders in women. Psychiatric Clin North Am 26:683–691, 2003a

Kafantaris V, Coletti DJ, Dicker R, et al: Adjunctive antipsychotic treatment of adolescents with bipolar psychosis. J Am Acad Child Adolesc Psychiatry 40:1448–1456, 2001

Kafantaris V, Coletti DJ, Dicker R, et al: Lithium treatment of acute mania in adolescents: a large open trial. J Am Acad Child Adolesc Psychiatry 42:1038–1045, 2003

Keating AM, Aoun SL, Dean CE: Ziprasidone-associated mania: a review and report of 2 additional cases. Clin Neuropharmacol 28:83–86, 2005

Keck PE Jr, Marcus R, Tourkodimitris S, et al: A placebo-controlled, double-blind study of the efficacy and safety of aripiprazole in patients with acute bipolar mania. Am J Psychiatry 160:1651–1658, 2003

Kowatch RA, Suppes T, Carmody TJ, et al: Effect size of lithium, divalproex sodium, and carbamazepine in children and adolescents with bipolar disorder. J Am Acad Child Adolesc Psychiatry 39:713–720, 2000

Kowatch RA, Sethuraman G, Hume JH, et al: Combination pharmacotherapy in children and adolescents with bipolar disorder. Biol Psychiatry 53:978–984, 2003

Kowatch RA, Fristad M, Birmaher B, et al: Treatment guidelines for children and adolescents with bipolar disorder. J Child Adolesc Psychopharmacol 44:213–235, 2005

Kudriakova TB, Sirtoa LA, Rozova GI, et al: Autoinduction and steady-state pharmacokinetics of carbamazepine and its major metabolites. Br J Clin Pharmacol 33:611–615, 1992

Marchand WR, Wirth L, Simon C: Quetiapine adjunctive monotherapy for pediatric bipolar disorder: a retrospective chart review. J Child Adolesc Psychopharmacol 14:405–411, 2004

Masi G, Mucci M, Millepiedi S: Clozapine in adolescent inpatients with acute mania. J Child Adolesc Psychopharmacol 12:93–99, 2002

National Institute of Mental Health: Abnormal Involuntary Movement Scale (AIMS). Psychopharmacol Bull 21:1077–1080, 1985

Nelson-DeGrave VL, Wickenheisser JK, Cockrell JE, et al: Valproate potentiates androgen biosynthesis in human ovarian theca cells. Endocrinology 145:799–808, 2004

Papatheodorou G, Kutcher SP, Katic M, et al: The efficacy and safety of divalproex sodium in the treatment of acute mania in adolescents and young adults: an open clinical trial. J Clin Psychopharmacol 15:110–116, 1995

Pavuluri MN, Henry DB, Carbray JA, et al: Open-label prospective trial of risperidone in combination with lithium or divalproex sodium in pediatric mania. J Affect Disord 82(suppl):S103–S111, 2004

Pavuluri MN, Henry DB, Carbray JA, et al: Divalproex sodium for pediatric mixed mania: a 6-month prospective trial. Bipolar Disord 7:266–273, 2005

Qin K, Ehrmann DA, Cox N, et al: Identification of a functional polymorphism of the human type 5 17beta-hydroxysteroid dehydrogenase gene associated with polycystic ovarian syndrome. J Clin Endocrinol Metab 91:270–276, 2006

Scheffer RE, Kowatch RA, Carmody T, et al: Randomized, placebo-controlled trial of mixed amphetamine salts for symptoms of comorbid ADHD in pediatric bipolar disorder after mood stabilization with divalproex sodium. Am J Psychiatry 162:58–64, 2005

Soutullo CA, Sorter MT, Foster KD, et al: Olanzapine in the treatment of adolescent acute mania: a report of seven cases. J Affect Disord 53:279–283, 1999

Soutullo CA, Díez-Suárez A, Figueroa-Quintana A: Adjunctive lamotrigine treatment for adolescents with bipolar disorder: retrospective report of five cases, J Child Adolesc Psychopharmacol 16:357–364, 2006

Staller JA: Intramuscular ziprasidone in youth: a retrospective chart review. J Child Adolesc Psychopharmacol 14:590–592, 2004

Teitelbaum M: Oxcarbazepine in bipolar disorder. J Am Acad Child Adolesc Psychiatry 40:993–994, 2001

Tohen M, Kryzhanovskaya L, Carlson G, et al: Olanzapine in the treatment of acute mania in adolescents with bipolar I disorder: a 3-week randomized double-blind placebo-controlled study. Neuropsychopharmacology 30(suppl):S176–S177, 2005

Tuzun U, Zoroglu SS, Savas HA: A 5-year-old boy with recurrent mania successfully treated with carbamazepine. Psychiatry Clin Neurosci 56:589–591, 2002

Wagner KD, Weller EB, Carlson GE, et al: An open-label trial of divalproex in children and adolescents with bipolar disorder. J Am Acad Child Adolesc Psychiatry 41:1224–1230, 2002

Wagner KD, Kowatch RA, Emslie GJ, et al: A double-blind, randomized, placebo-controlled trial of oxcarbazepine in the treatment of bipolar disorder in children and adolescents. Am J Psychiatry 163:1179–1186, 2006

Weller EB, Weller RA, Fristad MA: Lithium dosage guide for prepubertal children: a preliminary report. J Am Acad Child Adolesc Psychiatry 25:92–95, 1986

Wood JR, Nelson-DeGrave VL, Jansen E, et al: Valproate-induced alterations in human theca gene expression: clues to the association between valproate use and metabolic side effects. Physiol Genomics 20:233–243, 2005

Woolston JL: Case study: carbamazepine treatment of juvenile-onset bipolar disorder. J Am Acad Child Adolesc Psychiatry 38:335–338, 1999

7

Autism and Other Pervasive Developmental Disorders

Kimberly A. Stigler, M.D.

Craig A. Erickson, M.D.

David J. Posey, M.D.

Christopher J. McDougle, M.D.

This work was supported in part by a Research Unit on Pediatric Psychopharmacology Psychosocial Intervention grant (U10-MH66766) from the National Institute of Mental Health (NIMH) to Indiana University (Drs. McDougle, Stigler, and Posey), a Department of Housing and Urban Development grant (B-01-SP-IN-0200) (Dr. McDougle), a Daniel X. Freedman Psychiatric Research Fellowship Award (Dr. Stigler), a Research Career Development Award (K23-MH068627) from the NIMH (Dr. Posey), and a National Institutes of Health Clinical Research Center grant (M01-RR00750) to Indiana University.

In 1943, Leo Kanner presented 11 case histories illustrating a syndrome in which the "pathognomonic, fundamental disorder is the children's inability to relate themselves in the ordinary way to people and situations from the beginning of life" (Kanner 1943, p. 140). Several common characteristics were described, such as an autistic aloneness, impaired language development, stereotypies, literalness, and a need for sameness. In this compelling article, Kanner illustrated the clinical entity known today as *autistic disorder*.

Thirty-seven years later, the publication of DSM-III (American Psychiatric Association 1980) heralded the inclusion of infantile autism among its formal diagnoses. Many of Kanner's initial findings were reflected in the criteria of the DSM-III, as well as in subsequent revisions. The pervasive developmental disorders (PDDs), presently classified in DSM-IV-TR (American Psychiatric Association 2000), include autistic disorder (autism), Asperger's disorder, Rett's disorder, childhood disintegrative disorder, and pervasive developmental disorder not otherwise specified (PDD NOS). Similar to Kanner's observations, current criteria include severe impairments in social interaction and communication, as well as restricted interests and activities. In this chapter we focus on the pharmacotherapy of autism, Asperger's disorder, and PDD NOS—the most commonly diagnosed PDDs.

Epidemiological surveys of PDDs began in the 1960s in England (Lotter 1966). Since that time, numerous surveys have been conducted in many countries. Methodological differences existing among the studies make comparisons between the surveys difficult. From 1966 to 1993, the median prevalence rate for autism was 4.7/10,000 (Fombonne 2005). However, the median prevalence rate from 1994 to 2004 was higher, at 12.7/10,000. Currently, the working rate of autism is 13/10,000, and the rates of Asperger's disorder and PDD NOS are 2.6/10,000 and 20.8/10,000, respectively. A conservative estimate of 36.4/10,000 for all PDDs has been reported. However, other recent surveys have generated even higher rates (Bertrand et al. 2001; Chakrabarti and Fombonne 2005; Gurney et al. 2003; Scott et al. 2002), resulting in an overall estimate of 60/10,000 for all PDDs.

Autism is approximately four times more common in males than in females and is often associated with mental retardation (Fombonne 1999). The etiology of autism is unknown but appears to be multifactorial. Investigations into the pathophysiology of autism have involved studies in neurochemistry, neuroanatomy, genetics, neuroimmunology, and neuroendocrinology. Among these areas of exploration, twin and family studies robustly support a genetic factor (Wassink and Piven 2000).

The variability of outcome among individuals with PDDs was observed shortly after autism was first described (Kanner and Eisenberg 1956). Although much research into the variables contributing toward outcome has been conducted, two factors are consistently associated with prognosis: early language development and IQ. Lord and Bailey (2002) reported that the presence of useful speech by age 5 years was greatly predictive of a positive outcome. With regard to IQ, many studies have found an association between outcome and cognitive ability (Howlin et al. 2004; Rutter et al. 1967).

The therapeutic approach to the management of autism and related disorders is multimodal. Because approximately 75% of persons affected with autism have some degree of mental retardation, educational interventions are particularly important. In addition, many exhibit delays in language development, thus making speech therapy essential to improving outcome. Occupational therapy, social skills training, and physical therapy are also frequently necessary. Educating caregivers in behavioral management techniques can be very useful and may decrease the use of pharmacotherapy in this population.

In addition to nonpharmacological approaches, medication is often required to diminish severe maladaptive behaviors. The decision to prescribe medication to youth with PDDs can significantly impact their ability to benefit from behavioral and educational interventions. To date, risperidone is the only U.S. Food and Drug Administration (FDA)–approved drug in autism. Although no other medications have FDA approval for use in PDDs, a variety of drugs are utilized to treat interfering target symptoms in this population. In this chapter, we present evidence to date regarding the pharmacotherapy of PDDs (Table 7–1) and review the adverse effects of the medications used and practical management strategies.

Atypical Antipsychotics

Research into the pharmacotherapy of PDDs began in the 1960s, with the typical antipsychotics. Because of significant adverse effects associated with the low-potency antipsychotics, the high-potency antipsychotic haloperidol was systematically investigated in numerous well-designed studies (L. T. Anderson et al. 1989; Campbell et al. 1978; Cohen et al. 1980). However, haloperi-

Table 7–1. Selected published double-blind, placebo-controlled trials in pervasive developmental disorders

Drug	Study	N	Age	Design	Results
Antipsychotics					
Haloperidol	L. T. Anderson et al. 1989	45	2–7 years	12 weeks, crossover	Haloperidol > placebo
Risperidone	McDougle et al. 1998b	31	Adults	12 weeks, parallel groups	Risperidone > placebo (8/14 [57%] responders)
Risperidone	RUPP Autism Network 2002	101	5–17 years	8 weeks, parallel groups	Risperidone > placebo (34/49 [69%] responders)
Risperidone	Shea et al. 2004	79	5–12 years	8 weeks, parallel groups	Risperidone > placebo (35/40 [88%] responders)
Serotonin reuptake inhibitors					
Clomipramine	Gordon et al. 1993	30	6–23 years	10 weeks, crossover	Clomipramine > placebo; Clomipramine > desipramine (19/28 [68%] responders)
Clomipramine	Remington et al. 2001	36	10–36 years	7 weeks, crossover	Clomipramine > placebo
Fluvoxamine	McDougle et al. 1996a	30	Adults	12 weeks, parallel groups	Fluvoxamine > placebo (8/15 [53%] responders)
Fluvoxamine	Sugie et al. 2005	18	3–8 years	12 weeks, parallel groups	Fluvoxamine > placebo (10/18 [55%] responders)
Fluoxetine	Buchsbaum et al. 2001	6	Adults	16 weeks, crossover	Fluoxetine > placebo (3/6 [50%] responders)
Fluoxetine	Hollander et al. 2005	39	5–16 years	20 weeks, crossover	Fluoxetine > placebo

Table 7–1. Selected published double-blind, placebo-controlled trials in pervasive developmental disorders *(continued)*

Drug	Study	Subjects			Design	Results
		N	Age			
Alpha$_2$-adrenergic agonists						
Clonidine	Jaselskis et al. 1992	8	5–13 years		14 weeks, crossover	Clonidine > placebo by teacher and parent, but not clinician, ratings (6/8 [75%] responders)
Clonidine (transdermal)	Fankhauser et al. 1992	9	5–33 years		10 weeks, crossover	Clonidine > placebo (6/9 [67%] responders)
Psychostimulants						
Methylphenidate	Quintana et al. 1995	10	7–11 years		4 weeks, crossover	Methylphenidate > placebo
Methylphenidate	Handen et al. 2000	13	5–11 years		3 weeks, crossover	Methylphenidate > placebo (8/13 [62%] responders)
Methylphenidate	RUPP Autism Network 2005a	72	5–14 years		4 weeks, crossover	Methylphenidate > placebo (35/72 [49%] responders)

Note. RUPP = Research Units on Pediatric Psychopharmacology.

dol's potent dopamine D_2 receptor antagonism frequently led to acute dystonic reactions, as well as drug-induced and withdrawal-related dyskinesias (Campbell et al. 1997). Currently, the typical antipsychotics as a whole are reserved for individuals with severe treatment-resistant symptoms.

Concerns regarding the typical antipsychotics directed researchers toward the development of the atypical antipsychotics. These drugs, with their profile of potent antagonism at serotonin (5-hydroxytryptamine, 5-HT) and dopamine receptors, have a purported decreased risk of acute extrapyramidal symptoms (EPS) and tardive dyskinesia (TD).

Clozapine

Clozapine is an antagonist at the serotonin $5-HT_{2A}$, $5-HT_{2C}$, and $5-HT_3$ receptors and the dopamine D_1, D_2, D_3, and D_4 receptors (Baldessarini and Frankenburg 1991). There are three known reports on the use of this drug in autism (Chen et al. 2001; Gobbi and Pulverenti 2001; Zuddas et al. 1996). The lack of research on clozapine in PDDs is largely due to the drug's adverse-effect profile. The propensity of clozapine to lower the seizure threshold is troubling, particularly in a patient population predisposed to develop seizures. In addition, individuals with cognitive limitations and an impaired ability to communicate would have difficulty conveying symptoms associated with agranulocytosis and tolerating frequent venipuncture.

Risperidone

At present, risperidone is the only medication that is approved by the FDA for the treatment of irritability and associated dysfunctional behaviors in youth, ages 5–16 years, with autism. Risperidone has high affinities for serotonin $5-HT_{1D}$, $5-HT_{2A}$, and $5-HT_{2C}$ receptors; dopamine D_2, D_3, and D_4 receptors; α_1-adrenergic receptors; and H_1-histaminic receptors; and negligible affinities for muscarinic receptors (Leysen et al. 1988). There have been several open-label studies demonstrating risperidone to effectively target core and related symptoms of PDDs (Findling et al. 1997; Masi et al. 2001a; McDougle et al. 1997; Nicolson et al. 1998). The efficacy of risperidone was considered in a 12-week double-blind, placebo-controlled study of adults with autism ($n=17$) or PDD NOS ($n=14$) (McDougle et al. 1998b). Eight (57%) of 14 subjects randomly assigned to risperidone (mean dosage=2.9 mg/day), versus none in the placebo group, were deemed responders as measured by the Clinical Global Impression Improvement (CGI-I) scale. The most common adverse effect was transient somnolence. Weight gain was reported in only two of the subjects in the risperidone group.

The first double-blind, placebo-controlled study of risperidone in youth was conducted by the Research Units on Pediatric Psychopharmacology (RUPP) Autism Network (2002). In this short-term study, 101 children and adolescents (mean age=8.8 years) with target symptoms of tantrums, aggression, or self-injurious behavior were treated with risperidone or placebo. Risperidone treatment at a mean dosage of 1.8 mg/day (range=0.5–3.5 mg/day) was found to reduce the Irritability subscale score of the Aberrant Behavior Checklist (ABC) by 56.9% versus 14.1% with placebo. Overall, 69% of risperidone-treated subjects were judged responders, as compared with only 12% of those given placebo. Adverse effects of risperidone included weight gain (mean 2.7 kg vs. 0.8 kg with placebo), increased appetite, sedation, dizziness, and hypersalivation. Further analyses revealed the drug to be significantly more effective for reducing interfering stereotypical and repetitive behavior (McDougle et al. 2005).

The RUPP Autism Network subsequently published results of an open-label extension study to the aforementioned short-term study (Research Units on Pediatric Psychopharmacology Autism Network 2005b). This 16-week study involved 63 of the subjects who responded to risperidone in the 8-week trial. The mean risperidone dose remained stable. Subjects in this study continued to gain weight (mean=5.1 kg). Overall, only 8% discontinued the drug because of loss of efficacy; one subject discontinued the drug because of adverse effects. At the end of this phase, 32 subjects who were considered responders were then randomly assigned to receive continued risperidone versus gradual substitution with placebo over a duration of 4 weeks. A statistically significant difference in relapse rate was reported, with 10 (62.5%) of 16 subjects gradually switched to placebo relapsing versus 2 (12.5%) of 16 who continued on risperidone.

A second double-blind, placebo-controlled study of risperidone in children and adolescents with PDDs has been published (Shea et al. 2004). Seventy-nine youth, ages 5–12 years, were randomly assigned to receive risperidone at a mean dosage of 1.17 mg/day or placebo over a duration of 8 weeks. Overall, 87% of risperidone-treated subjects improved compared with 40%

of the subjects who were given placebo. In addition, there was a 64% reduction on the ABC Irritability subscale score versus 31% who received placebo. In regard to adverse effects, weight gain was more common in the risperidone group (2.7 kg vs. 1.0 kg with the placebo group), as was increased sedation, heart rate, and systolic blood pressure.

Olanzapine

Olanzapine has high affinity for dopamine D_1, D_2, D_4 receptors; serotonin 5-HT_{2A}, 5-HT_{2C}, and 5-HT_3 receptors; α_1-adrenergic receptors; H_1-histaminic receptors; and muscarinic receptors (Bymaster et al. 1996). Olanzapine has been found to be beneficial in PDDs in case reports, in an open-label trial, and in an open-label comparison with haloperidol (Malone et al. 2001). However, significant weight gain, along with its possible associated metabolic sequelae, has restricted its use in this population. The 12-week, open-label trial evaluated the use of olanzapine in eight patients, ages 5–42 years (Potenza et al. 1999). At a mean dosage of 7.8 ± 4.7 mg/day (range=5–20 mg/day), six (86%) of the seven patients who completed the trial were considered responders based on the CGI-I scale. Aggression, self-injurious behavior, irritability, hyperactivity, and overall symptoms of autism were found to be significantly improved. Despite the drug's positive effect, considerable weight gain was reported in six patients. The mean weight was found to increase from 62.5 ± 25.4 kg to 70.9 ± 25 kg at the 12-week endpoint. Sedation was also reported in three patients.

Quetiapine

Quetiapine has affinity for dopamine D_1 and D_2 receptors; serotonin 5-HT_{2A} and 5-HT_{1A} receptors; and H_1-histaminic receptors (Arnt and Skarsfeldt 1998). The drug has been investigated in an uncontrolled fashion, with mixed findings. A 16-week, open-label trial of the drug was conducted with six subjects (mean age=10.9 years) (Martin et al. 1999). Two youth who completed the trial were considered responders. Three withdrew because of sedation and lack of effectiveness, and one dropped out after a possible seizure. Overall, no statistically significant improvement was reported. A recent retrospective review was conducted of all patients in an outpatient PDD clinic (Corson et al. 2004). Patients who had received quetiapine for at least 4 weeks and who were not being concurrently treated with another antipsychotic or mood stabilizer were included in the study. Twenty patients, ages 5–28 years (mean age= 12.1±6.7 years), were included in the study and received a quetiapine trial (mean dosage=248.7±198.4 mg/day, range=25–600 mg/day) over a mean duration of 59.8 weeks (range=4–180 weeks). Of the 20 patients, 8 (40%) were considered responders to quetiapine. Adverse effects were reported in 50% of the patients, and 15% subsequently discontinued the drug.

Ziprasidone

Ziprasidone is a potent antagonist at dopamine D_1 and D_2 receptors and serotonin 5-HT_{2A} and 5-HT_{2C} receptors (Tandon et al. 1997). In addition, it is a 5-HT_{1A} receptor agonist that also inhibits serotonin and norepinephrine reuptake. A case series of ziprasidone in 12 patients, ages 8–20 years (mean age=11.6±4.4 years), with autism (n=9) or PDD NOS (n=3) has been published (McDougle et al. 2002). Six (50%) of the patients responded to the drug, as assessed by the CGI-I, at a mean dosage of 59.2±34.8 mg/day (range=20–120 mg/day) over a duration of at least 6 weeks. Treatment with ziprasidone resulted in improvement in symptoms of aggression, agitation, and irritability. The most common adverse effect was transient sedation. Mean weight change was −5.83 pounds (range=−35.5 to +6 pounds). No cardiovascular adverse effects were reported.

Aripiprazole

Aripiprazole is a partial dopamine D_2 and serotonin 5-HT_{1A} agonist, and a serotonin 5-HT_{2A} antagonist (Burris et al. 2002). In a prospective, open-label case series involving five children and adolescents with autism, ages 5–18 years (Stigler et al. 2004b). all five subjects were judged responders after a minimum of 8 weeks of treatment (range=8–16 weeks). At a mean dosage of 12 mg/day (range=10–15 mg/day), significant improvement was noted in a variety of interfering behaviors, including aggression, self-injury, and irritability. The drug was well tolerated. Two of the five case patients experienced mild transient sedation. No acute EPS or significant changes in heart rate or blood pressure were recorded. In this study, two patients lost weight, two had no change, and one gained 2.2 kg (mean=−3.7 kg; range=−13.6 to +2.2 kg). The weight loss was attributed to discontinuation of prior atypical antipsychotic treatments that had produced significant weight gain.

Serotonin Reuptake Inhibitors

Research into the pathophysiology of autism has often focused on the serotonergic system. Schain and Freedman (1961) first reported on elevated whole blood levels of serotonin in autistic children compared with control children. More recent reports have pointed to the possibility of abnormal maturational processes of the serotonergic system in autistic subjects, as exhibited by a lack of age-related serotonin decline in blood seen in normally developing subjects (G.M. Anderson et al. 1987; Leboyer et al. 1999).

Research into the genetic basis of a potential serotonergic abnormality in autistic disorder has yielded mixed results. Four studies have noted nominally significant excess transmission of alleles of the serotonin transporter gene, whereas three studies have reported no excess transmission (Conroy et al. 2004).

Other evidence suggesting the potential utility of drugs affecting serotonin in PDDs comes from findings of an exacerbation of behavioral symptoms in drug-free autistic adults undergoing acute dietary depletion of the serotonin precursor tryptophan (McDougle et al. 1996b).

Clomipramine

Clomipramine is a tricyclic agent that potently inhibits serotonin reuptake and also affects norepinephrine and dopamine reuptake. Clomipramine exhibits antiobsessional properties (Greist et al. 1995).

One open-label and two controlled studies have evaluated clomipramine in PDDs. In a 12-week open-label trial of clomipramine (mean dosage= 139.4 ± 50.4 mg/day) in 35 adults with PDDs, 18 (55%) of the 33 patients who completed the trial were judged, on the basis of the CGI-I, to have responded to treatment (Brodkin et al. 1997). Improvement was recorded in aggression, self-injurious behavior, repetitive phenomena, and social relatedness. Thirteen (39%) of the patients experienced significant adverse effects, including seizures (three patients), weight gain, constipation, sedation, and agitation.

Clomipramine (152 ± 56 mg/day) was found superior to the relatively selective norepinephrine reuptake inhibitor desipramine (127 ± 52 mg/day) and placebo in a 10-week, randomized, crossover study of 12 children with autism (mean age= 9.6 years) (Gordon et al. 1993). Improvement with clomipramine was associated with decreased anger and obsessive-compulsive symptoms. Adverse effects included prolongation of the cardiac-corrected (QTc) interval, tachycardia, and grand mal seizure. Similar tolerability issues were noted by Remington et al. (2001) in their report on a 7-week, double-blind, placebo-controlled trial of clomipramine (mean dosage = 128 mg/day), haloperidol (mean dosage = 1.3 mg/day), and placebo in 36 autistic patients (ages 10–36 years). Among patients who completed this trial, clomipramine and haloperidol were similarly effective in reducing irritability and stereotypy. However, significantly fewer individuals receiving clomipramine versus haloperidol were able to complete the trial (37.5% vs. 69.7%). Reasons for leaving the trial associated with clomipramine included lack of efficacy and the emergence of adverse effects, among which sedation and tremor were most prevalent. Because of tolerability issues, the use of clomipramine in PDDs remains limited.

Fluvoxamine

Fluvoxamine is a selective serotonin reuptake inhibitor (SSRI) that is FDA-approved for use in children and adolescents with obsessive-compulsive disorder (OCD). Fluvoxamine (mean dosage = 276.7 mg/day) reduced repetitive and maladaptive behavior in 8 (53%) of 15 autistic adults enrolled in a double-blind, placebo-controlled study (McDougle et al. 1996a). In these adults, fluvoxamine was generally well tolerated, with adverse effects including sedation and nausea. A double-blind, placebo-controlled study did not find fluvoxamine (mean dose = 107 mg/day) effective in 34 children and adolescents with PDDs (McDougle et al. 2000). In these younger patients, fluvoxamine was poorly tolerated, with 14 patients experiencing adverse effects, including hyperactivity, insomnia, aggression, and agitation. In an open-label report on 18 children (mean age = 11.3 ± 3.6 years) with PDDs who received low-dose fluvoxamine (1.5 mg/kg/day) for 10 weeks, fluvoxamine was similarly not associated with a significant treatment response (Martin et al. 2003). In a 12-week double-blind, placebo-controlled crossover study of fluvoxamine in 18 autistic children, Sugie et al. (2005) noted that 10 children (55%) had at least a mild treatment response, with 5 (28%) showing *excellent* drug response. In this report, fluvoxamine was generally well tolerated. Three children (17%) had to exit the study due to behavioral activation. Overall, although the findings are mixed, fluvoxamine appears to be better tolerated in adults as opposed to children with PDDs.

Fluoxetine

Fluoxetine is a SSRI approved for the treatment of OCD and major depressive disorder in youth. Two open-label and two controlled trials have evaluated the use of the SSRI fluoxetine in PDDs.

An open-label trial of fluoxetine (mean dosage = 37.1 mg/day) was conducted in seven persons with autism (ages 9–20 years) over a mean duration of 18 months (Fatemi et al. 1998). The authors recorded improvement in irritability, social relatedness, and stereotypy during the trial. Adverse effects included hyperactivity and decreased appetite. A second open-label trial enrolled 129 children (ages 2–8 years) with autism (DeLong et al. 2002). The patients received fluoxetine (0.15–0.5 mg/kg/day) over a mean duration of 34 months. Medication response was rated as *excellent* in 22 children (17%), *good* in 67 (52%), and *fair/poor* in 40 (31%). Aggression was the most prominent adverse effect noted in this trial.

A small, 16-week, placebo-controlled, crossover trial of fluoxetine in six adults with PDDs (five with autism, one with Asperger's disorder) noted significant drug-associated effect (Buchsbaum et al. 2001) as measured by the Yale-Brown Obsessive Compulsive Scale (Y-BOCS) (Goodman et al. 1989). A 20-week, placebo-controlled, crossover study of fluoxetine (mean dosage = 0.4 mg/kg/day, 9.9 mg/day, range = 2.4–20 mg/day) in 39 children (mean age = 8.2 years) with PDDs found the drug significantly better than placebo in reducing repetitive behaviors, as measured by the Children's Yale-Brown Obsessive Compulsive Scale (CY-BOCS) (Hollander et al. 2005; Scahill et al. 1997). No improvement on measures of speech or social interaction was noted, and adverse effects were not significantly different between fluoxetine and placebo.

Sertraline

Only open-label trials have described the use of the SSRI sertraline in PDDs. Sertraline is approved for the treatment of OCD in children.

McDougle et al. (1998a) found sertraline (mean dosage = 122 mg/day) effective at reducing aggression and repetitive behavior in a 12-week, open-label study of 42 adults with PDDs. Subjects with autism and PDD NOS showed significantly more improvement than those with Asperger's disorder. The authors attributed this response to the possibility that the patients with Asperger's disorder were less symptomatic at baseline. Three patients (7%) dropped out of the study because of worsening agitation and anxiety. An open-label trial of sertraline (25–50 mg/day for 2–8 weeks) was conducted in nine autistic children, ages 6–12 years (Steingard et al. 1997). Eight children (88%) showed improvement during the trial, manifesting reduced irritability, anxiety, and need for sameness.

Paroxetine

The SSRI paroxetine has been the subject of a few uncontrolled reports on PDDs. Two case reports have noted decreased irritable behavior associated with paroxetine use in a 15-year-old boy with autism (Snead et al. 1994) and a 7-year-old boy with autism (Posey et al. 1999). In a heterogeneous sample, 15 adults with mental retardation with or without a concomitant PDD received 16 weeks of open-label treatment with paroxetine (20–50 mg/day) (Davanzo et al. 1998). The drug was associated with reduced aggression after 1 month but not at the 4-month follow-up.

Citalopram

Two retrospective studies have evaluated the SSRI citalopram in PDDs. Citalopram has no approved indications for use in children.

In a retrospective case series, 17 youth with a PDD (ages 4–15 years) received citalopram (mean dosage = 19.7 ± 7.8 mg/day) over a mean duration of 7.4 months. Ten patients (59%) were responders as determined by the CGI-I (Couturier and Nicolson 2002). No improvements in social interaction or communication were noted. Four patients (24%) discontinued the drug due to adverse effects, including agitation, tics, and insomnia.

A retrospective review of citalopram (mean dosage = 16.9 ± 12.1 mg/day) was completed in 15 children and adolescents, ages 6–16 years, with PDDs over an average duration of 218.8 days (Namerow et al. 2003). Eleven patients (73%) were judged to be responders based on the CGI-I, with improvement in repetitive behaviors noted in 10 patients (66%), and irritability in 7 patients (47%). Of the responders, 9 of 10 reportedly had not responded to other SSRIs. Two of 5 patients experiencing adverse effects discontinued treatment. Side effects included headaches, sedation, agitation, and lip dyskinesias.

Escitalopram

Escitalopram, the *S*-enantiomer of citalopram, is not approved for any pediatric indication. A 10-week, open-label study of escitalopram (mean dosage = 11.1 mg/day) in 28 children and adolescents (mean age = 10.4 years) with PDDs found 17 (61%) were treatment responders, with response defined as a 50% reduction on the parent-rated ABC Irritability subscale (Owley et al. 2005). A wide variety of dose response was noted, with some patients unable to tolerate the drug at 10 mg/day, and others showing positive response at the lowest dosage, 2.5 mg/day.

Mirtazapine

Mirtazapine, a drug with both serotonergic and noradrenergic properties, has been evaluated in a single open-label trial in PDDs. Twenty-six individuals with PDDs were treated with mirtazapine (7.5–45 mg/day) over a mean duration of 150 days (Posey et al. 2001). Nine patients (35%) were considered treatment responders, as measured by the CGI-I, with reduced aggression, self-injury, irritability, hyperactivity, anxiety, insomnia, and depression. No effect on social relatedness or communication impairment was noted. Adverse effects were considered mild and included increased appetite, irritability, and sedation.

Venlafaxine

The antidepressant venlafaxine is a dual serotonin and norepinephrine reuptake inhibitor. Low-dose venlafaxine (18.75 mg/day) was associated with decreased hyperactivity and irritability in two adolescents and one young adult with autism over 6 months of treatment (Carminati et al. 2006). A retrospective review of 10 children, adolescents, and young adults with PDDs treated with venlafaxine (6.25–50 mg/day) found that 6 patients (60%) were responders, as defined by the CGI-I (Hollander et al. 2000). The medication was reportedly well tolerated, and improvement was noted in repetitive behaviors, socialization, communication, and inattention. One case report noted increased aggressive behavior when venlafaxine (37.5 mg increased to 75 mg/day) was added to the treatment regimen of an adolescent female with autism on a stable dose of olanzapine (10 mg/day) (Marshall et al. 2003).

Buspirone

Buspirone is a serotonin $5\text{-}HT_{1A}$ receptor partial agonist approved for the treatment of adult generalized anxiety disorder. Several case reports and small open-label studies have reported on the effectiveness of buspirone in patients with autism. Larger open-label studies have generated conflicting results. An open-label study of buspirone (30–60 mg/day for 28–413 days) found the drug to be ineffective in treating target symptoms including aggression and self-injury in 26 adults with mental retardation, which included nine patients with PDDs (King and Davanzo 1996). In another open-label study, 22 children and adolescents with PDDs were treated with buspirone (15–45 mg/day) for 6 to 8 weeks (Buitelaar et al. 1998). Nine patients (41%) showed significant improvement as measured by the CGI-I, addressing target symptoms of anxiety and irritability. During a continuation phase for treatment responders, one child developed an orofacial-lingual dyskinesia after 10 months of treatment that remitted after drug discontinuation. No controlled studies of buspirone in PDDs have been reported.

Alpha$_2$-Adrenergic Agonists

Clonidine

The α_2-adrenergic agonist clonidine has been evaluated in two small, controlled trials involving patients with autism. A double-blind, placebo-controlled, crossover trial (6-week treatment periods) of clonidine (4–10 µg/kg/day) was conducted in eight autistic boys (mean age=8.1 years) who demonstrated symptoms of inattention, impulsivity, and hyperactivity (Jaselskis et al. 1992). The drug was associated with decreased hyperactivity and irritability on teacher and parent ratings, but no treatment-associated differences were found on clinician ratings. Adverse effects of clonidine included hypotension, sedation, and irritability. Transdermal clonidine (5 µg/kg/day) was evaluated in a double-blind, placebo-controlled, crossover study (4-week treatment phases) involving nine males (ages 5–33 years) with autism (Fankhauser et al. 1992). Significant improvement in hyperactivity and anxiety was recorded. The most commonly reported adverse effects were sedation and fatigue.

Guanfacine

The α_2-adrenergic agonist guanfacine has been evaluated in one retrospective study of 80 youth, ages 3–18 years, with PDDs (Posey et al. 2004b). At a mean guanfacine dosage of 2.6 ± 1.7 mg/day, 19 children (23.8%) were judged responders, as assessed with the CGI-I over a mean duration of 334 days. Decreased symptoms of hyperactivity, inattention, and tics were reported. Guanfacine was generally well tolerated and did not alter blood pressure or heart rate. Sedation was the most commonly reported side effect.

Psychostimulants

Psychostimulants are considered first-line agents for the treatment of hyperactivity and inattention in patients diagnosed with attention-deficit/hyperactivity disorder (ADHD) (Greenhill et al. 2002b). Whereas early reviews concluded that stimulants were generally ineffective and associated with adverse effects in patients with PDDs (Aman 1982; Campbell 1975), other trials have suggested that stimulants may be effective in this population. A double-blind, crossover study (2-week treatment phases) of methylphenidate (10 or 20 mg twice daily) was conducted in 10 children with autism, ages 7–11 years (Quintana et al. 1995). Overall, a modest benefit of methylphenidate treatment over placebo was found. Adverse effects included decreased appetite, insomnia, and irritability. Another double-blind, placebo-controlled, crossover study of methylphenidate (0.3 and 0.6 mg/kg/day) found a 50% reduction on the Conners' Hyperactivity Index in 8 (62%) of 13 children with autism (ages 5–11 years) (Handen et al. 2000). Adverse effects, more common at the 0.6 mg/kg/day dosage, included social withdrawal and irritability.

A large retrospective medical record review of 195 patients, ages 2–19 years, found stimulants to be generally ineffective and poorly tolerated for the majority of patients (Stigler et al. 2004a). Individuals with Asperger's disorder, in contrast to those with autism or PDD NOS, were significantly more likely to respond to a stimulant. Use of concomitant medication was found to positively affect response, whereas no association was found between stimulant type or IQ and response. Adverse effects, such as irritability, agitation, and dysphoria, occurred in more than half of the patients.

The RUPP Autism Network recently completed the largest controlled trial of a psychostimulant in PDDs to date (Research Units on Pediatric Psychopharmacology Autism Network 2005a). This study involved 72 youth, ages 5–14 years, with target symptoms of moderate-to-severe hyperactivity. Subjects entered a 1-week test-dose phase in which placebo and three doses (low, medium, high) of methylphenidate were administered. The 66 subjects who tolerated the test dose received 1 week each of placebo and of methylphenidate at three different dosages in random order during a 4-week, double-blind, crossover phase. Those who responded to methylphenidate then entered an 8-week open-label phase. Overall, 35 (49%) of 72 enrolled subjects responded to methylphenidate. Discontinuation of study medication due to adverse effects occurred in 13 (18%) of 72 subjects. These results are consistent with the findings of a smaller study of methylphenidate in 13 youth with PDDs (Di Martino et al. 2004). Within 1 hour of a single test dose (0.4 mg/kg), five individuals developed increased hyperactivity, stereotypy, dysphoria, or tics and were unable to tolerate the drug. Six of the remaining eight subjects responded to the drug, resulting in an overall response rate of 46%.

In contrast to these findings, the National Institute of Mental Health (NIMH) Multimodal Treatment Study of Children With ADHD (MTA) found 69% of subjects responded to methylphenidate treatment, with only 1.4% discontinuing due to adverse effects (Greenhill et al. 2002a). When compared with typically developing children with ADHD, methylphenidate seems less effective and is associated with more frequent adverse effects in youth with PDDs.

Atomoxetine

The selective norepinephrine reuptake inhibitor atomoxetine is approved for the treatment of children and adolescents with ADHD. Results of a recent open-label study suggest that the drug may decrease symptoms of motor hyperactivity and inattention in higher-functioning children and adolescents with PDDs (Posey et al. 2005). In this study, 16 children and adolescents, ages 6 to 14 years, with autism ($n=7$), Asperger's disorder ($n=7$), or PDD NOS ($n=2$) received atomoxetine at a mean dosage of 1.2 mg/kg/day. Twelve (75%) of 16 subjects were deemed responders. The drug was well tolerated, aside from two subjects who discontinued atomoxetine due to irritability.

Beta-Adrenergic Antagonists

Beta-adrenergic blockers are drugs that block norepinephrine receptors, thus limiting norepinephrine neurotransmission. Eight hospitalized adults with autism were described as having improvement in speech and socialization after open-label treatment with propranolol or nadolol (mean dosage=225 mg/day over 14.2 months) (Ratey et al. 1987). All patients showed a marked decrease in aggression. Six patients (75%) showed improved social skills, and four (50%) developed improved speech during treatment. Seven of the patients were taking concomitant antipsychotics during this trial, with five able to decrease, and one able to discontinue, treatment during the trial. The authors felt the improvement noted was due to decreased hyperarousal.

Mood Stabilizers

Valproic Acid

The mood stabilizer and antiepileptic drug valproic acid (divalproex sodium) (mean dosage=768 mg/day, mean blood level=75.8 µg/mL) was investigated in an open-label trial in 14 persons, ages 5–10 years, with PDDs (Hollander et al. 2001). Over an average treatment duration of 10.7 months (range 0.5–43 months), significant improvement was noted in 10 patients (71%), as measured by the CGI-I. Improvement was recorded in affective instability, repetitive behavior, impulsivity, and aggression. Adverse effects included sedation, weight gain, hair loss, elevated liver enzymes, and behavioral activation. Two patients left the trial within the first 2 weeks of treatment because of severe behavioral activation.

In an 8-week, double-blind, placebo-controlled trial of valproic acid in 13 patients with autism and associated, interfering repetitive behavior, treatment was associated with a significant reduction in repetitive phenomena as measured by the CY-BOCS (Hollander et al. 2006). An 8-week, double-blind, placebo-controlled study of valproic acid (mean blood level=77.8 µg/mL at 8 weeks) was conducted in 30 subjects, ages 6–20 years, with PDDs and significant aggressive behavior (Hellings et al. 2005). In this trial, treatment was not associated with significant improvement in irritability as measured by the ABC or by global symptoms as measured by the CGI-I. One subject developed a rash, which remitted after drug discontinuation, and two subjects developed elevated serum ammonia while taking valproic acid.

Lithium

Three case reports have described the use of the mood stabilizer lithium in patients with PDDs. Two reports have noted reduced manic-like symptoms in individuals with autism and a family history of bipolar disorder (Kerbeshian et al. 1987; Steingard and Biederman 1987). A single report of lithium augmentation of fluvoxamine treatment in an adult with autism noted improvement in symptoms of aggression and irritability after 2 weeks of treatment, as measured by the CGI-I (Epperson et al. 1994).

Lamotrigine

Lamotrigine is an anticonvulsant and mood stabilizer that attenuates some forms of glutamate release via inhibition of sodium, calcium, and potassium channels. The use of lamotrigine (mean dosage = 4.5 mg/kg/day) over a mean duration of 14 months was described in 13 children, ages 3–13 years, with autism and intractable epilepsy (Uvebrant and Bauziene 1994). Eight subjects (62%) showed a decrease in autistic symptoms. Adverse effects included sleep disturbance and rash. A 4-week, double-blind, placebo-controlled trial of lamotrigine (5 mg/kg/day) in 14 children, ages 3–11 years, with autism reported no treatment-associated effect as measured by the ABC, Childhood Autism Rating Scale, and Pre-Linguistic Autism Diagnostic Observation Scale (Belsito et al. 2001). Insomnia and hyperactivity were the most common side effects reported.

Cholinesterase Inhibitors

Donepezil

The cholinesterase inhibitor donepezil has been evaluated in two open-label reports in patients with PDDs. Improved speech was noted in 25 boys (mean age = 6.6 years) taking donepezil (2.5 or 5 mg/day) over 12 weeks of open-label treatment (Chez et al. 2000). No improvements in social relatedness were noted. Adverse effects included aggression, irritability, sedation, and sleep disturbance. A retrospective review of open-label donepezil add-on treatment (mean dosage=9.37±1.76 mg/day) in eight autistic children taking other psychotropic medications (ages 7–19 years) noted that four children (50%) responded positively to treatment as measured by the CGI-I (Hardan and Handen 2002). Among all subjects, ABC scores decreased on the Hyperactivity and Irritability subscales. In this review, donepezil was generally well tolerated, with one patient developing nausea and vomiting and one patient reporting mild irritability.

Rivastigmine

The cholinesterase inhibitor rivastigmine was evaluated in one 12-week open-label trial in 32 autistic patients (Chez et al. 2004a). Treatment-associated improvement was noted in expressive speech and overall autistic behavior using standardized measures.

Glutamatergic Agents

Amantadine

Amantadine, a compound used to treat influenza, herpes zoster, and Parkinson's disease, has known noncompetitive N-methyl-D-aspartate (NMDA) antagonist activity (Kornhuber et al. 1994). In a four-week, double-blind, placebo-controlled trial in 39 youth with autism (ages 5–19 years) amantadine (final dosage=5 mg/kg/day) was associated with improved clinician-rated Aberrant Behavior Checklist—Community Version (ABC-CV) scores in the domains of hyperactivity and inappropriate speech (King et al. 2001). No significant treatment-associated improvements were noted on parent ratings. The drug was reportedly well tolerated.

Memantine

Memantine is an uncompetitive NMDA antagonist used in the treatment of Alzheimer's disease. The use of memantine (mean dosage=8.1 mg/day) was described in 30 children and adolescents (mean age=8.92 years) with PDDs over 8–40 weeks of treatment (Chez et al. 2004b). Although standardized assessments were not used, 16 (53.3%) of 30 patients showed significant improvement, and another 10 (33.3%) of 30 showed milder improvement. The improvement was reported in attention, motor planning, language function, and repetitive behavior. In a single case report, memantine (10 mg/day) was associated with decreased irritability during 32 weeks of treatment in a 23-year-old male with autistic disorder (Erickson and Chambers 2006).

D-Cycloserine

D-Cycloserine is an antibiotic traditionally used to treat tuberculosis. Additionally, the drug is an NMDA partial agonist that has been shown to reduce the negative symptoms associated with schizophrenia (Goff et al. 1999). In the only trial to date of D-cycloserine in PDDs, 10 drug-free autistic patients (mean age = 10.0 ± 7.7 years) participated in an 8-week trial (0.7, 1.4, 2.8 mg/ kg/day, 2 weeks at each dosage) that began with a 2-week placebo lead-in phase (Posey et al. 2004a). D-Cycloserine was associated with improvement on the Severity subscale of the Clinical Global Impression Scale and the Social Withdrawal subscale of the ABC. Four patients (40%) were considered responders based on CGI-I ratings of *much improved*. Two patients (20%) had to drop out of the study due to development of a transient motor tic and increased echolalia, respectively.

Naltrexone

The opiate receptor antagonist naltrexone has been evaluated in four controlled studies on patients with autism. This research was stimulated by findings of elevated endorphin levels in the blood (Weizman et al. 1984) and cerebrospinal fluid (Gillberg et al. 1985; Ross et al. 1987) of individuals with autism. Although initial reports were promising, subsequent, larger double-blind, placebo-controlled studies have not demonstrated significant efficacy regarding the core symptoms of autism (Campbell et al. 1993; Feldman et al. 1999; Leboyer et al. 1992; Willemsen-Swinkels et al. 1995). Overall, the majority of the evidence points toward naltrexone as ineffective in improving autistic symptoms and modestly effective in the treatment of hyperactivity.

Secretin

The gastrointestinal peptide secretin stimulates secretion of water and bicarbonate from the pancreas and supports the activity of cholecystokinin, which, in turn, further activates pancreatic secretion. Extensive study of this compound in autism occurred after an initial report of open-label treatment in three patients noted improvement in maladaptive behavior and core autistic symptoms (Horvath et al. 1998). After initial reports of secretin success were reported in the mainstream media, secretin use spread to the point that more than 500,000 doses had been administered to patients with autism by the year 1999 (Kaminska et al. 2002). Fifteen double-blind, placebo-controlled trials have evaluated the use of secretin in autistic disorder and none of the reports concluded that the drug was effective (Sturmey 2005). These reports included single-dose and multiple-dose trials of human or porcine secretin. Although secretin represents one of the most studied compounds in PDDs, no robust evidence exists to support its use in this diagnostic group.

Safety Issues

This portion of the chapter focuses on adverse effects for selected major groups of medications that are used in PDDs. The section is not meant to be an extensive review of all adverse effects for all drugs previously discussed, but rather to highlight major adverse effects of several commonly used classes of drugs that should be brought to the reader's attention. When selecting a medication, it is essential that the patient and caregivers are also educated regarding the potential adverse effects associated with a specific drug.

Atypical Antipsychotics

The use of atypical antipsychotics in PDDs is associated with a risk of several adverse events that warrant monitoring. Although the atypical antipsychotics purportedly have a decreased risk of TD and EPS in comparison with the typical agents, they have been reported in individuals with PDDs taking these drugs (Malone et al. 2002; Zuddas et al. 2000). Hyperprolactinemia is another potentially adverse effect that may occur during treatment with an atypical antipsychotic. Studies measuring prolactin levels found treatment with risperidone to be associated with significant elevation in prolactin levels in patients with PDDs, despite the fact that no participants showed clinical signs of hyperprolactinemia (Gagliano et al. 2004; Masi et al. 2001b, 2003). Chronic hyperprolactinemia can lead to disordered growth, sexual dysfunction, and osteoporosis (Saito et al. 2004).

In children and adolescents, olanzapine is associated with a considerable risk of weight gain, whereas quetiapine and risperidone are associated with a moderate risk (Stigler et al. 2004c). In contrast, published data in youth suggest that ziprasidone and aripiprazole may be associated with a decreased risk of weight gain. In trials of risperidone in PDDs, significant drug-associated weight gain was reported (Martin et al. 2004; Research Units on Pediatric Psychopharmacology Autism Network 2002; Shea et al. 2004). The association between weight gain and atypical antipsychotic use in patients with PDDs is troubling. Evidence has implicated the atypical antipsychotics in the onset or exacerbation of diabetes and hyperlipidemia (Stigler et al. 2004c). Regular monitoring of patient weight, as well as fasting glucose and lipids, is highly recommended. In addition, selection of a particular antipsychotic may warrant monitoring liver functions, blood count, and electrocardiogram (ECG).

SSRIs

In 2004, the FDA required manufacturers of SSRIs to include a black box warning describing the potential for increased suicidality in children and adolescents taking these drugs, especially during the first few months of treatment. With this risk in mind, regular assessment for suicidality must be part of the treatment plan for patients with PDDs taking any of these drugs. In addition, prepubertal patients with PDDs taking SSRIs may be at increased risk of behavioral activation and irritability during SSRI treatment (McDougle et al. 2000). It is therefore appropriate to begin with low doses of SSRIs and slowly titrate toward an effective dose.

Psychostimulants

As described earlier, stimulants may be less well tolerated in youth with PDDs in comparison with typically developing children with ADHD (Research Units on Pediatric Psychopharmacology Autism Network 2005a). Adverse effects that warrant close monitoring include increased irritability, agitation, hyperactivity, decreased appetite, exacerbation/development of tics, and psychosis (rarely).

Alpha$_2$-Adrenergic Agonists

This class of drugs is typically well tolerated, aside from possible adverse effects of sedation and hypotension. Depressive symptoms may worsen or be

induced as well. A baseline ECG prior to beginning this class of drugs is recommended whenever possible, particularly in persons with a significant history of cardiovascular problems.

Atomoxetine

In 2005, the FDA required manufacturers of atomoxetine to include a black
box warning regarding potential increased suicidal ideation in children and
adolescents treated with this drug. Because of this risk, regular assessment for
suicidality in patients taking this drug is warranted. In addition, rare cases of
hepatic dysfunction associated with atomoxetine warrant ongoing assessment
for signs and symptoms of liver failure in patients with PDDs taking this drug
(Formanek 2005).

Mood Stabilizers

Among the anticonvulsants, valproic acid is frequently used to treat persons
with PDDs. Drug levels should be monitored on a regular basis to ensure that
levels remain in the therapeutic range. Patients should be regularly assessed for
valproic acid toxicity symptoms, including nausea, vomiting, ataxia, tremor,
dizziness, headache, confusion, and somnolence. Hepatotoxicity is a possible
serious adverse effect associated with the drug, warranting periodic liver function tests (Dreifuss 1987). Pancreatitis is another rare but potentially life-
threatening complication. In addition, because of the risk of thrombocytopenia, a blood count including platelets should be obtained in all patients
receiving this drug.

Risks of another mood stabilizer, lithium, include impaired renal and thy-
roid function, thus warranting regular monitoring (Scahill et al. 2001). In addition, baseline ECGs are recommended. Lithium levels must be monitored
on a regular basis during treatment. Toxic levels of lithium are often close to the
therapeutic range (0.6–1.2 µg/mL), thus making it essential to monitor for
signs and symptoms of lithium toxicity during treatment. Signs of toxicity
include lethargy, nausea, vomiting, diarrhea, tremor, weakness, and seizures.

Practical Management Strategies

A multimodal approach to the management of autism and related disorders
is essential. This approach often incorporates speech therapy, occupational

therapy, physical therapy, educational interventions, and social skills training. Ongoing collaboration with the youth's educational team at school can ease transitions, decrease adverse behaviors, and optimize learning in the classroom setting. In addition, behavior therapy may be of particular significance in that it may decrease the need for pharmacotherapy in this population. Even with the use of such interventions, medication is often required to decrease the maladaptive behaviors commonly observed in youth with PDDs.

The pharmacotherapy of PDDs is based on a target symptom approach (Figure 7–1). As described in this chapter, a variety of medications may impact specific target symptom domains in this population. The algorithms provide an overview of drug treatment strategies for three symptom domains commonly encountered in PDDs: aggression and self-injury, motor hyperactivity and inattention, and interfering repetitive phenomena.

Children and adolescents presenting with mild symptoms of aggression or self-injury may derive benefit from an initial trial of an α_2-adrenergic agonist. The emergence of more severe symptoms often requires treatment with an atypical antipsychotic. From a clinical standpoint, mood stabilizers may also be efficacious, primarily in postpubertal individuals. However, controlled studies supporting their use in this population have not been published.

Symptoms of hyperactivity and inattention are also frequently observed in children with PDDs. Emerging evidence suggests that the stimulants, as well as the α_2-adrenergic agonists may be effective in this population. However, it is important to weigh the risks and benefits involved with the use of these drugs. Whereas the α_2-adrenergic agonist guanfacine is generally well tolerated, stimulants can be associated with a worsening of behavior. As a result, a trial of guanfacine is generally recommended prior to a trial of a stimulant.

Youth suffering from interfering repetitive phenomena frequently benefit from treatment with SSRIs. Because of potential activation that may be associated with this drug class in prepubertal individuals, use of small dosages and a slow titration schedule are recommended. In general, the atypical antipsychotics should be considered for treatment-resistant symptoms of hyperactivity and inattention, as well as for interfering repetitive behaviors.

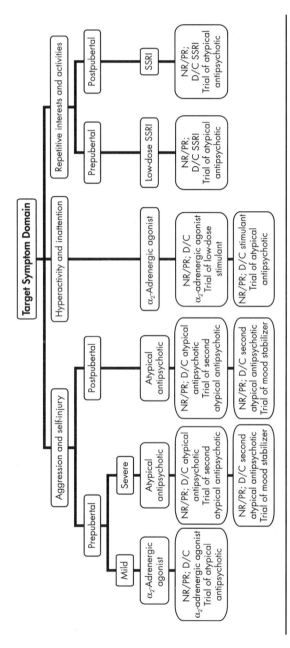

Figure 7-1. A target symptom approach to the pharmacotherapy of pervasive developmental disorders.

This algorithm provides an overview of drug treatment strategies for three symptom domains commonly encountered in PDDs: aggression and self-injury, motor hyperactivity and inattention, and interfering repetitive phenomena. It is recommended that behavior therapy also be considered at each treatment juncture.

D/C = discontinue; NR/PR = nonresponse/partial response; SSRI = selective serotonin reuptake inhibitor.

Conclusions

Research into the pharmacotherapy of pervasive developmental disorders will continue to explore the efficacy and tolerability of currently available drugs, as well as the use of novel agents, to address specific interfering target symptoms. Recent preliminary investigations into glutamatergic agents for addressing core social impairment are of particular interest. Although youth with PDDs often present with interfering symptoms in several domains, research to date has focused on the use of one drug to treat a specific group of symptoms. Studies of coactive pharmacological treatment strategies targeting more than one symptom domain are needed to better understand the effectiveness, tolerability, and safety of using more than one agent in the treatment of PDDs.

Clinical Pearls

- The therapeutic approach to the management of pervasive developmental disorders (PDDs) is multimodal.
- Medication use can reduce maladaptive behavior, allowing youth with PDDs to maximize benefit from therapy and educational services.
- Pharmacotherapy of PDDs is based on a target symptoms approach.
- Three major target symptom domains in PDDs are aggression/self-injury, hyperactivity/inattention, and repetitive interests/activities.
- Youth with mild aggression or self-injury may receive benefit from treatment with an α_2-adrenergic agonist, whereas more severe symptoms often require an atypical antipsychotic.
- Risperidone is the only medication approved by the U.S. Food and Drug Administration for the treatment of irritability in youth with autism, ages 5–16 years.
- Prepubertal patients with PDDs may be at increased risk of behavioral activation and irritability during selective serotonin reuptake inhibitor treatment for interfering repetitive phenomena.

- Stimulants appear less well tolerated in youth with PDDs in comparison with typically developing children with attention-deficit/hyperactivity disorder.

- A trial of guanfacine prior to a stimulant is generally recommended for symptoms of hyperactivity and inattention in PDDs.

- Studies of coactive pharmacological treatment strategies targeting more than one symptom domain are needed in children and adolescents with PDDs.

References

Aman MG: Stimulant drug effects in developmental disorders and hyperactivity: toward a resolution of disparate findings. J Autism Dev Disord 12:385–398, 1982

American Psychiatric Association: Diagnostic and Statistical Manual of Mental Disorders, 3rd Edition. Washington, DC, American Psychiatric Association, 1980

American Psychiatric Association: Diagnostic and Statistical Manual of Mental Disorders, 4th Edition, Text Revision. Washington, DC, American Psychiatric Association, 2000

Anderson GM, Freedman DX, Cohen DJ, et al: Whole blood serotonin in autistic and normal subjects. J Child Psychol Psychiatry 28:885–900, 1987

Anderson LT, Campbell M, Adams P, et al: The effects of haloperidol on discrimination learning and behavioral symptoms in autistic children. J Autism Dev Disord 19:227–239, 1989

Arnt J, Skarsfeldt M: Do novel antipsychotics have similar pharmacological characteristics: a review of the evidence. Neuropsychopharmacology 18:63–101, 1998

Baldessarini RJ, Frankenburg FR: Clozapine: a novel antipsychotic agent. N Engl J Med 14:746–754, 1991

Belsito KM, Law PA, Kirk KS, et al: Lamotrigine therapy for autistic disorder: a randomized, double-blind, placebo-controlled trial. J Autism Dev Disord 31:175–181, 2001

Bertrand J, Mars A, Boyle C, et al: Prevalence of autism in a United States population: the Brick Township, New Jersey, investigation. Pediatrics 108:1155–1161, 2001

Brodkin ES, McDougle CJ, Naylor ST, et al: Clomipramine in adults with pervasive developmental disorders: a prospective open-label investigation. J Child Adolesc Psychopharmacol 7:109–121, 1997

Buchsbaum MS, Hollander E, Hazender MM, et al: Effects of fluoxetine on regional cerebral metabolism in autistic spectrum disorder: a pilot study. Int J Neuropsychopharmacol 4:119–125, 2001

Buitelaar JK, van der Gaag RJ, van der Hoeven J: Buspirone in the management of anxiety and irritability in children with pervasive developmental disorders: results of an open-label trial. J Clin Psychiatry 59:56–59, 1998

Burris KD, Molski TF, Xu C, et al: Aripiprazole, a novel antipsychotic, is a high-affinity partial agonist at human dopamine D_2 receptors. J Pharmacol Exp Ther 302:381–389, 2002

Bymaster FP, Hemrick-Luecke SK, Perry KW, et al: Neurochemical evidence for antagonism by olanzapine of dopamine, serotonin, alpha 1-adrenergic and muscarinic receptors in vivo in rats. Psychopharmacology 124:87–94, 1996

Campbell M: Pharmacotherapy in early infantile autism. Biol Psychiatry 10:399–423, 1975

Campbell M, Anderson LT, Meier M, et al: A comparison of haloperidol and behavior therapy and their interaction in autistic children. J Am Acad Child Psychiatry 17:640–655, 1978

Campbell M, Anderson LT, Small AM, et al: Naltrexone in autistic children: behavioral symptoms and attentional learning. J Am Acad Child Adolesc Psychiatry 32:1283–1291, 1993

Campbell M, Armenteros JL, Malone PR, et al: Neuroleptic-related dyskinesias in autistic children: a prospective, longitudinal study. J Am Acad Child Adolesc Psychiatry 36:835–843, 1997

Carminati GG, Deriaz N, Bertschy G: Low-dose venlafaxine in three adolescents and young adults with autistic disorder improves self-injurious behavior and attention deficit/hyperactivity disorder (ADHD)–like symptoms. Prog Neuropsychopharmacol Biol Psychiatry 30:312–315, 2006

Chakrabarti S, Fombonne E: Pervasive developmental disorders in preschool children: confirmation of high prevalence. Am J Psychiatry 162:1133–1141, 2005

Chen NC, Bedair HS, McKay B, et al: Clozapine in the treatment of aggression in an adolescent with autistic disorder. J Clin Psychiatry 62:479–480, 2001

Chez MG, Nowinski CV, Buchanan CP, et al: Donepezil (Aricept) use in children with autistic spectrum disorders. Ann Neurol 48:541, 2000

Chez MG, Aimonovitch M, Buchanan T, et al: Treating autistic spectrum disorders in children: utility of the cholinesterase inhibitor rivastigmine tartrate. J Child Neurol 19:165–169, 2004a

Chez MG, Hung PC, Chin K, et al: Memantine experience in children and adolescents with autistic spectrum disorders (abstract). Ann Neurol 56:C10, 2004b

Cohen IL, Campbell M, Posner D, et al: Behavioral effects of haloperidol in young autistic children. J Am Acad Child Adolesc Psychiatry 19:665–677, 1980

Conroy J, Meally E, Kearney G, et al: Serotonin transporter gene and autism: a haplotype analysis in an Irish autistic population. Mol Psychiatry 9:587–593, 2004

Corson AH, Barkenbus JE, Posey DJ, et al: A retrospective analysis of quetiapine in the treatment of pervasive developmental disorders. J Clin Psychiatry 65:1531–1536, 2004

Couturier JL, Nicolson R: A retrospective assessment of citalopram in children and adolescents with pervasive developmental disorders. J Child Adolesc Psychopharmacol 12:243–248, 2002

Davanzo PA, Belin TR, Widawski MH, et al: Paroxetine treatment of aggression and self-injury in persons with mental retardation. Am J Ment Retard 102:427–437, 1998

DeLong GR, Ritch CR, Burch S: Fluoxetine response in children with autistic spectrum disorders: correlation with familial major affective disorder and intellectual achievement. Dev Med Child Neurol 44:652–659, 2002

Di Martino A, Melis G, Cianchetti C, et al: Methylphenidate for pervasive developmental disorders: safety and efficacy of acute single dose test and ongoing therapy: an open-pilot study. J Child Adolesc Psychopharmacol 14:207–218, 2004

Dreifuss FE, Santilli N, Langer DH, et al: Valproic acid hepatic fatalities: a retrospective review. Neurology 37:379–385, 1987

Epperson CN, McDougle CJ, Anand A: Lithium augmentation of fluvoxamine in autistic disorder: a case report. J Child Adolesc Psychopharmacol 4:201–207, 1994

Erickson CA, Chambers JE: Memantine for disruptive behavior in autistic disorder. J Clin Psychiatry 67:1000, 2006

Fankhauser MP, Karumanchi VC, German ML, et al: A double-blind, placebo-controlled study of the efficacy of transdermal clonidine in autism. J Clin Psychiatry 53:77–82, 1992

Fatemi SH, Realmuto GM, Khan L, et al: Fluoxetine in treatment of adolescent patients with autism: a longitudinal open-label trial. J Autism Dev Disord 28:303–307, 1998

Feldman HM, Koman BK, Gonzaga AM: Naltrexone and communication skills in young children with autism. J Am Acad Child Adolesc Psychiatry 38:587–593, 1999

Findling RL, Maxwell K, Wiznitzer M: An open clinical trial of risperidone monotherapy in young children with autistic disorder. Psychopharmacol Bull 33:155–159, 1997

Fombonne E: The epidemiology of autism: a review. Psychol Med 29:769–786, 1999

Fombonne E: Epidemiological studies of pervasive developmental disorders, in Handbook of Autism and Pervasive Developmental Disorders, 3rd Edition, Vol 1. Edited by Volkmar F, Paul R, Klin A, et al. Hoboken, NJ, Wiley, 2005, pp 42–69

Formanek R: New warning about ADHD drug. FDA Consum 39:3, 2005

Gagliano A, Germano E, Pustorino G, et al: Risperidone treatment of children with autistic disorder: effectiveness, tolerability, and pharmacokinetic implications. J Child Adolesc Psychopharmacol 14:39–47, 2004

Gillberg C, Terenius L, Lonnerholm G: Endorphin activity in childhood psychosis. Arch Gen Psychiatry 42:780–783, 1985

Gobbi G, Pulvirenti L: Long-term treatment with clozapine in an adult with autistic disorder accompanied by aggressive behavior. J Psych Neurol 26:340–341, 2001

Goff DC, Tsai G, Levitt J, et al: A placebo-controlled trial of D-cycloserine added to conventional neuroleptics in patients with schizophrenia. Arch Gen Psychiatry 56:21–27, 1999

Goodman WK, Price LH, Rasmussen SA, et al: The Yale-Brown Obsessive Compulsive Scale, I: development, use and reliability. Arch Gen Psychiatry 46:1006–1011, 1989

Gordon CT, State RC, Nelson JE, et al: A double-blind comparison of clomipramine, desipramine, and placebo in the treatment of autistic disorder. Arch Gen Psychiatry 50:441–447, 1993

Greenhill L, Beyer DH, Finkleson J, et al: Guidelines and algorithms for the use of methylphenidate in children with attention-deficit/hyperactivity disorder. J Atten Disord 6(suppl):S89–S100, 2002a

Greenhill LL, Pliszka S, Dulcan MK, et al: American Academy of Child and Adolescent Psychiatry. Practice parameter for the use of stimulant medications in the treatment of children, adolescents, and adults. J Am Acad Child Adolesc Psychiatry 41:26S–49S, 2002b

Greist JH, Jefferson JW, Kobak KA, et al: Efficacy and tolerability of serotonin transport inhibitors in obsessive-compulsive disorder. Arch Gen Psychiatry 52:53–60, 1995

Gurney JG, Fritz MS, Ness KK, et al: Analysis of prevalence trends of autism spectrum disorder in Minnesota. Arch Pediatr Adolesc Med 157:622–627, 2003

Handen BL, Johnson CR, Lubetsky M: Efficacy of methylphenidate among children with autism and symptoms of attention-deficit hyperactivity disorder. J Autism Dev Disord 30:245–255, 2000

Hardan AY, Handen BL: A retrospective open trial of adjunctive donepezil in children and adolescents with autistic disorder. J Child Adolesc Psychopharmacol 12:237–241, 2002

Hellings JA, Weckbaugh M, Nickel EJ, et al: A double-blind, placebo controlled study of valproate for aggression in youth with pervasive developmental disorder. J Child Adolesc Psychopharmacol 15:682–692, 2005

Hollander E, Kaplan A, Cartwright C, et al: Venlafaxine in children, adolescents and young adults with autism spectrum disorders: an open retrospective clinical report. J Child Neurol 15:132–135, 2000

Hollander E, Dolgoff-Kaspar R, Cartwright C, et al: An open trial of divalproex sodium in autism spectrum disorders. J Clin Psychiatry 62:530–534, 2001

Hollander E, Phillips A, Chaplin W, et al: A placebo controlled crossover trial of liquid fluoxetine on repetitive behaviors in childhood and adolescent autism. Neuropsychopharmacology 30:582–589, 2005

Hollander E, Soorya L, Wasserman S, et al: Divalproex sodium vs. placebo in the treatment of repetitive behaviours in autism spectrum disorder. Int J Neuropsychopharmacol Aug 9:209–213, 2006

Horvath K, Stefanatos G, Sokolaki KN, et al: Improved social and language skills after secretin administration in patients with autism spectrum disorders. J Assoc Acad Minor Phys 9:9–15, 1998

Howlin P, Goode S, Hutton J, et al: Adult outcomes for children with autism. J Child Psychol Psychiatry 45:212–229, 2004

Jaselskis CA, Cook EH Jr, Fletcher KE, et al: Clonidine treatment of hyperactive and impulsive children with autistic disorder. J Clin Psychopharmacol 12:322–327, 1992

Kaminska B, Czaja M, Kozielska E, et al: Use of secretin in the treatment of childhood autism. Med Sci Monit 8:RA22–RA26, 2002

Kanner L: Autistic disturbances of affective contact. Nerv Child 2:217–250, 1943

Kanner L, Eisenberg L: Early infantile autism 1943–1955. Am J Orthopsychiatry Psychiatry 26:55–65, 1956

Kerbeshian J, Burd L, Fisher W: Lithium carbonate in the treatment of two patients with infantile autism and atypical bipolar symptomatology. J Clin Psychopharmacol 7:401–405, 1987

King BH, Davanzo P: Buspirone treatment of aggression and self-injury in autistic and nonautistic persons with severe mental retardation. Dev Brain Dysfunc 9:22–31, 1996

King BH, Wright DM, Handen BL, et al: Double-blind, placebo-controlled study of amantadine hydrochloride in the treatment of children with autistic disorder. J Am Acad Child Adolesc Psychiatry 40:658–665, 2001

Kornhuber J, Weller M, Schoppmeyer K, et al: Amantadine and memantine are NMDA receptor antagonists with neuroprotective properties. J Neurol Transm Suppl 43:91–104, 1994

Leboyer M, Bouvard MP, Launey JM, et al: Brief report: a double-blind study of naltrexone in infantile autism. J Autism Dev Disord 22:309–319, 1992

Leboyer M, Philippe A, Bouvard M, et al: Whole blood serotonin and plasma beta-endorphin in autistic probands and their first-degree relatives. Biol Psychiatry 45:158–163, 1999

Leysen JE, Gommeren W, Eens A, et al: Biochemical profile of risperidone, a new antipsychotic. J Pharmacol Exp Ther 247:661–670, 1988

Lord C, Bailey A: Autism spectrum disorders, in Child and Adolescent Psychiatry, 4th Edition. Edited by Rutter M, Taylor E. Oxford, England, Blackwell, 2002, pp 636–663

Lotter V: Epidemiology of autistic conditions in young children, I: prevalence. Soc Psychiatry 1:124–137, 1966

Malone RP, Cater J, Sheikh RM, et al: Olanzapine versus haloperidol in children with autistic disorder: an open pilot study. J Am Acad Child Adolesc Psychiatry 40:887–894, 2001

Malone RP, Maislin G, Choudhury MS, et al: Risperidone treatment in children and adolescents with autism: short- and long-term safety and effectiveness. J Am Acad Child Adolesc Psychiatry 41:140–147, 2002

Marshall BL, Napolitano DA, McAdam DB, et al: Venlafaxine and increased aggression in a female with autism. J Am Acad Child Adolesc Psychiatry 42:383–384, 2003

Martin A, Koenig K, Scahill L, et al: Open-label quetiapine in treatment of children and adolescents with autistic disorder. J Child Adolesc Psychopharmacol 9:99–107, 1999

Martin A, Koenig K, Anderson GM, et al: Low-dose fluvoxamine treatment of children and adolescents with pervasive developmental disorder: a prospective, open-label study. J Autism Dev Disord 33:77–85, 2003

Martin A, Scahill L, Anderson GM, et al: Weight and leptin changes among risperidone-treated youths with autism: 6-month prospective data. Am J Psychiatry 161:1125–1127, 2004

Masi G, Cosenza A, Mucci M, et al: Open trial of risperidone in 24 young children with pervasive developmental disorders. J Am Acad Child Adolesc Psychiatry 40:1206–1214, 2001a

Masi G, Cosenza A, Mucci M: Prolactin levels in young children with pervasive developmental disorders. J Child Adolesc Psychopharmacol 11:389–394, 2001b

Masi G, Cosenza A, Mucci M, et al: A 3-year naturalistic study of 53 preschool children with pervasive developmental disorders treated with risperidone. J Clin Psychiatry 64:1039–1047, 2003

McDougle CJ, Naylor ST, Cohen DJ, et al: A double-blind, placebo-controlled study of fluvoxamine in adults with autistic disorder. Arch Gen Psychiatry 53:1001–1008, 1996a

McDougle CJ, Naylor ST, Cohen DJ, et al: Effects of tryptophan depletion in drug-free adults with autism. Arch Gen Psychiatry 53:993–1000, 1996b

McDougle CJ, Holmes JP, Bronson MR, et al: Risperidone treatment of children and adolescents with pervasive developmental disorders: a prospective, open-label study. J Am Acad Child Adolesc Psychiatry 36:685–693, 1997

McDougle CJ, Brodkin ES, Naylor ST, et al: Sertraline in adults with pervasive developmental disorder: a prospective open-label investigation. J Clin Psychopharmacol 18:62–66, 1998a

McDougle CJ, Holmes JP, Carlson DC, et al: A double-blind, placebo-controlled study of risperidone in adults with autistic disorder and other pervasive developmental disorders. Arch Gen Psychiatry 55:633–41, 1998b

McDougle CJ, Kresch LE, Posey DJ: Repetitive thoughts and behavior in pervasive developmental disorders: treatment with serotonin reuptake inhibitors. J Autism Dev Disord 30(5):425–433, 2000

McDougle CJ, Kem DL, Posey DJ: Case series: use of ziprasidone for maladaptive symptoms in youth with autism. J Am Acad Child Adolesc Psychiatry 41:921–927, 2002

McDougle CJ, Scahill L, Aman MG, et al: Risperidone for the core symptom domains of autism: results from the RUPP Autism Network Study. Am J Psychiatry 162:1142–1148, 2005

Namerow LB, Thomas P, Bostic JQ, et al: Use of citalopram in pervasive developmental disorder. J Dev Behav Pediatr 24:104–108, 2003

Nicolson R, Awad G, Sloman L: An open trial of risperidone in young autistic children. J Am Acad Child Adolesc Psychiatry 37:372–376, 1998

Owley T, Walton L, Salt J, et al: An open-label trial of escitalopram in pervasive developmental disorders. J Am Acad Child Adolesc Psychiatry 44:343–348, 2005

Posey DJ, Litwiller M, Koburn A, et al: Paroxetine in autism. J Am Acad Child Adolesc Psychiatry 38:111–112, 1999

Posey DJ, Guenin KD, Kohn AE, et al: A naturalistic open-label study of mirtazapine in autistic and other pervasive developmental disorders. J Child Adolesc Psychopharmacol 11:267–277, 2001

Posey DJ, Kem DL, Swiezy NB, et al: A pilot study of D-cycloserine in subjects with autistic disorder. Am J Psychiatry 161:2115–2117, 2004a

Posey DJ, Puntney JI, Sasher TM, et al: Guanfacine treatment of hyperactivity and inattention in pervasive developmental disorders: a retrospective analysis of 80 cases. J Child Adolesc Psychopharmacol 14:233–241, 2004b

Posey DJ, Wiegand RE, Wilkerson J, et al: A prospective, open-label study of atomoxetine for ADHD symptoms associated with higher-functioning pervasive developmental disorders. Neuropsychopharmacology 31:S156, 2005

Potenza MN, Holmes JP, Kanes SJ, et al: Olanzapine treatment of children, adolescents, and adults with pervasive developmental disorders: an open-label pilot study. J Clin Psychopharmacol 19:37–44, 1999

Quintana H, Birmaher B, Stedge D, et al: Use of methylphenidate in the treatment of children with autistic disorder. J Autism Dev Disord 25:283–294, 1995

Ratey JJ, Bemporad J, Sorgi J, et al: Brief report: open trial effects of beta-blockers on speech and social behaviors in 8 autistic adults. J Autism Dev Disord 17:439–446, 1987

Remington G, Sloman L, Konstantareas M, et al: Clomipramine versus haloperidol in the treatment of autistic disorder: a double-blind, placebo-controlled, crossover study. J Clin Psychopharmacol 21:440–444, 2001

Research Units on Pediatric Psychopharmacology Autism Network: Risperidone in children with autism and serious behavioral problems. N Engl J Med 347:314–321, 2002

Research Units on Pediatric Psychopharmacology Autism Network: Randomized, controlled, crossover trial of methylphenidate in pervasive developmental disorders with hyperactivity. Arch Gen Psychiatry 62:1266–1274, 2005a

Research Units on Pediatric Psychopharmacology Autism Network. Risperidone treatment of autistic disorder: longer-term benefits and blinded discontinuation after 6 months. Am J Psychiatry 162:1361–1369, 2005b

Ross DL, Klykylo WM, Hitzemann R: Reduction of elevated CSF beta-endorphin by fenfluramine in infantile autism. Pediatr Neurol 3:83–86, 1987

Rutter M, Greenfeld D, Lockyer L: A five to fifteen year follow-up of infantile psychosis, II: social and behavioral outcome. Br J Psychiatry 113:1183–1189, 1967

Saito E, Correll C, Gallelli K, et al: A prospective study of hyperprolactinemia in children and adolescents treated with atypical antipsychotic agents. J Child Adolesc Psychopharmacol 14:350–358, 2004

Scahill L, Riddle MA, McSwiggin-Hardin M, et al: Children's Yale-Brown Obsessive Compulsive Scale: reliability and validity. J Am Acad Child Adolesc Psychiatry 36:844–852, 1997

Scahill L, Farkas L, Hamrin V: Lithium in children and adolescents. J Child Adolesc Psychiatr Nurs 14:89–93, 2001

Schain RJ, Freedman DX: Studies on 5-hydroxyindole metabolism in autistic and other mentally retarded children. J Pediatr 58:315–320, 1961

Scott FJ, Baron-Cohen S, Bolton P, et al: Brief report: prevalence of autism spectrum conditions in children aged 5–11 years in Cambridgeshire, UK. Autism 6:231–237, 2002

Shea S, Turgay A, Carroll A, et al: Risperidone in the treatment of disruptive behavioral symptoms in children with autistic and other pervasive developmental disorders. Pediatrics 114:634–641, 2004

Snead RW, Boon F, Presberg J: Paroxetine for self-injurious behavior. J Am Acad Child Adolesc Psychiatry 33:909–910, 1994

Steingard R, Biederman J: Lithium responsive manic-like symptoms in two individuals with autism and mental retardation. J Am Acad Child Adolesc Psychiatry 26:932–935, 1987

Steingard RJ, Zimnitsky B, DeMaso DR, et al: Sertraline treatment of transition-associated anxiety and agitation in children with autistic disorder. J Child Adolesc Psychopharmacol 7:9–15, 1997

Stigler KA, Desmond LA, Posey DJ, et al: A naturalistic retrospective analysis of psychostimulants in pervasive developmental disorders. J Child Adolesc Psychopharmacol 14:49–56, 2004a

Stigler KA, Posey DJ, McDougle CJ: Aripiprazole for maladaptive behavior in pervasive developmental disorders. J Child Adolesc Psychopharmacol 14:455–463, 2004b

Stigler KA, Potenza MN, Posey DJ, et al: Weight gain associated with atypical antipsychotic use in children and adolescents: prevalence, clinical relevance, and management. Paediatr Drugs 6:33–44, 2004c

Sturmey P: Secretin is an ineffective treatment for pervasive developmental disabilities: a review of 15 double-blind randomized controlled trials. Res Dev Disabil 26:87–97, 2005

Sugie Y, Sugie H, Fukuda T, et al: Clinical efficacy of fluvoxamine and functional polymorphism in a serotonin transporter gene. J Autism Dev Disord 35:377–385, 2005

Tandon R, Harrigan E, Zorn SH: Ziprasidone: a novel antipsychotic with unique pharmacology and therapeutic potential. J Serotonin Res 4:159–177, 1997

Uvebrant P, Bauziene R: Intractable epilepsy in children. The efficacy of lamotrigine treatment, including non-seizure related benefits. Neuropediatrics 25:284–288, 1994

Wassink TH, Piven J: The molecular genetics of autism. Curr Psychiatry Rep 2:170–175, 2000

Weizman R, Weizman A, Thano S, et al: Humoral-endorphin blood levels in autistic, schizophrenic and healthy subjects. Psychopharmacology 82:368–370, 1984

Willemsen-Swinkels SHN, Buitelaar JK, Nijhof GJ, et al: Failure of naltrexone hydrochloride to reduce self-injurious and autistic behavior in mentally retarded adults: double-blind placebo-controlled studies. Arch Gen Psychiatry 52:766–773, 1995

Zuddas A, Ledda MG, Fratta A, et al: Clinical effects of clozapine on autistic disorder. Am J Psychiatry 153:738, 1996

Zuddas A, Dimartino A, Muglia P, et al: Long-term risperidone for pervasive developmental disorder: efficacy, tolerability, and discontinuation. J Child Adolesc Psychopharmacol 10:79–90, 2000

8

Tic Disorders

Lawrence Scahill, M.S.N., Ph.D.

Tic disorders, including Tourette's syndrome, are movement disorders that begin in childhood and are defined by the presence of enduring motor tics, phonic tics, or both. The tics of Tourette's syndrome (TS) show an extraordinary range from mild to severe across patients and a fluctuating course within patients (Leckman 2002; Lin et al. 2002). In addition to association with tics, TS is frequently connected with obsessive-compulsive symptoms, hyperactivity, impulsive behavior, and inattention (Jankovic 2001). Therefore, the assessment and treatment of children and adolescents with TS correctly include consideration of these multiple sources of impairment. Indeed, although the referral question may be about tics, the presence of attention-deficit/hyperactivity disorder (ADHD) or obsessive-compulsive disorder (OCD) may be more

Supported by National Institute of Mental Health Grants U10 MH066764 and R03MH67845–01A1 to Dr. Scahill and National Institute of Nursing Research Grants R15NR007637–01 and M01RR00125 (Yale University).

pressing than the tic symptoms. In addition to the sources of impairment, assessment and treatment planning must also take into account the domains of functioning that may be adversely affected. For example, TS or one of the closely associated conditions may contribute to maladaptive, even volatile, family interactions, may interfere with educational progress, and may contribute to unstable peer relationships. This chapter is a review of the diagnosis and treatment of tic disorders and the assessment of ADHD and OCD that may co-occur in children with TS. Although the treatments considered in this chapter focus primarily on pharmacological interventions, emerging behavioral and surgical interventions will also be considered briefly. Before addressing the issues of diagnosis and treatment, the chapter includes a brief review of the epidemiology of tic disorders to underscore their public health importance.

Epidemiology

Transient tics are relatively common in school-age children, affecting 6%–12% (Scahill et al. 2005). Tic disorders, in which the tics endure over time, affect an estimated 4% of children (Costello et al. 1996). Tic disorders are defined in DSM-IV-TR (American Psychiatric Association 2000) by the duration and types of tics present. DSM-IV-TR also stipulates that the tics must begin before the age of 18 years. In practice, however, tics usually begin in early school age, between the ages of 5 and 7 years.

Until recently, TS was considered a rare and uniformly severe condition. However, prior estimates of prevalence were typically based on counts of clinically ascertained cases. This method resulted in a systematic undercount because it failed to include cases that had not come to clinical attention— perhaps milder cases or cases with poor access to care. To correct this problem, recent studies have surveyed community samples. Not surprisingly, this strategy has resulted in higher estimates of prevalence. Recent studies have also relied on detailed parent interviews and, in some instances, direct observation of the child to confirm the presence of tics. This approach also promotes the identification of milder cases. Furthermore, the recognition of milder cases has encouraged the view that tic disorders, including TS, reside on a continuum from mild to severe forms. Finally, as in other areas of psychiatry, the introduction of DSM-III (American Psychiatric Association 1980) specified and broadened the diagnostic criteria. For example, Rutter et al. (1970) evaluated a sample of 3,000 children between 10 and 12 years of age in the Isle of Wight study. In that sample, 4.4% of the children were identified as having tics, but no cases of TS were identified. By contrast, using DSM-III-R (American Psychiatric Association 1987) criteria, Costello et al. (1996) reported a prevalence of 4.2% for all tic disorders combined (transient tic disorder, chronic tic disorder, and TS) in a similar age group of children in the Great Smoky Mountains Study. The differences in diagnostic classification across these two studies appear to be due to differences in definitions rather than true differences in prevalence of tic disorders.

Over the past decade, there have been 10 community surveys on the prevalence of tic disorders in children. The prevalence of TS has been estimated from a lower bound of 1 per 1,000 to an upper bound of 30 per 1,000. This level of imprecision is not ideal for judging public health importance and service need. In a recent critical review of the literature, Scahill et al. (2005) noted that several methodologically sound studies agree on a narrower range of 3 to 8 cases per 1,000 for TS. As noted above, the combined prevalence of transient tic disorder and chronic tic disorders is likely to be 4% in school-age children.

Diagnosis and Assessment

The assessment of a child suspected of having TS begins with a review of tic symptoms and exploration of associated problems, particularly inattention, impulsiveness and hyperactivity, and obsessive-compulsive symptoms. The review of tic symptoms includes the age at onset and course of symptoms, current severity of motor and phonic tics, presence of premonitory sensations and capacity for tic suppression, overall burden caused by the tics, and treatment approaches implemented to date. Tics tend to be rapid movements or brief vocalizations that are performed in a stereotyped manner. Tics also tend to occur in bouts—brief or extended clusters of tics followed by a period of relative quiescence. In mild cases, the bouts of tics are brief, with relatively long tic-free periods (an hour to several hours), and may go unnoticed by casual observers. By contrast, individuals with moderate or marked severity may have bouts of forceful tics consisting of multiple movements and vocalization with only brief tic-free periods. Frequent and forceful movements or vocalizations may be easily noticeable across settings and may interfere with everyday activities.

Many patients with TS describe a warning or urge prior to the performance of a tic. This may be described as a vague feeling of tension or a physical feeling occurring in a specific body region. In fact, the body region involved may be the same muscle group inherent in tic expression (Leckman et al. 1993). Patients with TS also describe an ability to suppress their tics—at least momentarily. The relationship between premonitory sensations and tic suppression is intriguing, though poorly understood. First, young children (between the ages of 7 and 10 years) may not spontaneously report either of these phenomena. However, by age 10 years, most children with TS describe both the warning before some of their tics and at least a fleeting capacity to suppress tics. Second, children and adults often report that the act of suppressing tics intensifies the urge to perform the tic. This accentuation pushes the tic urge to a crescendo and ultimately makes the tic irresistible (Leckman et al. 1993). Third, although many patients describe the capacity to suppress tics, at least momentarily, few can describe how this is accomplished. Data from a functional magnetic resonance imaging study (Peterson et al. 1998) suggest that the tic suppression involves activation of frontal cortex. This increase in cortical activity may reflect an effort to exert voluntary control of dysregulated subcortical output or simply increased attention to the tics (Peterson et al. 1998; Woods et al. 2005). Fourth, the effort to suppress tics may reflect the child's gradual awareness that the tics can have social consequences. In other words, as children with TS begin to understand that the tics can have social consequences, they increase their vigilance about the tics and recruit conscious effort to suppress them. The increased vigilance may promote the evolution of premonitory sensations as the child becomes more aware of the earliest signs of tic behavior. This conceptualization has not been specifically tested and remains speculative.

The differential diagnosis of TS and tic disorders is based on the type of tics present (motor or vocal) and the duration of symptoms (American Psychiatric Association 2000). Transient tic disorder is defined by the presence of motor or vocal tics for less than a year. The diagnosis of chronic tic disorder (CTD) is made when the child has motor or vocal tics (but not both) for longer than a year. TS is defined by the presence of both motor and phonic tics for more than a year. It is not required that both motor and phonic tics be present at the same time—just that there is clear history that both were present during the course of illness. Other key elements in the diagnosis include onset before the age of 18 years and exclusion of other causes for the tics, such as medication or another medical condition. For example, a child who only showed tics while being treated with a psychostimulant would not be diagnosed with TS. Although the diagnosis of TS is based on history, the diagnosis of TS is more convincing when the tics are actually observed by an experienced clinician.

Although there are no laboratory tests for the diagnosis of TS, selective laboratory tests can help to rule out rare medical problems such as neuroacanthocytosis, Huntington's disease, and Wilson's disease (Jankovic 2001).

The physical and neurological examinations of most children with TS are unremarkable. An abnormal physical examination or positive neurological findings may signal the need for further evaluation in search of other conditions. For example, repetitive eye blinking with momentary loss of conscious awareness may prompt referral for an electroencephalogram (EEG). Referrals for a neurology consultation or an EEG are usually not necessary. Differences in brain volumes on magnetic resonance imaging (MRI) such as larger volumes in prefrontal regions and smaller caudate volumes have been observed in research studies comparing TS patients with normal control subjects (Peterson et al. 2001, 2003). In addition, although findings are not consistent across studies, an increased number of dopamine receptors and enhanced dopamine innervation in patients with TS compared with controls have been demonstrated in several functional neuroimaging studies (see Frey and Albin 2006). Computed tomography, MRI, positron emission tomography, and single-photon emission computed tomography are not part of the routine diagnostic evaluation of TS at the present time.

Developmental history and medical history may be informative in the differential diagnosis of TS. A child with a history of social disability, language delay, and stereotypic hand flapping may point to an autism spectrum disorder rather than TS. A thorough evaluation of how the symptoms affect family, interpersonal relationships, and school performance is essential for treatment planning through the identification of priorities for intervention. Similarly, a review of family history for tics, ADHD, and obsessive-compulsive symptoms is warranted as an aid to making the diagnosis and as part of family education. For example, a family with a paternal uncle afflicted with severe TS may need to be reassured that most cases are mild to moderate and that it is unlikely that their newly diagnosed child will be as severely affected as the uncle.

There are several tic symptom checklists and clinician interviews for the assessment of tic severity. Two commonly used instruments include the Tic

Symptom Self-Report (TSSR) (Allen et al. 2005; Scahill et al. 2003b) and the Yale Global Tic Severity Scale (YGTSS) (Leckman et al. 1989). The TSSR can be used as a self-report in children over the age of 10 years, though some orientation for the child may be needed on first administration. It can also be completed by parents or teachers to gather information across settings. The reliability of the TSSR has not been formally studied, but the TSSR performed similarly to the YGTSS as a change measure in two placebo-controlled trials (Allen et al. 2005; Scahill et al. 2003b).

The TSSR contains 20 items for motor tics and 20 items for phonic tics. Each item is rated 0 to 3 for frequency and intensity. The primary advantage of the TSSR is its ease of completion and scoring. The YGTSS is a clinician-rated instrument that surveys the number, frequency, intensity, complexity, and interference of motor and phonic tics separately. Each dimension is rated from 0 to 5. Thus, across the five dimensions, the total motor score can range from 0 to 25; likewise, the phonic tic score can range from 0 to 25. The Total Tic score (combined total of motor and phonic tic scores ranging from 0 to 50) is commonly used as an outcome measure in treatment studies. The YGTSS also has an overall Impairment score ranging from 0 to 50, with a higher score reflecting greater impairment. This scale is meant to capture the impairment and distress experienced by the patient that is due to tics. Although the correlation of the Impairment score and the Total Tic score is statistically significant in group analysis, some patients may show high degrees of impairment in the presence of mild tics. Other patients may show the opposite pattern: high tic severity with lower impairment. The YGTSS has well-established reliability and validity. One of the strengths of the YGTSS is that it allows the rater to incorporate reports of multiple informants (e.g., parent and child) and observation during the interview into the scoring. For example, when asking about the forcefulness of tics, the rater can ask the child and parent to contrast the average tic intensity over the past week to the observed intensity during the interview.

Treatment of Tics in Children With Tourette's Syndrome

The first-line treatment for tics in children with TS is *education*, especially the following points:

1. TS is not a progressive condition.
2. In most cases, the tics are mild to moderate in severity.
3. Treating tics may not improve symptoms of ADHD or disruptive behavior.
4. Tics have a fluctuating course, even when a child is taking a tic-suppressing medication.
5. Most children with TS will show a decline in tics by early adulthood (Bloch et al. 2006).

Understandably, parents and children may overfocus on the child's tics. The role of the clinician is to help refocus the parents on the child's most pressing problems and to keep the parents mindful of the child's overall development. All of these educational needs may extend to teachers and other school personnel.

Antipsychotics

Early randomized trials demonstrated that the potent dopamine D_2 receptor antagonists haloperidol and pimozide are superior to placebo for suppressing tics (Ross and Moldofsky 1978; A.K. Shapiro and Shapiro 1984). Two randomized clinical trials (RCTs) compared pimozide with haloperidol, showing better results with haloperidol in one study (E. Shapiro et al. 1989) and no difference in another (Sallee et al. 1997). However, the trial by Sallee et al. (1997) indicated that pimozide was better tolerated than haloperidol at equivalent doses. Compared with current practice, the early studies used these agents at high dosages (up to 20 mg/day for haloperidol and up to 48 mg/day for pimozide). In contemporary clinical practice, the trend is clearly toward the use of lower dosages, such as 1–4 mg/day for haloperidol and 2–6 mg/day for pimozide (R.A. King et al. 2003). Fluphenazine, a phenothiazine antipsychotic with dopamine D_1- and D_2-blocking properties, is used in clinical practice, though it has not been well studied. In an open-label trial with subjects that included children and adults, at dosages ranging from 2 to 15 mg/day given in two divided doses, fluphenazine was effective in 17 of 21 patients. A majority of the subjects with previous experience with haloperidol preferred fluphenazine (Goetz et al. 1984).

The atypical antipsychotics available in the United States include risperidone, olanzapine, ziprasidone, quetiapine, paliperidone, and clozapine, which have serotonin-blocking effects and variable D_2-blocking properties (Table 8–1).

Table 8–1.   Dosing guidelines for antipsychotic drugs used in the treatment of children with tics of moderate or greater severity

Medication[a]	Starting dose (mg)	Usual dosage range (mg/day)	Placebo-controlled trial?
Haloperidol	0.25–0.5	1–4	Yes[b]
Pimozide	0.5–1.0	2–6	Yes[b]
Risperidone	0.25–0.5	1.0–3.0	Yes[b]
Fluphenazine	0.5–1.0	1.5–10	No
Ziprasidone	5–10	10–80	Yes[c]
Olanzapine	2.5–5.0	2.5–12.5	No
Quetiapine	25–50	75–150	No
Aripiprazole	5–10	10–20	No

[a]Clozapine is not listed because of its complexity of use and failure to show efficacy.
[b]Superior to placebo in more than one study.
[c]Superior to placebo in one study.

The more recently released antipsychotic aripiprazole is a partial dopamine agonist that is believed to act as antagonist in hyperdopaminergic state. Clozapine, which has low affinity for D_2 receptors, was no better than placebo for the treatment of tics (Caine et al. 1979). Considered in light of the effectiveness of haloperidol and pimozide, the failure of clozapine suggests that D_2 blockade is an important mechanism in tic suppression. To date, the best-studied atypical antipsychotic is risperidone, which is a relatively potent D_2 receptor blocker. It was superior to placebo for tic reduction in two trials (Dion et al. 2002; Scahill et al. 2003b) and equally as effective as pimozide (Bruggeman et al. 2001; Gilbert et al. 2004) and clonidine (Gaffney et al. 2002). Two open-label trials of olanzapine in a total of 30 adult patients have yielded encouraging results for the treatment of tics (Budman et al. 2001; Stamenkovic et al. 2000). Ziprasidone was well tolerated and superior to placebo in a randomized trial of 28 children with TS (Sallee et al. 2000). To date, only case reports are available for quetiapine (Mukaddes and Abali 2003) and aripiprazole (Kastrup et al. 2005).

The appeal of the atypical antipsychotic drugs is their demonstrated lower probability for neurological side effects such as dystonia, dyskinesia, tremor, and parkinsonism. There is also a presumption that the atypical antipsychotics are less likely to cause tardive dyskinesia in the long term. After more than a decade of experience with the newer antipsychotics, they indeed appear to have a lower likelihood of neurological side effects in the short term. The relative risk of tardive dyskinesia also appears to be lower, but we may need more person-years of exposure to confirm this assumption.

Although the neurological side-effect burden appears to be lower with the atypical antipsychotics, other adverse effects have emerged in recent years. Chief among the emerging concerns are increased appetite, weight gain, and the potential for metabolic abnormalities (Meyer and Koro 2004). Based on reports from non-TS clinical populations, clozapine appears to be associated with the highest risk of weight gain, followed in order by olanzapine, quetiapine, risperidone, and ziprasidone (Allison and Casey 2001). Other adverse events reported in children and adolescents include social phobia, constipation, drooling, sedation, and cognitive blunting (Aman et al. 2005; Scahill et al. 2003b).

Clinical concerns have also been raised about alterations in cardiac conduction times such as QTc prolongation. This issue is not new, given that similar concerns have been expressed about pimozide for several years. Although the occurrence of prolonged QTc is presumed to be rare in the dose ranges used in the treatment of tics, an electrocardiogram (ECG) is recommended before starting treatment with pimozide, during the dose adjustment phase, and annually during ongoing treatment (R.A. King et al. 2003). Pimozide also appears to be vulnerable to interaction with drugs such as clarithromycin that inhibit cytochrome P450 (CYP) 3A4 (Desta et al. 1999). Of the atypical antipsychotics, ziprasidone appears to increase the QTc to a mild degree. In a series of 20 children with various psychiatric conditions, there was a modest increase in QTc during treatment with ziprasidone (Blair et al. 2005). Unlike pimozide, however, ziprasidone does not appear to be vulnerable to drug-drug interaction because it does not rely on a single hepatic pathway. Following a delay in U.S. Food and Drug Administration (FDA) approval for the treatment of adults with schizophrenia, ziprasidone is now approved with no specific warnings regarding cardiac monitoring. The package insert mentions that ziprasidone is contraindicated in patients with a known history of QTc prolongation. Until more data are available to inform practice, guidelines similar to those used for pimozide have been recommended (R.A. King et al. 2003).

Nonantipsychotic Medications

Several nonantipsychotic medications have been tried for the treatment of tics, including clonidine, guanfacine, pergolide, nicotine, tetrabenazine, botulinum toxin, fluoxetine, ondansetron, and baclofen. Most have not been well studied. A detailed review of each of these compounds is beyond the scope of this chapter (see Scahill et al. 2006). Results from studies with pergolide, botulinum toxin, and ondansetron will be presented briefly. Guanfacine and clonidine will be reviewed in the section on treating ADHD in children with TS.

Pergolide is a dopamine agonist with action at dopamine D_1, D_2, and D_3 receptors that was developed for the treatment of Parkinson's disease. In Parkinson's, pergolide is presumed to enhance dopaminergic function. Given the proposed heightened dopaminergic tone in TS, pergolide is hypothesized to improve tics by turning down presynaptic synthesis of dopamine. Two double-blind, placebo-controlled studies with pergolide showed superiority to placebo, though the results of both studies are somewhat difficult to interpret (Gilbert et al. 2000, 2003). The first study used a crossover design and showed evidence of an order effect. Subjects who received pergolide followed by placebo did better than the subjects who received placebo followed by pergolide (Gilbert et al. 2000). The second study used a parallel design in 51 subjects. After 8 weeks of treatment at doses ranging from 300 to 450 µg, pergolide was no better than placebo on the clinician-rated measure of tic severity (i.e., the Total Tic score of the YGTSS). Superiority to placebo was demonstrated only when tic-related impairment was included in the analysis (Gilbert et al. 2003). Pergolide is an ergot derivative. Several case reports of ergot-induced pleural, retroperitoneal, or pericardial fibrosis, vasospasm, and cardiotoxicity are likely to limit the use of pergolide in Parkinson's disease and TS. There are limited data on other dopamine agonists such as pramipexole and ropinirole, which are not ergot derivatives.

The injection of botulinum toxin is now a standard treatment for dystonia. Following encouraging results in three open studies on TS (Jankovic 1994; Kwak et al. 2000). Marras et al. (2001) conducted a placebo-controlled trial in TS. In this study, there was about a 40% difference between active drug and placebo. Treatment with botulinum toxin involves direct injection into the selected muscle of the motor tic or the laryngeal folds, in the case of vocal tic (Porta et al. 2004). In open-label studies, the botulinum toxin injections appeared to reduce the premonitory sensations as well as the tic at the injection site. Adverse effects include transient soreness at the injection site, weakness of the injected muscle, and loss of voice volume if the vocal cords are the target of treatment. Because benefit is generally confined to the injected muscle group, botulinum toxin should only be considered in cases with a prominent and interfering tic. The dose and frequency of repeat injections have not been standardized. More study is needed to answer these critical issues.

Ondansetron is a selective serotonin 5-HT$_3$ receptor antagonist that was developed as an antiemetic. A placebo-controlled trial provided encouraging, though inconclusive results (Toren et al. 2005). In this study, 30 subjects were randomly assigned to receive ondansetron 24 mg/day (8 mg three times per day) or placebo for the 3-week trial. On one measure of tic severity, there was a significant difference between active drug and placebo. On the more frequently used YGTSS Total Tic score, there was no difference between drug and placebo. In addition to the small sample size, two limitations qualify these findings. First, the duration of trial was only 3 weeks, which may not have been long enough to detect a treatment effect. Second, there was a significant difference in the YGTSS scores at baseline across treatment groups. Ondansetron was well tolerated, and only 1 of 15 subjects randomly assigned to receive active drug withdrew because of an adverse effect. This subject reported gastrointestinal complaints. One major drawback of ondansetron treatment is cost. Ondansetron is an expensive medication, and, given that it is generally not used for open-ended treatment, insurance companies may balk at its use for TS.

Future Treatments

Several novel medications are of interest for the treatment of tics in children and adults with TS. For example, there is an ongoing RCT with an over-the-counter omega-3 fatty acid preparation, and a planned multisite trial of the dopamine-depleting agent tetrabenazine. When available, the results of these trials may provide guidance for clinicians on the optimal use of these compounds. Anticonvulsant medications such as topiramate and levetiracetam are also of interest for the treatment of tics. To date, however, these drugs have only been tested in open-label trials (Abuzzahab and Brown 2001; Awaad et al. 2005). Dosages of topiramate are likely to range from 75 to 150 mg/day, and dosages of levetiracetam range from 1,000 to 2,000 mg/day. Enthusiasm for topiramate has diminished because of reports of acute angle-closure glaucoma and short-term memory problems associated with its use (Fraunfelder and Fraunfelder 2004). Both compounds warrant further study to provide better guidance for clinical practice.

There is also tremendous interest in the potential for repetitive transcranial magnetic stimulation (rTMS) (Orth et al. 2005) and an even more invasive procedure, deep brain stimulation (Ackermans et al. 2006; Temel and Visser-Vandewalle 2004), for treatment in severe, refractory cases. rTMS uses a magnetic coil to generate a current that can be directed into the cortex in a noninvasive manner. In fact, the handheld magnetic coil does not come in contact with the skull. The amplitude of the current can be varied and the procedure appears safe when used appropriately. When the frequency and intensity of the stimuli are varied, it is presumed possible to increase or decrease cortical excitability. Orth et al. (2005) were unable to show benefit with rTMS in five subjects with prominent tics. The authors suggested that focusing on different targets and different intensity settings of the magnetic pulse may prove more successful. Deep brain stimulation, which involves the placement of an electrode into the brain, is emerging as a standard treatment in Parkinson's disease, and several reports in extremely severe cases of TS have shown some promise (Ackermans et al. 2006). There is ongoing debate about the anatomical placement (thalamus or globus pallidus interna) of the electrodes, as well as the amplitude and frequency of the stimulation that are most advantageous for treatment effect.

Deep brain stimulation and rTMS are interventions that are currently being pursued with agreement in the field that only patients with refractory conditions should be treated with these methods. Behavioral interventions have also garnered interest in recent years. Perhaps most attention has been focused on habit reversal training (HRT; Piacentini and Chang 2006; Wilhelm et al. 2003). HRT is a cognitive-behavioral intervention that appears to rely on awareness training and competing response as the active ingredients. The aim of awareness training is to increase the chance of initiating a voluntary, competing movement prior to the execution of the tic. The patient is asked to engage in the competing response until the urge to tic subsides. Preliminary studies are positive, and there are two ongoing multisite trials (one in children and one in adults) that should provide important new information on the effectiveness of HRT in reducing tics.

Conclusions: Pharmacotherapy for Tics

For children and adolescents with mild tics, medications aimed at reducing tics may not be necessary. For children who have tics that are frequent, forceful, and interfere with activities of daily living, medication is likely to be indicated. The goal of medication treatment should be to reduce, not eliminate, the tics. The antipsychotic medications haloperidol, pimozide, risperidone, ziprasidone, and fluphenazine appear to be the most effective. Although it is considered effective, haloperidol has fallen out of use because of concerns about short- and long-term adverse effects. Pimozide is effective and generally well tolerated at low doses, but requires cardiac monitoring and is vulnerable to drug-drug interaction. On balance, fluphenazine may be the best choice among the traditional antipsychotic medications. Risperidone is the best studied of the newer atypical antipsychotic, and is superior to placebo. Although there is a lower risk of neurological side effects, weight gain is an important clinical concern. Ziprasidone also appears to be effective. Botulinum toxin may be considered in patients with a single, interfering tic. However, treatment guidelines on dose and frequency of injection remain somewhat uncertain. Finally, for tics of moderate severity, but not for tics of greater severity, guanfacine or clonidine may also be considered as first-line treatments, given the favorable safety margin of these medications.

Treatment of OCD in Children With Tourette's Syndrome

Diagnosis and Assessment

Obsessive-compulsive disorder is characterized by recurrent, unwanted worries; thoughts or impulses (obsessions) that are difficult to dislodge; and/or repetitive behavior that the person feels driven to perform (compulsions). Patients report that attempts to resist the performance of compulsions increases anxiety as well as the urge to perform the compulsion. According to DSM-IV-TR, the obsessions or compulsions must expend at least an hour per day and be the source of distress or impairment. Adolescents and adults acknowledge that their obsessions or compulsions are excessive. This realization may not be present in younger children.

The lifetime prevalence of OCD is estimated to be 2%–3% in adults (Karno et al. 1988), with similar estimates in adolescents (Valleni-Basile et al. 1994). The prevalence in preadolescents, however, appears to be lower, with estimates in the range of 2 per 1,000 in children under the age of 13 years (Costello et al. 1996).

Common obsessions in children and adolescents include contamination worries, fears about harm coming to self or family members, worry about acting on unwanted aggressive impulses, and concern about order and symmetry (Scahill et al. 2003a). Although many children and adolescents report that their obsessions come "out of the blue," careful discussion usually reveals that the obsessive worries occur in specific events and situations. Common compulsions include hand washing, cleaning rituals, repetitive requests for reassurance about disease or harm, arranging objects in patterns, checking, counting, and repeating routine activities (e.g., opening and closing a door, going back and forth across a doorway). In many cases, there is a close relationship between the obsession and the repetitive behavior, as exemplified by fears of contamination and hand washing. By contrast, other patients state that the ritual is done to achieve a sense of completion. In either model, the ritual is associated with at least a temporary relief in anxiety, which reinforces the compulsive habit.

In the assessment of children with tic disorders and OCD, it may be difficult to distinguish between tics and compulsive behaviors. For example, some children may describe a recurring concern that "something bad will happen" if a specific touching ritual is not completed. Another child may perform a similar-appearing ritual but will describe a need or an urge to carry out the behavior that is similar to the premonitory sensations preceding tic. Children with these behaviors, who are driven by a sensation or urge, will often describe a need to "get it right" or achieve a sense of completion. In milder cases, the ritual achieves its aim quickly and the child moves on without much notice. In more severe cases, the child gets caught in multiple repetitions, seemingly unable to achieve a sense of completion. Still other children may describe experiences that contain a mixture of "just right" elements and harm reduction. In a series of 80 children and adolescents, we observed differences in the OCD symptom picture according to the presence or absence of chronic tics (Scahill et al. 2003a). Children with OCD without tics tend to perform rituals to prevent harm. By contrast, children with chronic tics and OCD appear to carry out repetitive behaviors to achieve a sense of completion rather than harm reduction. These findings suggest that assessment should consider what seems to drive the repetitive behavior—harm reduction or a sense of the need to achieve completion.

There is another type of repetitive urge and behavioral sequence that warrants mention. Some children describe an intense urge to touch potentially harmful objects such as a flame, the tip of a knife, or a hot stove. These urges and the actions that may follow are probably best viewed as impulsive behaviors rather than compulsive behaviors and do not arise from self-injurious intent. Children may be reluctant to describe these urges, but upon careful inquiry, they may feel some relief to learn that others have had such experiences.

Several clinician ratings, self-reports, and parent reports have been developed for assessing obsessive-compulsive symptoms in children with TS. A commonly used clinician rating is the Children's Yale-Brown Obsessive Compulsive Scale (CY-BOCS) (Scahill et al. 1997b), which was derived from the original adult instrument, the Yale-Brown Obsessive-Compulsive Scale (Y-BOCS; Goodman et al. 1989). The CY-BOCS rates time spent, interference, distress, level of resistance and degree of control over the obsessions and compulsions. The CY-BOCS interview may also assist with charting the phenomenology of the obsessive-compulsive symptoms.

Serotonin Reuptake Inhibitors

To date, the only effective pharmacological treatment for children with OCD is the serotonin reuptake inhibitors (SRIs). There are currently seven SRIs marketed in the United States: clomipramine, fluoxetine, sertraline, paroxetine, fluvoxamine, citalopram, and escitalopram. With the exception of clomipramine, these drugs are called *selective* serotonin reuptake inhibitors (SSRIs), indicating the specificity of the mechanism. The reuptake blockade at the presynaptic transporter site begins to occur with the first dose. However, beneficial effects are often delayed for several weeks, suggesting that reuptake inhibition begins a cascade of events that ultimately leads to enhanced serotonergic function.

Twelve RCTs of OCD pharmacotherapy in pediatric populations have been published over the past two decades (Scahill et al., in press). Of these, eight were placebo controlled and used the CY-BOCS as the primary outcome measure. The total sample size across these studies was 750 subjects (range=14–207). Taken together, the results of these studies indicate that clomipramine, fluoxetine, fluvoxamine, sertraline, and paroxetine were superior to placebo in at least one study. The magnitude of effect was modest, with a range of 10%–25% improvement over placebo. Children with TS were often excluded from these trials. Furthermore, the distinct phenomenology of obsessive-compulsive symptoms in tic-related forms of OCD versus other forms of OCD indicates that the beneficial effects of the SSRIs in children with OCD may not extend to children with OCD and TS.

Fluoxetine was evaluated in two small placebo-controlled studies in children with Tourette's syndrome (Kurlan et al. 1993; Scahill et al. 1997a). The results of these studies showed that fluoxetine provided only modest benefit in reducing repetitive behavior in these populations. Table 8–2 presents dosing guidelines for the SRIs for children and adolescents with OCD.

Augmentation Strategies

Given the modest benefit, on average, for the SSRIs and clomipramine in children with OCD, it follows that only a partial response or no benefit may be seen in an estimated 30%–40% of cases. Several pharmacological augmentation strategies have been examined in adults, though few have been tested in children and adolescents (Scahill et al., in press). Although several augmentation approaches have been tried in order to improve partial response to the SSRIs in OCD, the most consistently effective approach has been the addition of an antipsychotic medication. For example, McDougle et al. (1994) showed that the addition of haloperidol to fluvoxamine was superior to placebo in subjects who showed a partial response or no benefit with fluvoxamine only. This finding has been replicated with the addition of risperidone, quetiapine, and olanzapine, though the findings with quetiapine and olanzapine have not been consistently positive (see Scahill et al., in press, for a review). Across these augmentation trials, a positive response was seen with the addition of the antipsychotic drug in approximately half of the cases of OCD refractory to SSRI monotherapy.

To date, only two open-label SSRI augmentation studies have been conducted in the pediatric population. Both studies involved the addition of risperidone (dosage range=0.25–2.0 mg/day). Fitzgerald et al. (1999) reported improvement following the addition of risperidone to SSRI treatment in four children ages 8–13 years. In a sample of 17 subjects ages 15–19 years, Thomsen (2004) observed an average improvement of 4.3% on the Y-BOCS after

Table 8–2. Dosing guidelines for medications used in the treatment of children with obsessive-compulsive disorder

Medication	Starting dose (mg)	Usual dosage range (mg/day)	Placebo-controlled trial?
Clomipramine	25–50	100–200	Yes
Fluoxetine	5–10	10–40	Yes
Sertraline	25–50	50–200	Yes
Fluvoxamine	25–50	50–200	Yes
Paroxetine	5–10	10–40	Yes
Citalopram	5–10	20–40	No
Escitalopram	5–10	10–20	No

the addition of risperidone to ongoing treatment with an SSRI. Although the level of improvement in these pediatric studies appears to be modest, these preliminary results are generally consistent with findings from controlled risperidone addition studies in adults.

An alternative to the addition of an antipsychotic medication for the treatment of refractory OCD is the introduction of cognitive-behavioral therapy (CBT). CBT, based on the principles of exposure and response prevention, has been shown to be effective in controlled studies in adults and in several open studies in children. A three-site, randomized trial compared sertraline, CBT, and the combination of sertraline and CBT with placebo in 112 children (mean age = 11.5 years) (Pediatric OCD Treatment Study [POTS] Team 2004). Sertraline alone was superior to placebo; CBT was also superior to placebo. In addition, the group that received CBT plus sertraline showed greater improvement than the sertraline-alone group. There was no difference between combined treatment and CBT alone. The 15% difference between sertraline alone and placebo was similar to the magnitude of positive response in the pediatric SSRI placebo-controlled trials described earlier. By contrast, the improvement level above placebo was nearly 40% for the combined treatment group (drug plus CBT) and 30% for the CBT-only group. Also of interest in this study was the difference in sertraline dose. The combined treatment group received sertraline at an average dosage of 133 mg/day compared with 170 mg/day for the sertraline-only group. These results suggest that CBT should be strongly considered in the treatment plan for children with

OCD. However, it must be noted that studies showing the effectiveness of exposure and response prevention in children with a tic-related form of OCD have not been undertaken.

Adverse Effects

Despite the evidence showing efficacy, clomipramine is generally not used as a first-line treatment for children with OCD. Its relegation to second-line status is due to concern about adverse effects and the need to monitor blood levels and cardiac conduction during treatment. Common adverse events of clomipramine include dry mouth, somnolence, fatigue, constipation, tachycardia, dizziness, and sweating. Clomipramine can also increase the QTc interval and, although uncommon, may produce cardiac arrhythmia. It can also lower the seizure threshold. Finally, clomipramine can be fatal on overdose and is vulnerable to drug-drug interactions.

The SSRIs rarely cause serious medical side effects. A common adverse effect, termed *behavioral activation*, is characterized by insomnia, overactivity, restlessness, talkativeness, irritability, and impulsiveness. Behavioral activation tends to occur early in treatment or with dose increases. Not surprisingly, then, the risk of behavioral activation appears to increase when the dose is increased quickly There are also hints that the risk of activation is higher in younger children. Other common adverse effects associated with the use of SSRIs include nausea, heartburn, tremor, fatigue, weight loss, and palpitations, which are often self-limited.

Drug Interactions

As noted above, clomipramine is vulnerable to drug interaction. Drugs that inhibit CYP3A4, such as erythromycin, can cause a dramatic rise in the clomipramine level into the toxic range. Drug interaction issues for the SSRIs are quite different than for clomipramine. To varying degrees, the SSRIs inhibit one or more hepatic CYP isoenzymes. Therefore, the concern with the SSRIs is their potential impact on the metabolism of other drugs, leading to higher rates of adverse effects for these other drugs. For example, fluoxetine and paroxetine are potent inhibitors of CYP2D6, which is the metabolic pathway used by antipsychotics such as risperidone. As monotherapy, risperidone is unlikely to cause dystonia in children in the usual dose range. When added to ongoing treatment with paroxetine, however, hepatic inhibition increases the level of risperidone and the risk of drug-induced dystonia.

Conclusion: Pharmacotherapy for OCD

Ironically, most randomized trials of SRIs in children and adolescents with OCD have excluded subjects with TS. In addition, there is evidence in children and adults that tic-related OCD may be a distinct subtype of OCD (Leckman et al. 1995; Scahill et al. 2003a). Thus, it is not at all clear that SRIs will be effective in children and adolescents with tic-related OCD.

Before treatment with an SRI is initiated for repetitive behavior in a child with TS, a careful inventory of the repetitive behaviors, including the differentiation of rituals from tics, as well as documentation of the impairment, is warranted. As in the treatment of children with OCD who do not have TS, the medication should be started at a low dose, and the dosage should be increased slowly, with attention to therapeutic and adverse effects. Children treated with clomipramine need an ECG to assess heart rate and QTc interval prior to starting treatment, during dose adjustment, and when the maintenance dose is achieved, as well as annually thereafter. Parents need to be educated about the potential for drug interaction and encouraged to call before starting any concomitant treatment while the patient is taking clomipramine.

Treatment of ADHD in Children With Tourette's Syndrome

Diagnosis and Assessment

ADHD is characterized by the early childhood onset of an enduring pattern of inattention and/or hyperactivity and impulsive behavior (American Psychiatric Association 2000). Establishing the diagnosis of ADHD to measure symptom severity in children and adolescents requires information from parents, teachers, and the child. The use of multiple informants is necessary to show that the behavioral pattern is consistent across settings. Clinic observation is also important, but some children are able to maintain behavioral control during a clinic visit. ADHD affects 2%–10% of school-age children, depending on the definition and sampling methods used (Scahill and Schwab-Stone 2000). ADHD affects as many as two-thirds of children from TS clinical samples (Spencer et al. 2001). The presence of ADHD is associated with substantial impairment unrelated to the severity of the tics (Sukhodolsky et al. 2003). Because the symptoms of ADHD, such as impulsiveness, overactivity, disruptiveness, and distractibility, are likely to interfere with family life, peer relationships, and academic progress, aggressive treatment of ADHD in children with TS is warranted.

A practical method of collecting information from multiple informants across settings and measuring change with treatment is through the use of parent and teacher rating scales. The parent and teacher questionnaires developed by Conners (Goyette et al. 1978); the ADHD Rating Scale (DuPaul et al. 1998); and the Swanson, Nolan, and Pelham rating scale (SNAP-IV) (Swanson et al. 1999) are examples of reliable and valid behavior scales. Each of these scales is scored from 0 (symptom not present) to 3 (severe). The ADHD Rating Scale and the SNAP-IV have one-to-one correspondence to DSM-IV (American Psychiatric Association 1994) symptoms of ADHD. Both scales have also been shown to be sensitive to change with treatment ("A Fourteen-Month Randomized Clinical Trial of Treatment Strategies for Attention-Deficit/Hyperactivity Disorder" 1999; Michelson et al. 2001; Scahill et al. 2001). Based on clinical and population data on the SNAP-IV and the ADHD Rating Scale, an average per item score of 2.0 on these scales is predictive of ADHD. Despite their practical value, these scales cannot be relied upon as the only means of making the diagnosis.

Medications for ADHD

Stimulants

Stimulants are the first-line agents for the treatment of ADHD ("A Fourteen-Month Randomized Clinical Trial" 1999; see Chapter 2, Attention-Deficit/Hyperactivity Disorder," this volume). However, because of lack of efficacy or adverse effects, stimulants fail in 10%–20% of children with ADHD (Elia et al. 1991). Case reports over the past three decades suggest that stimulants may induce the emergence of tics or an increase in preexisting tics in children with ADHD (Erenberg et al. 1985; Golden 1974; Lipkin et al. 1994; Lowe et al. 1982; Riddle et al. 1995; Varley et al. 2001). Two placebo-controlled trials that *excluded* children with tic disorders (Barkley et al. 1992; Borcherding et al. 1990) also reported the emergence of tics in a small percentage of children treated with stimulants.

This body of evidence has had an enormous impact on clinical practice until recently. Over the past decade, three short-term, placebo-controlled studies in children with ADHD and tic disorders reported no significant increase in tics among stimulant-treated subjects compared with placebo (Castellanos et al. 1997; Gadow et al. 1995; Tourette Syndrome Study Group 2002). Two naturalistic studies also provide information on the longer-term effects of stimulants in children with TS (Gadow et al. 1999; Law and Schachar 1999). Although most children in these longer-term studies did not show an increase in tics, acute exacerbations did occur in a few children resulting in discontinuation of the stimulant or addition of a tic-suppressing medication. Taken together, these findings suggest that stimulants should be considered in the treatment of children with ADHD and tics.

In the 16-week Treatment of ADHD in Children With Tic Disorders (TACT) trial conducted by the Tourette Syndrome Study Group (2002), 136 children with ADHD and a tic disorder were randomly assigned to placebo, clonidine alone, methylphenidate alone, or clonidine plus methylphenidate. Although the effect was modest, tics declined in all active treatment groups. Monotherapy with clonidine or methylphenidate was effective in reducing teacher-rated ADHD symptoms, but the magnitude was small (40% and 38%, respectively) compared with the level of improvement documented for methylphenidate in the multisite Multimodal Treatment Study of Children With ADHD (MTA) (56% for the medication-only group) ("A Fourteen-Month Randomized Clinical Trial" 1999). By contrast, subjects randomly assigned to clonidine plus methylphenidate showed a 59% improvement on ADHD outcomes. Compared with doses given in the MTA study, the dose of methylphenidate in the TACT study was relatively low in this study (25.7 mg in two divided doses compared with a range of 31–38 mg in three divided doses in the MTA study). The more conservative approach in the TACT study may explain the lower level of improvement observed in the methylphenidate group. The level of improvement for monotherapy with clonidine in this study is consistent with the results of other nonstimulant medications in ADHD (see below). Taken together, the results of the TACT trial indicate that methylphenidate can be used safely in children with TS. Given the conservative dosing for methylphenidate in the TACT study, clinicians may decide against the more aggressive approach described in the MTA study. Although the more conservative approach may be associated with a lower magnitude of effect, it may also be associated with a lower likelihood of adverse effects, including tics. For example, in the TACT trial, approximately one-quarter of the subjects in the methylphenidate-only group showed an increase in tics, which was only slightly higher than the rate observed in the placebo group.

Nonstimulants

A range of nonstimulant medications have been used in the treatment of children with ADHD, including selective noradrenergic reuptake inhibitors (atomoxetine and desipramine), the novel antidepressant bupropion, α_2-adrenergic agonists, modafinil, and selegiline. Table 8–3 shows the starting dose and usual maintenance dosage of nonstimulant medications that have been evaluated in the treatment of ADHD. This section will examine the nonstimulants listed in the table that have been evaluated in children with ADHD and a chronic tic disorder (see Chapter 2, "Attention-Deficit/Hyperactivity Disorder," for description of other nonstimulants used in the treatment of ADHD).

Atomoxetine is the only nonstimulant medication that is approved for the treatment of children with ADHD. It has been shown to be safe and effective in several randomized, placebo-controlled trials in children and adolescents (Kelsey et al. 2004; Michelson et al. 2001, 2002). The revised Texas Algorithm positions atomoxetine as a second-line treatment for ADHD. Although not strongly supported by evidence, the algorithm further suggests that atomoxetine may be useful in children with ADHD and anxiety (Pliszka et al. 2006).

An 18-week, placebo-controlled study by Allen et al. (2005) evaluated the efficacy and safety of atomoxetine in 148 children (mean age=11.2 years) with ADHD and a chronic tic disorder. Atomoxetine showed a 28% improvement on a clinician-rated measure of ADHD symptoms compared with 14% for placebo. This level of improvement in ADHD symptoms is similar, though slightly lower, than that seen with guanfacine, clonidine, and desipramine in this population. There was no difference in tic severity across the atomoxetine and placebo groups, suggesting that atomoxetine neither improves nor worsens tics. The adverse effects in this study were also similar to reports on atomoxetine in children with ADHD. Nausea, vomiting, decreased appetite, and weight loss were significantly more frequent in the atomoxetine group compared with placebo. Insomnia, which has been reported in other pediatric ADHD studies, was no different from placebo in this study.

The tricyclic antidepressant desipramine has been used in the treatment of ADHD for the past two decades. Placebo-controlled trials in the 1980s and

Table 8–3. Dosing guidelines for nonstimulant medications used in the treatment of children with tics and attention-deficit/hyperactivity disorder

			Placebo-controlled trial?	
Medication[a]	Starting dose (mg)	Usual dosage range (mg/day)	ADHD[b]	ADHD + tics[c]
Atomoxetine	18–25	36–100	Yes	Yes
Bupropion	25–50	75–150	Yes	No
Clonidine	0.025–0.05	0.2–0.3	Yes	Yes
Guanfacine	0.25–0.5	2–3	No	Yes
Modafinil	50–100	200–400	Yes	No
Pindolol	5–10	15–40	Yes	No
Selegiline	5	5–10	No	Yes

[a]Desipramine not listed, falling out of use due to concerns about QTc prolongation.
[b]Children with ADHD without a tic disorder.
[c]Children with ADHD plus a chronic tic disorder.

1990s showed that it was effective for the treatment of ADHD in children without co-occurring tic disorders (Biederman et al. 1989), and in children with ADHD and tic disorders (Singer et al. 1995). Spencer et al. (2002) conducted a 6-week, placebo-controlled study in 41 children with ADHD and a chronic tic disorder. At total daily doses averaging 3.4 mg/kg given in two divided doses, desipramine was superior to placebo on an ADHD symptom rating scale. The desipramine group improved by 42% compared with little change in the placebo group. Tics improved by 30% on average in the desipramine group compared with no change in the placebo group. Adverse effects included decreased appetite, insomnia, and dry mouth. The investigators detected a significant increase in pulse and blood pressure in the desipramine group, but no ECG abnormalities. Despite these overall positive results, desipramine is falling out of use because of concerns about prolonged cardiac conduction times and reports of sudden death.

Selegiline is a selective monoamine oxidase inhibitor that directly enhances dopamine function in the brain. In addition, it is metabolized to an amphetamine compound in the brain, which may further enhance central catecholamine function. To date, there are two controlled studies of selegiline in children with ADHD. Mohamaddi et al. (2004) compared selegiline with methylphenidate in a double-blind, randomized trial involving 40 children with ADHD without co-occurring tics. The subjects ranged in age from 6 to 15 years. After 60 days of treatment at a maximum total daily dose of 40 mg of methylphenidate or 10 mg of selegiline (both dispensed in two divided doses), there was a 54% decrease in the teacher rating for methylphenidate and a 50% improvement for selegiline. Results on parent ratings were slightly more favorable for both medications than teacher ratings. Headache and decreased appetite were more frequent in the methylphenidate group, otherwise both medications were well tolerated.

Using a double-blind, crossover design, Feigin et al. (1996) studied selegiline in 24 children with TS and ADHD. In the crossover design, subjects were randomly assigned to receive selegiline followed by placebo, or placebo followed by selegiline. Despite the 6-week washout between phases, the study design poses serious problems to the interpretation of the results. First, over one-third of the sample dropped out of the study. Second, there was a clear order effect, in that the subjects who received selegiline first showed benefit compared with placebo. By contrast, the subjects who received selegiline second actually showed a mean worsening of ADHD symptoms. Overall, selegiline was no better than placebo. However, a secondary analysis showed a significant effect for selegiline in the first phase. There was no apparent impact of selegiline on tics. Selegiline appears to be well tolerated. At low doses, there are no dietary restrictions with selegiline, and drug interaction is not a major concern. However, given the inconsistent results to date, more study is needed to demonstrate its efficacy for ADHD symptoms.

The α_2-adrenergic agonists clonidine and guanfacine are also used to treat children with ADHD and co-occurring tic disorders. Indeed, this class of medications is perhaps the most commonly used for the treatment of tics and ADHD in tic disorder clinics (Freeman et al. 2000). Although there is some evidence that clonidine and guanfacine can reduce tics (Leckman et al. 1991; Scahill et al. 2001), these drugs are more often used in the treatment of ADHD in children who also have a tic disorder. The use of clonidine in children with tic disorders has been evaluated in a number of small studies (e.g., Hunt et al. 1985). The randomized, placebo-controlled trial of desipramine by Singer et al. (1995) involving 34 children also included a clonidine arm in the crossover design. In that study, clonidine was deemed no better than placebo.

As noted earlier, the Tourette Syndrome Study Group (2002) conducted a multisite, randomized trial with four groups: clonidine alone, methylphenidate alone, clonidine plus methylphenidate, and placebo. The clonidine-alone group showed a 40% improvement on the 10-item Conners Abbreviated Symptom Questionnaire for Teachers compared with 38% for the methylphenidate group and 59% for combined treatment. The combined treatment with clonidine and methylphenidate also attenuated side effects associated with each monotherapy. For example, sedation was less of a problem with the combined treatment compared with clonidine only and insomnia was less of a problem for the combined treatment than for methylphenidate only.

Adverse effects of clonidine include sedation, dry mouth, headache, irritability, and midsleep awakening. Blood pressure and pulse should be measured at baseline and monitored during dose adjustment, though blood pressure is generally not a problem with clonidine. Nonetheless, patients and families should be educated about the potential for rebound increases in blood pressure, tics, and anxiety with abrupt discontinuation (Leckman et al. 1986).

Guanfacine is another α-adrenergic antihypertensive that has entered into clinical practice. Interest in guanfacine emerged following animal studies showing that it may be more specific in its action (see Arnsten and Li 2005 for a review). Traditionally, the α_2 agonists were presumed to enhance prefrontal function by decreasing the firing of presynaptic noradrenergic receptors in the locus coeruleus. This reduced firing by locus coeruleus neurons regulates norepinephrine function and decreases arousal. Via long axons projecting from the locus coeruleus, it is now clear that guanfacine has direct effects on prefrontal function by mimicking norepinephrine at α_2 receptors in this region. This pharmacological effect appears to explain the improvements in distractibility, impulsiveness, and overactivity (Arnsten and Li 2005). To date, there are two placebo-controlled trials of guanfacine in TS populations (Cummings et al. 2002; Scahill et al. 2001). Guanfacine was associated with a 30% decrease in tics from baseline in both studies. However, these results are difficult to interpret because the tic severity at baseline in these trials was mild. Whether guanfacine would be effective for the treatment of moderate-to-severe tics remains unanswered.

The trial by Scahill et al. (2001) evaluated 34 children (ages 7–14 years) with ADHD and a chronic tic disorder in a randomized, placebo-controlled trial. After 8 weeks of treatment with dosages ranging from 1.5 to 3.0 mg/day given in three divided doses, there was a 37% improvement for the guanfacine group compared with 8% for placebo on the teacher-rated ADHD Rating Scale. Sedation led to discontinuation in only one subject. Other adverse effects included a slight drop in the mean blood pressure and pulse and mid-sleep awakening in a few subjects. The three-times-per-day dosing may have been protective against hypotensive effects by minimizing the fluctuation of the medication level across the day. For example, in a case series of 200 children from a TS clinic who were treated with guanfacine, 4 subjects had syncopal episodes (A. King et al. 2006). In this case series, guanfacine was administered in a single bedtime dose. A recent review indicated that cardiac monitoring with routine ECGs is not necessary when treating children with clonidine or guanfacine (Scahill et al. 2006). Clearly, blood pressure and pulse should be monitored during dose adjustment and during the maintenance phase.

Conclusion: Pharmacotherapy of ADHD

Atomoxetine and the α_2 agonists are rational choices for the treatment of ADHD in children with chronic tic disorders, especially if an adequate stimulant trial has been unsuccessful. The α_2 agonists may also be used as an adjunct to stimulants. For patients with prominent tics at baseline or for families who decline treatment with a stimulant, the α agonists may also be a rational alternative.

There are theoretical and practical reasons to select guanfacine over clonidine for treatment of ADHD, but the evidence does not clearly favor one of the α_2 agonists over the other. The α_2-adrenergic agonists can also be considered as a first-line treatment for tics independent of ADHD, though the magnitude of improvement is unlikely to exceed 30%. The findings with selegiline are inconclusive.

Clinical Pearls

- Tourette's syndrome is not as rare as it once was believed to be.
- Tourette's syndrome is frequently associated with obsessive-compulsive symptoms as well as hyperactivity, impulsivity, and inattention.
- The first-line treatment for tics in children with Tourette's syndrome is education.
- For children and adolescents with mild tics, pharmacotherapy specifically targeted at reducing tics may not be needed.
- Psychostimulants, particularly methylphenidate, may be considered as a treatment option for children with attention-deficit/hyperactivity disorder and tics.

References

Abuzzahab FS, Brown VL: Control of Tourette's syndrome with topiramate. Am J Psychiatry 158:968, 2001

Ackermans L, Temel Y, Cath D, et al: Deep brain stimulation in Tourette's syndrome: two targets? Mov Disord 21:709–713, 2006

Allen AJ, Kurlan RM, Gilbert DL, et al: Atomoxetine treatment in children and adolescents with ADHD and comorbid tic disorders. Neurology 65:1941–1949, 2005

Allison DB, Casey DE: Antipsychotic-induced weight gain: a review of the literature. J Clin Psychiatry 62:22–31, 2001

Aman MG, Arnold LE, McDougle CJ, et al: Acute and long-term safety and tolerability of risperidone in children with autism. J Child Adoles Psychopharmacology 15:869–884, 2005

American Psychiatric Association: Diagnostic and Statistical Manual of Mental Disorders, 3rd Edition. Washington, DC, American Psychiatric Association, 1980

American Psychiatric Association: Diagnostic and Statistical Manual of Mental Disorders, 3rd Edition, Revised. Washington, DC, American Psychiatric Association, 1987

American Psychiatric Association: Diagnostic and Statistical Manual of Mental Disorders, 4th Edition. Washington, DC, American Psychiatric Association, 1994

American Psychiatric Association: Diagnostic and Statistical Manual of Mental Disorders, 4th Edition, Text Revision. Washington, DC, American Psychiatric Association, 2000

Arnsten AF, Li BM: Neurobiology of executive functions: catecholamine influences on prefrontal cortical functions. Biol Psychiatry 57:1377–1384, 2005

Awaad Y, Michon AM, Minarik S: Use of levetiracetam to treat tics in children and adolescents with Tourette's syndrome. Mov Disord 20:714–718, 2005

Barkley RA, McMurray MB, Edelbrock CS, et al: Side effects of methylphenidate in children with attention deficit hyperactivity disorder: a systematic, placebo-controlled evaluation. Pediatrics 86:184–192, 1992

Biederman J, Baldessarini RJ, Wright V, et al: A double-blind placebo controlled study of desipramine in the treatment of ADD, I: efficacy. J Am Acad Child Adolesc Psychiatry 28:777–784, 1989

Blair J, Scahill L, State M, et al: Electrocardiographic changes in children and adolescents treated with ziprasidone: a prospective study. J Am Acad Child Adolesc Psychiatry 44:73–79, 2005

Bloch MH, Peterson BS, Scahill L, et al: Adulthood outcome of tic and obsessive-compulsive symptom severity in children with Tourette's syndrome. Arch Pediatr Adolesc Med 160:65–69, 2006

Borcherding BG, Keysor CS, Rapoport JL, et al: Motor/vocal tics and compulsive behaviors on stimulant drugs: is there a common vulnerability? Psychiatry Res 33:83–94, 1990

Bruggeman R, van der Linden C, Buitelaar GS, et al: Risperidone versus pimozide in Tourette's syndrome: a comparative double-blind parallel group study. J Clin Psychiatry 62:50–56, 2001

Budman CL, Gayer A, Lesser M, et al: An open-label study of the treatment efficacy of olanzapine for Tourette's disorder. J Clin Psychiatry 62:290–294, 2001

Caine ED, Polinsky RJ, Kartzinel R, et al: The trial use of clozapine for abnormal involuntary disorders. Am J Psychiatry 136:317–320, 1979

Castellanos FX, Geidd JN, Elia J: Controlled stimulant treatment of ADHD and comorbid Tourette's syndrome: effects of stimulant and dose. J Am Acad Child Adolesc Psychiatry 36:589–596, 1997

Costello EJ, Angold A, Burns BJ, et al: The Great Smoky Mountains Study of Youth: goals, design, methods, and the prevalence of DSM-III-R disorders. Arch Gen Psychiatry 53:1129–1136, 1996

Cummings DD, Singer HS, Krieger M, et al. Neuropsychiatric effects of guanfacine in children with mild Tourette's syndrome: a pilot study. Clin Neuropharmacol 25:325–332, 2002

Desta Z, Kerbusch T, Flockhart DA: Effect of clarithromycin on the pharmacokinetics and pharmacodynamics of pimozide in healthy poor and extensive metabolizers of cytochrome P450 2D6 (CYP2D6). Clin Pharmacol Ther 65:10–20, 1999

Dion Y, Annable L, Sandor P, et al. Risperidone in the treatment of Tourette's syndrome: a double-blind, placebo-controlled trial. J Clin Psychopharmacol 22:31–39, 2002

DuPaul GJ, Power TJ, McGoey KE, et al: Reliability and validity of parent and teacher ratings of attention-deficit/hyperactivity disorder symptoms. Journal of Psychoeducation Assessment 16:55–68, 1998

Elia J, Borcherding BG, Rapoport JL, et al: Methylphenidate and dextroamphetamine treatments of hyperactivity: are there true non-responders? Psychiatry Res 36:141–155, 1991

Erenberg G, Cruse RP, Rothner AD: Gilles de la Tourette's syndrome: effects of stimulant drugs. Neurology 35:1346–1348, 1985

Feigin A, Kurlan R, McDermott MP, et al. A controlled trial of deprenyl in children with Tourette's syndrome and attention deficit hyperactivity disorder. Neurology 46:965–968, 1996

Fitzgerald KD, Stewart CM, Tawile V, et al. Risperidone augmentation of serotonin reuptake inhibitor treatment of pediatric obsessive compulsive disorder. J Child Adolesc Psychopharmacol 9:115–123, 1999

A 14-month randomized clinical trial of treatment strategies for attention-deficit/hyperactivity disorder. The MTA Cooperative Group. Multimodal Treatment Study of Children With ADHD. Arch Gen Psychiatry 56:1073–1086, 1999

Fraunfelder FW, Fraunfelder FT: Adverse ocular drug reactions recently identified by the National Registry of Drug-Induced Ocular Side Effects. Ophthalmology 111:1275–1279, 2004

Freeman RD, Fast DK, Burd L, et al: An international perspective on Tourette's syndrome: selected findings from 3,500 individuals in 22 countries. Dev Med Child Neurol 42:436–447, 2000

Frey KA, Albin RL: Neuroimaging of Tourette's syndrome. J Child Neurol 21:672–677, 2006

Gadow KD, Sverd J, Sprafkin J, et al: Efficacy of methylphenidate for attention-deficit hyperactivity disorder in children with tic disorder. Arch Gen Psychiatry 52:444–455, 1995

Gadow KD, Sverd J, Sprafkin J, et al: Long-term methylphenidate therapy in children with comorbid attention-deficit hyperactivity disorder and chronic multiple tic disorder. Arch Gen Psychiatry 56:330–336, 1999

Gaffney GR, Perry PJ, Lund BC, et al: Risperidone versus clonidine in the treatment of children and adolescents with Tourette's syndrome. J Am Acad Child Adolesc Psychiatry 41:330–336, 2002

Gilbert DL, Sethuraman G, Sine L, et al: Tourette's syndrome improvement with pergolide in a randomized, double-blind, crossover trial. Neurology 54:1310–1315, 2000

Gilbert DL, Dure L, Sethuraman G, et al: Tic reduction with pergolide in a randomized controlled trial in children. Neurology 60:606–611, 2003

Gilbert DL, Batterson JR, Sethuraman G, et al: Tic reduction with risperidone versus pimozide in a randomized, double-blind, crossover trial. J Am Acad Child Adolesc Psychiatry 43:206–214, 2004

Goetz CG, Tanner CM, Klawans HL: Fluphenazine and multifocal tic disorders. Arch Neurol 41:271–272, 1984

Golden GS: Gilles de la Tourette's syndrome following methylphenidate administration. Dev Med Child Neurol 16:76–78, 1974

Goodman WK, Price LH, Rasmussen SA, et al: The Yale-Brown Obsessive Compulsive Scale, II: validity. Arch Gen Psychiatry 46:1012–1016, 1989

Goyette CH, Conners CK, Ulrich RF: Normative data on revised Conners Parent and Teacher Rating Scales. J Abnorm Child Psychol 6:221–236, 1978

Hunt RD, Minderaa RB, Cohen DJ: Clonidine benefits children with attention deficit disorder and hyperactivity: report of a double-blind placebo-crossover therapeutic trial. J Am Acad Child Psychiatry 24:617–629, 1985

Jankovic J: Botulinum toxin in the treatment of dystonic tics. Mov Disord 9:347–349, 1994

Jankovic J: Tourette's syndrome. N Engl J Med 345:1184–1192, 2001

Karno M, Golding JM, Sorenson SB, et al: The epidemiology of obsessive-compulsive disorder in five US communities. Arch Gen Psychiatry 45:1094–1098, 1988

Kastrup A, Schlotter W, Plewnia C, et al: Treatment of tics in Tourette's syndrome with aripiprazole. J Clin Psychopharmacol 25:94–96, 2005

Kelsey DK, Sumner CR, Casat CD, et al: Once-daily atomoxetine treatment for children with attention-deficit/hyperactivity disorder, including an assessment of evening and morning behavior: a double-blind, placebo-controlled trial. Pediatrics 114:e1–e8, 2004

King A, Harris P, Fritzell J, et al: Syncope in children with Tourette's syndrome treated with guanfacine. Mov Disord 21:419–420, 2006

King RA, Scahill L, Lombroso PJ, et al: Tourette's syndrome and other tic disorders, in Pediatric Psychopharmacology: Principles and Practice. Edited by Martin A, Scahill L, Charney DS, et al. New York, Oxford University Press, 2003, pp 526–542

Kurlan R, Como PG, Deeley C, et al: A pilot controlled study of fluoxetine for obsessive compulsive symptoms in children with Tourette's syndrome. Clin Neuropharmacol 16:167–172, 1993

Kwak CH, Hanna PA, Jankovic J: Botulinum toxin in the treatment of tics. Arch Neurol 57:1190–1193, 2000

Law SF, Schachar RJ: Do typical clinical doses of methylphenidate cause tics in children treated for attention-deficit hyperactivity disorder? J Am Acad Child Adolesc Psychiatry 38:944–951, 1999

Leckman JF: Tourette's syndrome. Lancet 360:1577–1586, 2002

Leckman JF, Ort S, Caruso KA, et al: Rebound phenomena in Tourette's syndrome after abrupt withdrawal of clonidine. Arch Gen Psychiatry 43:1168–1176, 1986

Leckman JF, Riddle MA, Hardin MT, et al: The Yale Global Tic Severity Scale: initial testing of a clinician-rated scale of tic severity. J Am Acad Child Adolesc Psychiatry 28:566–573, 1989

Leckman JF, Hardin MT, Riddle MA, et al: Clonidine treatment of Gilles de la Tourette's syndrome. Arch Gen Psychiatry 48:324–328, 1991

Leckman JF, Walker DE, Cohen DJ: Premonitory urges in Tourette's syndrome. Am J Psychiatry 150:98–102, 1993

Leckman JF, Grice DE, Barr LC, et al: Tic-related vs. non-tic-related obsessive compulsive disorder. Anxiety 1:208–215, 1995

Lin H, Yeh CB, Peterson BS, et al: Assessment of symptom exacerbations in a longitudinal study of children with Tourette's syndrome or obsessive-compulsive disorder. J Am Acad Child Adolesc Psychiatry 41:1070–1077, 2002

Lipkin PH, Goldstein IJ, Adesman AR: Tics and dyskinesias associated with stimulant treatment in attention-deficit hyperactivity disorder. Arch Pediatr Adolesc Med 148:859–861, 1994

Lowe TL, Cohen DJ, Detlor J, et al: Stimulant medications precipitate Tourette's syndrome. JAMA 26:1729–1731, 1982

Marras C, Andrews D, Sime E, et al: Botulinum toxin for simple motor tics: a randomized, double-blind, controlled clinical trial. Neurol 56:605–610, 2001

McDougle CJ, Goodman WK, Leckman JF, et al: Haloperidol addition in fluvoxamine-refractory obsessive-compulsive disorder: a double-blind, placebo-controlled study in patients with and without tics. Arch Gen Psychiatry 51:302–308, 1994

Meyer JM, Koro CE: The effects of antipsychotic therapy on serum lipids: a comprehensive review. Schizophr Res 70:1–17, 2004

Michelson D, Faries D, Wernicke J, et al: Atomoxetine in the treatment of children and adolescents with attention-deficit/hyperactivity disorder: a randomized, placebo-controlled, dose-response study. Pediatrics 108:E83, 2001

Michelson D, Allen AJ, Busner J, et al: Once-daily atomoxetine treatment for children and adolescents with attention deficit hyperactivity disorder: a randomized, placebo-controlled study. Am J Psychiatry 159:1896–1901, 2002

Mohammadi MR, Ghanizadeh A, Alaghband-Rad J: Selegiline in comparison with methylphenidate in attention deficit hyperactivity disorder children and adolescents in a double-blind, randomized clinical trial. J Child Adolesc Psychopharmacol 14:418–425, 2004

Mukaddes NM, Abali O: Quetiapine treatment of children and adolescents with Tourette's disorder. J Child Adolesc Psychopharmacol 13:295–299, 2003

Orth M, Kirby R, Richardson MP, et al: Subthreshold rTMS over pre-motor cortex has no effect on tics in patients with Gilles de la Tourette's syndrome. Clin Neurophysiol 116:764–768, 2005

Pediatric OCD Treatment Study (POTS) Team: Cognitive-behavior therapy, sertraline, and their combination for children and adolescents with obsessive-compulsive disorder: the Pediatric OCD Treatment Study (POTS) randomized controlled trial. JAMA 292:1969–1976, 2004

Peterson BS, Skudlarski P, Anderson AW, et al: A functional magnetic resonance imaging study of tic suppression in Tourette's syndrome. Arch Gen Psychiatry 55:326–333, 1998

Peterson BS, Staib L, Scahill L, et al: Regional brain and ventricular volumes in Tourette's syndrome. Arch Gen Psychiatry 58:427–440, 2001

Peterson BS, Thomas P, Kane MJ, et al: Basal ganglia volumes in patients with Gilles de la Tourette's syndrome. Arch Gen Psychiatry 60:415–424, 2003

Piacentini JC, Chang SW: Behavioral treatments for tic suppression: habit reversal training. Adv Neurol 99:227–233, 2006

Pliszka SR, Crismon ML, Hughes CW, et al: The Texas Children's Medication Algorithm Project: revision of the algorithm for pharmacotherapy of attention-deficit/hyperactivity disorder. J Am Acad Child Adolesc Psychiatry 45:642–657, 2006

Porta M, Maggioni G, Ottaviani F, et al: Treatment of phonic tics in patients with Tourette's syndrome using botulinum toxin type A. Neurol Sci 24:420–423, 2004

Riddle MA, Lynch KA, Scahill L, et al: Methylphenidate discontinuation and re-initiation during long-term treatment of children with Tourette's disorder and attention-deficit hyperactivity disorder. J Child Adolesc Psychopharmacol 5:205–214, 1995

Ross MS, Moldofsky H: A comparison of pimozide and haloperidol in the treatment of Gilles de la Tourette's syndrome. Am J Psychiatry 135:585–587, 1978

Rutter M, Tizard J, Whitmore K: Education, Health, and Behavior. London, Longman, 1970

Sallee FR, Nesbitt L, Jackson C, et al: Relative efficacy of haloperidol and pimozide in children and adolescents with Tourette's disorder. Am J Psychiatry 154:1057–1062, 1997

Sallee FR, Kurlan R, Goetz CG, et al: Ziprasidone treatment of children and adolescents with Tourette's syndrome: a pilot study. J Am Acad Child Adolesc Psychiatry 39:292–299, 2000

Scahill L, Schwab-Stone M: Epidemiology of ADHD in school-age children. Child Adolesc Psychiatr Clin N Am 9(3):541–555, 2000

Scahill L, Riddle MA, King RA, et al: Fluoxetine has no marked effect on tic symptoms in patients with Tourette's syndrome: a double-blind placebo-controlled study. J Child Adolesc Psychopharmacol 7:75–85, 1997a

Scahill L, Riddle MA, McSwiggin-Hardin M, et al: Children's Yale-Brown Obsessive Compulsive Scale: reliability and validity. J Am Acad Child Adolesc Psychiatry, 36:844–852, 1997b

Scahill L, Chappell PB, Kim YS, et al: Guanfacine in the treatment of children with tic disorders and ADHD: a placebo-controlled study. Am J Psychiatry 158:1067–1074, 2001

Scahill L, Kano Y, King RA, et al: Influence of age and tic disorders on obsessive-compulsive disorder in a pediatric sample. J Child Adolesc Psychopharmacol 13 (suppl):7–18, 2003a

Scahill L, Leckman JF, Schultz RT, et al: A placebo-controlled trial of risperidone in Tourette's syndrome. Neurology. 60:1130–1135, 2003b

Scahill L, Sukhodolsky D, Williams S, et al: The public health importance of tics and tic disorders. Adv Neurol 96:240–248, 2005

Scahill L, Erenberg G, Berlin CM, et al: Contemporary assessment and pharmacotherapy of Tourette's syndrome. NeuroRx 3:192–206, 2006

Scahill L, Kim YS, Lettinga J: Assessment and pharmacological treatment of children with obsessive-compulsive disorder. J Clin Psychopharmacol (in press)

Shapiro AK, Shapiro E: Controlled study of pimozide vs. placebo in Tourette's syndrome. J Am Acad Child Adolesc Psychiatry 23:161–173, 1984

Shapiro E, Shapiro AK, Fulop G, et al: Controlled study of haloperidol, pimozide, and placebo for the treatment of Gilles de la Tourette's syndrome. Arch Gen Psychiatry 46:722–730, 1989

Singer HS, Brown J, Quaskey S, et al: The treatment of attention-deficit hyperactivity disorder in Tourette's syndrome: a double-blind placebo-controlled study with clonidine and desipramine. Pediatrics 95:74–81, 1995

Spencer T, Biederman J, Coffey B, et al: Tourette's disorder and ADHD. Adv Neurol 85:57–77, 2001

Spencer T, Biederman J, Coffey B, et al: A double-blind comparison of desipramine and placebo in children and adolescents with chronic tic disorder and comorbid attention-deficit/hyperactivity disorder. Arch Gen Psychiatry 59:649–656, 2002

Stamenkovic M, Schindler SD, Aschauser HN, et al: Effective open-label treatment of Tourette's disorder with olanzapine. Int Clin Psychopharmacol 15:23–28, 2000

Sukhodolsky D, Scahill L, Zhang H, et al: Disruptive behavior in children with Tourette's syndrome: association of ADHD comorbidity, tic severity, and functional impairment. J Am Acad Child Adolesc Psychiatry 42:98–105, 2003

Swanson J, Lerner M, March J, et al: Assessment and intervention for attention-deficit/hyperactivity disorder in the schools: lessons from the MTA study. Pediatr Clin North Am 46:993–1009, 1999

Temel Y, Visser-Vandewalle V: Surgery in Tourette's syndrome. Mov Disord 19:3–14, 2004

Thomsen PH: Risperidone augmentation in the treatment of severe adolescent OCD in SSRI-refractory cases: a case-series. Ann Clin Psychiatry 16:201–207, 2004

Toren P, Weizman A, Ratner S, et al: Ondansetron treatment in Tourette's disorder: a 3-week, randomized, double-blind, placebo-controlled study. J Clin Psychiatry 66:499–503, 2005

Tourette Syndrome Study Group: Treatment of ADHD in children with tics: a randomized controlled trial. Neurology 58:527–536, 2002

Valleni-Basile LA, Garrison CZ, Jackson KL, et al: Frequency of obsessive-compulsive disorder in a community sample of young adolescents, J Am Acad Child Adolesc Psychiatry 33:782–791, 1994

Varley CK, Vincent J, Varley P, et al: Emergence of tics in children with attention deficit hyperactivity disorder treated with stimulant medications. Compr Psychiatry 42:228–233, 2001

Wilhelm S, Deckersbach T, Coffey BJ, et al: Habit reversal versus supportive psychotherapy for Tourette's disorder: a randomized controlled trial. Am J Psychiatry 160:1175–1177, 2003

Woods DW, Piacentini J, Himle MB, et al: Premonitory Urge for Tics Scale (PUTS): initial psychometric results and examination of the premonitory urge phenomenon in youths with tic disorders. J Dev Behav Pediatr 26:397–403, 2005

9

Schizophrenia and Psychotic Illnesses

Judith L. Rapoport, M.D.

Nitin Gogtay, M.D.

Phillip Shaw, M.D., Ph.D.

By virtually every clinical and neurobiological measure, childhood or very-early-onset schizophrenia, defined as the onset of psychotic symptoms before the thirteenth birthday, is continuous with the adult disorder. Clinically, childhood-onset schizophrenia (COS) resembles the adult form in its cardinal positive symptoms of hallucinations, delusions, and thought disorder and the constellation of negative symptoms, such as lack of drive and a flattened affect. Neurobiologically, it shares many of the same neuroanatomical anomalies, risk genes, and neuropsychological deficits as adult-onset schizophrenia (for a review, see Rapoport et al. 2005). The disorder is rare, and as is often the case with very early-onset illnesses, psychotic disorders in children are usually more severe than in their adult counterparts (Childs and Scriver 1986). COS is thus associated with a particularly severe disruption of cognitive and social development, and the burden to the family can be devastating. The term *early-onset schizophrenia* has been used to describe an onset before the eighteenth birthday (American Academy of Child and Adolescent Psychiatry 2001), and most studies considered in this chapter include patients with an onset of symptoms in adolescence, although we will emphasize studies among patients with the very early-onset form of the disorder.

History and Classification of Psychosis in Children

Although the existence of childhood schizophrenia was recognized early in the twentieth century (Kraepelin 1919), the term *psychosis* was used so broadly in children that a spectrum of behavioral disorders and autism were grouped under the category of childhood schizophrenia (Volkmar 1996). The landmark studies of Kolvin first established the clinical distinction between autism and other psychotic disorders of childhood (Kolvin 1971). However, even today, high rates of initial misdiagnosis remain because of symptom overlap, particularly for mood disorders, and the presence of relatively fleeting hallucinations and delusions in nonpsychotic pediatric patients. Anxiety and stress are probably the most common causes of hallucinations in preschool children, and the prognosis of these phenomena is usually benign. Psychotic phenomena in school-age children generally tend to be more persistent and are more likely to be associated with significant mental illness. Data from a large birth-cohort indicate that self-reported psychotic symptoms at age 11 predicted a very high risk (odds ratio = 16.4) of schizophreniform diagnosis by age 26 (Poulton et al. 2000).

The transient psychotic symptoms and multiple developmental abnormalities found in a sizable, heterogeneous group of children referred to the NIMH COS study over the past 15 years were not adequately characterized by existing DSM-IV categories (American Psychiatric Association 1994) (the diagnosis of psychosis not otherwise specified would probably be made). We have used the term *multidimensionally impaired* to capture the mix of stress-related transient episodes of psychosis, emotional lability, impaired interpersonal skills, and information-processing deficits these children exhibit (Frazier et al. 1994; Kumra et al. 1998).

Epidemiology

Because of the rarity of the disorder, large-scale epidemiological studies of COS are not feasible, although findings in retrospective studies all show that the condition is extremely rare. For example, a Canadian study of diagnoses on drug prescriptions indicated that the rate of schizophrenia under the age of 15 is 1/50 the rate in adults (Beitchman 1985). A study of hospital admissions of 312 psychotic youth over a 13-year period in Denmark found only 4 patients who were younger than 13 years (Thomsen 1996). Our own experience at the NIMH indicates that most children receiving the diagnosis of schizophrenia do not meet criteria for schizophrenia. At our screening, they received other diagnoses, resulting in only 5% of the 1,500 patients initially referred to our project being considered to have schizophrenia. The most common other diagnosis was mood disorder with psychotic features.

Course and Outcome

Long-term follow-up of early-onset cases indicates chronic illness and impairment. In a comparison with nonschizophrenic psychoses, Hollis found that a large cohort diagnosed with early-onset schizophrenia (mean age at onset = 14 years) had significantly worse outcomes at a mean follow-up of 11 years, characterized by a chronic illness course and severe impairments in social relationships (Hollis 2000). An even longer follow-up of 42 years found that earlier age at onset among 44 patients retrospectively meeting diagnostic criteria for COS was associated with a much poorer clinical outcome and high levels of disability (Eggers and Bunk 1997). We recently reported on a prospective follow-up study over a mean of 5 years with 32 children in an NIMH cohort, and noted that despite optimal pharmacotherapy there was evidence of high levels of disability and residual psychotic symptoms (Sporn et al., in press). Thus, all these studies converge to suggest a particularly malignant course.

Our group has conducted a follow-up of 32 patients in the psychosis not otherwise specified or multidimensionally impaired populations. None of the patients have developed schizophrenia, but 12 (38%) met the criteria for bipolar I disorder within 2–8 years of follow-up (Gogtay et al., in press; Nicolson et al. 2001). Our number was not sufficient to discuss their treatment separately, and they were excluded from double-blind trials at the NIMH (which included only children meeting the criteria for COS).

Rationale for Psychopharmacological Treatment

The severity and chronicity of COS necessitates early and aggressive treatment, including family education and special education. The mainstay of pharmacological treatment in COS is antipsychotic medication. Most classifications of antipsychotics divide the medication into typical, or first-generation, antipsychotic drugs and atypical, or second-generation, antipsychotics. The typical antipsychotics are all high-affinity antagonists of dopamine D_2 receptors, a property that remains the most plausible explanation for their therapeutic effects. Dopamine D_2 receptor antagonism also explains, in part, one of the other key features of typical antipsychotics: the high rate of unwanted side effects, particularly extrapyramidal signs and tardive dyskinesia (which will be considered later). Atypical or second-generation antipsychotics differ pharmacologically from previous antipsychotic agents in their lower affinity for D_2 receptors and greater affinities for other neuroreceptors. They are also thought to have a lower incidence of extrapyramidal side effects (EPS), tardive dyskinesia, and hyperprolactinemia, although there is considerable variation among the atypicals in their side-effect profiles. In clinical practice, atypical agents have become the treatment of choice in patients with COS. For example, in a review of practices in the United States, the prescription of atypical antipsychotics increased by nearly 500% between 1995 and 2000, and accounted for the majority of antipsychotic prescriptions among children and adolescents (Patel et al. 2002). Indeed, the ratio of atypical antipsychotics to traditional antipsychotics used is greater among child (2.7:1) and adolescent (3.8:1) patients than among adults (1.6:1) (IMS Health 2002).

In evaluating the efficacy of antipsychotics in patients with COS, double-blind studies are discussed in depth. We include summaries of the larger prospective open trials of atypicals to reflect current practices and share our experience with newer medications. It should be stressed here that antipsychotics have a wide use in childhood disorders and that information about use of both typical and atypical medications is presented throughout this manual.

Pharmacotherapy

Typical Antipsychotics

Are Typical Antipsychotics More Efficacious Than Placebo in COS?

Some of the first studies in patients with COS addressed the important question of whether antipsychotics have any treatment efficacy through a comparison with placebo (Table 9–1). In one of the earliest such studies, Pool et al. (1976) conducted a double-blind, placebo-controlled trial comparing haloperidol (mean dosage=9.8 mg/day) with loxapine (mean dosage=200 mg/day) in 75 hospitalized adolescents. All three groups, including placebo, showed significant improvement, as assessed with the Clinical Global Impression (CGI) Scale. Although there was no difference among the groups overall, patients who were rated as severely or very severely ill at baseline did show a trend toward more improvement on the active treatments (87.5% for loxapine and 70% for haloperidol, compared with 37% for placebo). There are several limitations to this trial. First, the criteria for diagnosis of schizophrenia rested on clinical consensus, and it is unclear whether all of these subjects would meet contemporary DSM-IV-TR (American Psychiatric Association 2000) criteria for schizophrenia. The exact age at onset of first symptoms is not given, so not all of the subjects may have had an onset of symptoms by age 13, and the degree of prior treatment resistance is also not provided. Despite these caveats, it remains a landmark study establishing the efficacy of typical antipsychotics in COS.

Spencer and colleagues (1992), in a double-blind, placebo-controlled study with a crossover design, randomly assigned 12 children with DSM-III-R (American Psychiatric Association 1987) schizophrenia to receive either haloperidol for 4 weeks followed by placebo for 4 weeks, or placebo for 4 weeks followed by haloperidol for 4 weeks (Spencer et al. 1992). It is likely that most of these subjects had at least partially treatment-resistant illness, as most were hospitalized and had prior exposure to psychotropics, although exact details of prior antipsychotic response were not given. In the primary outcome measures (CGI Scale) and ratings of positive psychotic symptoms, the haloperidol group alone showed a significant improvement (with a fall from a baseline score of 5.15 to 2.99 in the haloperidol group [$P<0.001$]) with no significant change in the placebo group. The authors note that a relatively small dosage of haloperidol, with a range of 0.5–3.5 mg/day, was optimal.

Table 9–1. Controlled trials of typical antipsychotics in patients with childhood-onset schizophrenia

Study	Medication	Mean dosage	N	Age (years)	Design	Criteria	Response rate
Engelhardt et al. 1973	Fluphenazine	10 mg/day	15	10	Randomized, double-blind	CGI *much* or *very much* improved	93% (14/15)
	Haloperidol	10 mg/day	15				87% (13/15)
Pool et al. 1976	Loxapine	90 mg/day	26	15	Randomized, double-blind	CGI *much* or *very much* improved	88% (23/26)
	Haloperidol	10 mg/day	25				72% (18/25)
	Placebo		24				38% (9/24)
Versiani et al. 1977	Loxapine	70 mg/day	25	16	Randomized, double-blind	CGI *much* or *very much* improved	64% (16/25)
	Haloperidol	8 mg/day	25				60% (15/25)
Realmuto et al. 1984	Thiothixene	0.26 mg/kg/day	13	15	Randomized, single-blind	CGI *much* or *very much* improved	54% (7/13)
	Thioridazine	2.57 mg/kg/day	8				63% (5/8)
Spencer et al. 1992	Haloperidol	8.8 mg/day	12	9	Randomized, double-blind, crossover	Marked improvement on clinical judgment	75% (9/12)
	Placebo		12				0% (0/12)

Note. CGI = Clinical Global Impression Scale.

The importance of such placebo-controlled studies has been emphasized recently by a demonstration that the degree of improvement in active-controlled trials of antipsychotics was nearly double that seen with the same drugs and dosages in placebo-controlled studies (Woods et al. 2005). It should be noted that there are no recent studies of antipsychotics (and specifically atypical agents) in COS, with a placebo wing being a limitation that should inform the interpretation of recent trials.

Are All Typical Antipsychotic Agents Equivalent?

Several studies have directly compared the efficacy of two antipsychotics in the absence of a placebo wing, including two double-blind comparisons of fluphenazine and haloperidol (Engelhardt et al. 1973), thiothixene and thioridazine (Realmuto et al. 1984), and loxapine and haloperidol (Versiani et al. 1977) (see Table 9–1).

All studies reported high rates of response (based on the CGI), ranging from 57% to over 90%, and on nearly all outcome measures the antipsychotics did not differ significantly. However, in some of these earlier studies the criteria used to define schizophrenia were not clear, and change in specific psychotic symptoms was not reported, limiting the applicability to current practice. Indeed, given current prescribing practices, most comparisons of typical agents are of historical interest. However, given the recent results of the NIMH Clinical Antipsychotic Trials of Intervention Effectiveness (CATIE) project, which demonstrated equal efficacy in adults with chronic schizophrenia for the typical perphenazine with four atypical antipsychotics, it is possible that there may be renewed interest in the use of low-dose typical antipsychotics for psychosis (Lieberman et al. 2005).

Atypical Antipsychotics

Mechanisms of Action

The advent of so-called atypical agents appeared to herald an era of treatment for schizophrenia with possibly more efficacious agents and more favorable side-effect profiles (Kane et al. 1988). Several reviews have considered the issue of what makes an atypical agent atypical (Kapur and Remington 2001). Most agree upon a lower risk of EPS and a lack of prolactin level elevation, with some additionally claiming that the atypicals are more effective in ameliorating the negative symptoms of schizophrenia, although this differential effect is likely to be small (with an effect size on the order of 0.1 [Cohen's *d*]). In terms of pharmacological properties, most atypicals have a higher affinity for serotonin receptors, specifically the 5-HT$_{2A}$ family, and, to a lesser extent, the dopamine D$_4$ receptor. However neither property is necessary for atypicality. Amisulpride is a relatively pure D$_2$/D$_3$ antagonist lacking serotonin receptor antagonism, and several typicals, including haloperidol, have high affinity for D$_4$ receptors. More recently, it has been proposed that atypical antipsychotics may have a faster rate of dissociation from the D$_2$ receptor, allowing the drug to be more responsive to endogenous dopamine, thus allowing an antipsychotic effect while avoiding EPS and prolactin elevation.

Efficacy of Atypical Antipsychotics: What Do Open-Label Studies Tell Us?

Risperidone.   A 6-week open-label study of risperidone (mean dosage=3.14 mg/day) in 11 treatment-naive adolescents who met DSM-IV criteria for schizophrenia reported significant improvements in outcome measures: CGI, Brief Psychiatric Rating Scale (BPRS), and Positive and Negative Syndrome Scale (PANSS) (positive but not negative symptoms) (Zalsman et al. 2003). Another study reported a categorical response rate of 60% (response defined with the CGI) among 10 adolescents (Armenteros et al. 1997). The dosages of risperidone in this study were higher (mean dosage=6.6 mg/day), perhaps reflecting the inclusion of a large proportion of subjects with a history of treatment resistance.

Olanzapine.   In one of the earliest studies at the NIMH, only modest improvement was noted among subjects receiving open-label olanzapine, with a reported 17% improvement on the BPRS but only a 6% improvement in positive symptoms and no significant change in Clinical Global Impression Improvement (CGI-I) scores. These only modest gains may reflect the treatment-refractory nature of the illnesses in most of the NIMH cohort. However, among a group of nine children with similarly treament-refractory schizophrenia, Mozes et al. (2003) found an overall more impressive response in a 12-week open-label study, with significant improvement on all outcome measures. Studies that include a treatment-naive population or those involving subjects with minimal prior exposure to antipsychotics show more robust effects. For example, Findling et al. (2003) found robust responses in both negative and positive symptoms among patients in an outpatient study. Similarly, Ross et al. (2003) reported 37% full response and 32% partial response rates. Notably, this significant improvement was observed only at the 1-year mark, and there was evidence of an increasing amelioration of negative symptoms with time, emphasizing the need for such longer-term studies.

Other agents: quetiapine, ziprasidone, and aripiprazole. Quetiapine, ziprasidone, and aripiprazole have not been specifically studied among patients with COS, although reports of efficacy are mentioned among children and adolescents with a range of largely nonschizophrenia psychotic disorders. Like clozapine, quetiapine has a higher affinity for $5\text{-}HT_{2A}$ receptors relative to D_2 receptors and affinity for α_1-adrenergic and dopamine D_1 receptors, but relatively little muscarinic action. Quetiapine has emerged as a potential treatment for COS through demonstrations of its efficacy in two open-label studies—one lasting 8 weeks, and the other lasting 88 weeks—among adolescents with a range of psychotic disorders (McConville et al. 2003; J.A. Shaw et al. 2001). Ziprasidone has a complex pharmacology, acting as an agonist at $5\text{-}HT_{1A}$ receptors and an antagonist at $5\text{-}HT_{1D}$ and $5\text{-}HT_{2C}$ receptors—properties that may confer antidepressant effects. It has not been studied in COS patients, although efficacy in a small open-label study of children with bipolar affective disorder has been reported (Barnett 2003). Aripiprazole has a unique receptor profile, with partial agonist action at D_2 and $5\text{-}HT_{1A}$ receptors. A double-blind study comparing aripiprazole with risperidone at the NIMH was stopped early when the first two patients randomly assigned to receive aripiprazole showed precipitous declines in mental state. Given the treatment-resistant nature of the NIMH cohort, this does not mean the agent will not be of use in a treatment-naive population, although there are as yet no reports of its usefulness in that population.

Efficacy of Atypical Antipsychotics: Are Atypical Antipsychotics Superior to Typical Antipsychotics in the Treatment of COS?

A direct comparison between two atypical antipsychotics, olanzapine and risperidone, and the most commonly prescribed typical agent, haloperidol, has been made in a double-blind, parallel, treatment study (Sikich et al. 2004). The 8-week study included 75 children and adolescents with psychotic symptoms stemming from a wide range of underlying diagnoses. All three treatments were associated with marked and significant reductions in the total Brief Psychiatric Rating Scale for Children (BPRS-C) scores, falling to 50% of the baseline scores in the risperidone group, 44% of the baseline score in the olanzapine group, and 67% of the baseline score in the haloperidol group. The categorical response rates, like most outcome measures, did not differ significantly, but there was a trend toward better response rates for the atypicals: 74% (14/19) with risperidone, 88% (14/16) with olanzapine, and 53% (8/15) with haloperidol.

Although this is one of the very few controlled studies comparing typical and atypical agents in the field, there are several important limitations to its applicability to a patient group with COS. Most importantly, the study included a diagnostically heterogeneous group, and only half of the subjects had a diagnosis of schizophrenia. A large proportion of the subjects were receiving other psychotropic medications, although there were no differences in response rates between the different treatment groups detected among participants who were treated exclusively with an antipsychotic.

The findings of the study are congruent with an 8-week open-label, nonrandomized comparison of olanzapine, risperidone, and haloperidol in 43 adolescents with schizophrenia, which found all three agents were equally efficacious (Gothelf et al. 2003).

In conclusion, the atypical antipsychotics olanzapine and risperidone are likely to be at least as effective as typical agents in the treatment of patients with COS and are thus appropriate as first-line agents. Among other atypicals, quetiapine and ziprasidone appear to be promising treatment candidates.

Use of Clozapine in Treating COS

Clozapine has emerged as the gold standard antipsychotic in the treatment of adult-onset schizophrenia, particularly for psychosis that has not responded to other agents (Kane et al. 1988). Most, but not all, meta-analyses suggest that clozapine is more efficacious than typical and possibly most atypical antipsychotics in the short term (Davis et al. 2003; Geddes et al. 2000; Leucht et al. 2003; Moncrieff 2003). Unfortunately, the benefits of clozapine must be weighed against its severe adverse side effects, particularly agranulocytosis, which led to temporary withdrawal of the drug.

The clinical trials of clozapine in COS have all incorporated the criteria of treatment resistance, which is a requirement of current routine clinical use. Thus, there are no data on the efficacy of clozapine as a first-line agent in COS (unlike in the adult literature; see Lieberman et al. 2003). With this in mind, it is striking that all open trials found clear efficacy for clozapine in children who were not helped by other medications. Frazier et al. (1994) reported on 11 adolescents from the NIMH cohort and found that 9 of 11 children showed greater than a 33% reduction in BPRS ratings and only one patient showed clinical deterioration. Turetz et al. (1997) demonstrated a similar reduction of approximately 50% on all psychopathology scales in a report of 11 children who had shown no response to neuroleptic agents. It was noted that the response occurred relatively early in treatment, between weeks 2 and 8, and was sustained at a 4-month follow-up.

Clozapine has been compared with both atypical and typical antipsychotics. The first study compared haloperidol, probably the most widely used typical antipsychotic at the time of the study (1990–1996), with clozapine, randomly assigning 21 children to receive treatment for 6 weeks (Kumra et al. 1996). Clozapine was markedly superior on all components of the BPRS and overall ratings of clinical improvement—a striking finding, given the small sample and the severity of illness at baseline. The mean dosage of haloperidol used was 16.8 mg/day, which is at the upper end of the contemporary treatment range. Such relatively high doses have been implicated in an excess of side effects that mimic the negative symptoms of schizophrenia and lead to an underestimation of antipsychotic efficacy (Geddes et al. 2000). However, given the history of previous resistance to antipsychotics among the patients in this study, high doses would have been expected and were guided by clinical judgment.

Kumra et al. (1997) further reported on an open trial of clozapine involving all of the 21 patients who initially had been randomly assigned to receive haloperidol (and who had generally shown a poor response). Of these patients, 2 (9.5%) were rated as *very much improved* on the CGI, 11 (52.4%) as *improved*, 7 (33%) as *minimally improved*, and 1 (4.8%) as *worse*—results that are in line with the response to clozapine seen in the double-blind phase of the study. The results of the study helped establish the efficacy of clozapine in treatment-resistant COS and strongly suggested that the agent is superior to haloperidol.

The introduction of atypical antipsychotics in the late 1990s has led to a marked shift in prescribing practices, resulting in the vast majority of children with psychotic disorder receiving atypicals. We thus compared the efficacy and safety of olanzapine, a widely used atypical, with the gold standard, clozapine. In a 8-week double-blind randomized controlled trial with a 2-year follow-up, 25 patients with COS were randomly assigned to receive treatment

(12 to clozapine and 13 to olanzapine). Using intent-to-treat analyses, we found that clozapine was associated with a significant reduction in all outcome measures, with olanzapine showing a rather less impressive improvement (Figure 9–1).

A direct comparison of treatment efficacy showed that there was generally no significant difference between the groups, but a significant advantage for clozapine did emerge in the alleviation of negative symptoms of schizophrenia (producing a 45% greater reduction in Scale for the Assessment of Negative Symptoms ratings, $P=0.04$, effect size$=0.89$). The size of the differential effect on negative symptoms is therefore large and in marked contrast to studies in adults with schizophrenia, which report no significant difference between olanzapine and clozapine in treating negative symptoms, despite a larger sample size and power to detect smaller effects (Bitter et al. 2004; Tollefson et al. 2001; Volavka et al. 2002). The improvement in negative symptoms is unlikely to have been an epiphenomenon of improvement in mood or extrapyramidal symptoms, given that there was no correlation between change in these indices and change in negative symptoms. Although the study is limited by its small size and the unique features of its tertiary research setting, it is the first comparison of two of the most widely used atypical antipsychotics in children and adolescents. It provides further high-quality evidence to support recommendations for the use of clozapine in treatment-resistant COS.

Data on the effectiveness and tolerability of antipsychotics in the longer term are of importance, but, with some significant exceptions, such data are scarce in the pediatric literature (Findling et al. 2004; Ross et al. 2003). We thus included data from a 2-year follow-up period during which all patients had returned to the care of the referring physician and received open-label treatment according to clinical judgment. By the 2-year stage, 15 of the 18 patients were being treated with clozapine, because olanzapine produced sustained treatment response for only 2 patients. The patients receiving clozapine showed modest but no significant improvement in clinical ratings from the end of the double-blind trial to the 2-year assessment.

It is difficult to give a quantitative summary of the various studies on the use of clozapine in COS, because meta-analyses are complicated by the multiple sources of heterogeneity (e.g., treatment design, double-blind vs. open, different dosing schedules, inclusion criteria). However, the impression of the narrative synthesis and conclusion of the double-blind direct comparison of

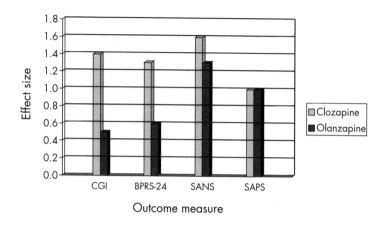

Figure 9–1. Effect sizes of clozapine and olanzapine in a double-blind trial in 25 patients with childhood-onset schizophrenia.
BPRS-24 = Brief Psychiatric Rating Scale (24-item); CGI = Clinical Global Impression Scale; SANS = Scale for the Assessment of Negative Symptoms; SAPS = Scale for the Assessment of Positive Symptoms.

clozapine with olanzapine suggests that is it is a highly efficacious choice in a treatment-resistant population.

There has been considerable interest in determining what attributes afford clozapine its efficacy. Among 54 patients with COS, we found outcome at 2 years (measures using the Children's Global Assessment Scale) was associated with a less severe illness at baseline and a greater initial clinical response to clozapine during the first 6 weeks of treatment, as has been reported in studies of adults with schizophrenia (Pickar et al. 1994; Sporn et al., in press). Intriguingly, the ratio of one of the metabolites of clozapine, *N*-desmethylclozapine (NDMC), to clozapine, was the only variable that was significantly associated with response at 6 weeks. This result replicated a finding in an adult-onset schizophrenia study, which indicated that greater NDMC-clozapine ratio, but not the concentrations of clozapine and NDMC themselves, is associated with better response. The higher NDMC-clozapine ratio in responders may suggest a higher rate of clozapine metabolism, with the metabolite of clozapine proving to be more efficacious than the parent compound, perhaps through its unique feature of muscarinic M_1 receptor agonism (Weiner et al. 2004).

Clozapine Augmentation

Even when receiving clozapine, a substantial proportion of children have residual psychotic symptoms that impair functioning. This raises the issue of possible adjunctive medication to boost partial response to clozapine. A systematic review of the adult literature showed best evidence for augmentation with sulpiride, lamotrigine, and ethyl-eicosapentaenoic acid; lithium was shown to benefit only schizoaffective patients (Kontaxaki and Roukas 2005). In our experience, there is generally little benefit to treatment with more than one antipsychotic agent in the pediatric population. A focus on psychosocial interventions, particularly adequate support in education and appropriate placement, may be more helpful in improving the child's quality of life.

Although the course of COS is difficult, the high overall response rates found among patients treated with clozapine are encouraging. Moreover, we have consistently not found any correlation between age at onset and poor response in double-blind settings. In fact, some studies even report significantly *greater* improvement in *younger* subjects (Sholevar et al. 2000).

Treatment of Comorbid Conditions

Patients with COS have a very high rate of comorbid conditions. Among 76 children from the NIMH cohort, the most frequent comorbid diagnosis at NIMH screening was depression (54%), followed by obsessive-compulsive disorder (21%), and generalized anxiety disorder (15%). A particularly challenging comorbid condition is attention-deficit/hyperactivity disorder (present in 15% of our sample). Psychiatrists have often been reluctant to treat these symptoms with stimulants for fear of worsening psychosis. However, we found that five children showed a significant improvement in the Brief Conners' Teachers Rating Scale of inattentive symptoms following stabilization with an antipsychotic—without any initial worsening of psychosis (Tossell et al. 2004). This reflects a more general principle of treatment of comorbidity in the psychotic child: The treatment of the coexisting condition should be modeled on the evidence for each disorder and should follow the stabilization of psychosis.

Side Effects

The chronic course of COS necessitates long-term treatment, and thus a consideration of side effects is vital. In addition, although most clinicians will be aware of the range of EPS, there may be less familiarity with some of the metabolic side effects strongly associated with newer atypical antipsychotics. Knowledge of the differential profile of side effects is also of practical use: The choice of medication for an obese psychotic child is likely to differ from the choice being made for a child with schizophrenia and comorbid obsessional-compulsive disorder.

Extrapyramidal Side Effects

EPS are among the most troublesome and distressing unwanted sequelae of treatment with antipsychotic drugs. Pathophysiologically, the blockade of nigrostriatal dopaminergic tracts mimics the neurochemical deficits seen in Parkinson's disease and exhibits a similar clinical profile. The mechanisms underlying tardive dyskinesias are less clear but may stem from the development of supersensitivity to dopamine resulting from chronic blockade. As mentioned earlier, atypical antipsychotics have a high serotonin-dopamine receptor blockade ratio in the brain. The serotonergic blockade leads to increased dopamine release, which may partially offset the postsynaptic dopaminergic blockade, resulting in fewer EPS (Glazer 2000).

Abnormal movements that arise in the first few hours or days of treatment are typically acute dystonic reactions, manifesting as spasms of the orofacial muscles or oculogyric crises with involuntary upward rotation of the eyes. Dyskinetic movements can affect any body part: in the face there is frequently tongue protrusion and lip smacking; the trunk and limbs can show continuous writhing or athetoid and choreiform movements. *Pseudoparkinsonism* refers to the classic triad of bradykinesia (slowed or reduced voluntary movements), muscular rigidity, and tremor (although the classic pill-rolling tremor is very rare in neuroleptic-induced parkinsonism). Akathisia refers to an intensely dysphoric sensation of restlessness associated with an intense need for movement. Several ratings scales have been developed to assess abnormal movements, including the Abnormal Involuntary Movement Scale (AIMS) (Guy 1976), the Barnes Akathisia Rating Scale (Barnes 1989), and the Simpson-Angus Extrapyramidal Side Effects Scale (Simpson and Angus 1970).

A comparison of rates of EPS in various studies suggests that typical antipsychotics are associated with high levels of EPS (58%–80%) in patients with COS—a rate higher than that reported in patients with adult-onset schizophrenia (Table 9–2).

By contrast, five open-label studies of olanzapine and quetiapine, involving patients with varying treatment histories and a range of ages at illness onset, found no significant change in ratings of EPS from baseline (Findling et al. 2003; McConville et al. 2003; Mozes et al. 2003; Ross et al. 2003; J.A. Shaw et al. 2001). Three open-label studies of risperidone suggest that this atypical is associated with more EPS, akathisia, and acute dystonic reactions, especially at higher doses. One study reported increases in all measures of movement disorders over a 6-week period. Other studies reported a 19% EPS rate and a 40% rate of dystonic reactions (Armenteros et al. 1997; Grcevich et al. 1996; Zalsman et al. 2003). These findings are supported by direct comparisons of typical and atypical antipsychotics. For example, Sikich et al. (2004) found that haloperidol, but not olanzapine or risperidone, was associated with a significant increase in EPS over an 8-week treatment period.

The management of EPS in children follows the principles derived from adult populations. The antipsychotic is reduced to as low a dose as possible, with awareness that this may be associated with some temporary increase in abnormal movements. Some clinicians also recommend regular "drug holidays" to observe for the development of EPS, although clearly this has to be weighed against the risk of a recurrence of psychosis. Alternatively, the child can be switched to an agent with a lower potential for EPS, such as quetiapine or olanzapine. For pseudoparkinsonism, anticholinergics are frequently used to good effect. For tardive dyskinesia, two controlled studies in adults suggest that clozapine may be the best overall option, given its ability to treat both the psychosis and the movement disorder, although the risks and attendant intensive monitoring make this a less attractive option. Other medications that carry a lower risk of complications can be used in tardive dyskinesia, with vitamin E having the best evidence base in adult efficacy studies.

Akathisia

Akathisia has been described in the adult medical literature mostly in association with typical neuroleptics, but also with olanzapine and risperidone (at rates

Table 9–2. Rates of extrapyramidal side effects (EPS) in controlled studies of antipsychotics in treatment of childhood-onset schizophrenia

Study	Drug	Mean dosage (mg/day)	Measures	Results
Typical antipsychotics				
Engelhardt et al. 1973	Fluphenazine	10.4	Clinical	8/15 EPS, 1/15 acute dystonia, 0/15 akathisia
	Haloperidol	10.4		4/15 EPS, 0/15 acute dystonia, 1/15 akathisia
Pool et al. 1976	Loxapine	87.5	Clinical, muscular rigidity of parkinsonian type	19/26 EPS
	Haloperidol	9.8		18/25 EPS
	Placebo	—		1/24 EPS
Spencer et al. 1992	Haloperidol	8.8	AIMS	3/12 parkinsonian, 2/12 orofacial dyskinesia, 2/12 acute dystonia
	Placebo	—		0/12
Comparisons of typicals and atypicals				
Kumra et al. 1996	Haloperidol	16	AIMS, SAS	No significant increase from baseline
	Clozapine	176		No significant increase from baseline
Sikich et al. 2004	Olanzapine	12.3	AIMS, SAS	No significant increase from baseline, but 56% taking anticholinergics; no acute dystonia; 2/16 akathisia
	Risperidone	4		No significant increase from baseline, but 53% taking anticholinergics; no acute dystonia; no akathisia
	Haloperidol	5		Significant increase from baseline, and significantly greater than with atypicals; 67% taking anticholinergics; 2/15 acute dystonia, 2/15 akathisia

Table 9–2.   Rates of extrapyramidal side effects (EPS) in controlled studies of antipsychotics in treatment of childhood-onset schizophrenia (*continued*)

Study	Drug	Mean dosage (mg/day)	Measures	Results
Comparisons of typicals and atypicals (*continued*)				
Gothelf et al. 2003	Olanzapine	12.9	AIMS, UKU	3/19 EPS, 0/19 dystonia, 0/19 akathisia
	Risperidone	3.3		4/17 EPS, 1/17 dystonia, 1/17 akathisia
	Haloperidol	8.3		4/7 EPS, 2/7 dystonia, 3/7 akathisia
P. Shaw et al. 2006	Olanzapine	18.1	AIMS, BAS, SAS	No significant change from baseline
	Clozapine	327		No significant change from baseline

Note.   AIMS=Abnormal Involuntary Movement Scale; BAS=Barnes Akathisia Rating Scale; SAS=Simpson-Angus Rating Scale; UKU=Udvalg for Kliniske Undersøgelser Side Effect Rating Scale.

of about 13%) and least with clozapine (about 7%) (Chengappa et al. 1994; Leucht et al. 1999). In the NIMH cohort of children, 2 out of 40 children treated with clozapine developed akathisia, which was misinterpreted as a worsening of psychotic symptoms in one case and led to a temporary increase in clozapine dose and a concomitant worsening of symptoms (Gogtay et al. 2002). However, when the diagnosis was made, propranolol was initiated and ameliorated symptoms greatly, allowing continued treatment with clozapine. Other useful agents include benzodiazepines and, perhaps, anticholinergics.

Neuroleptic Malignant Syndrome

Neuroleptic malignant syndrome is a rare but potentially life-threatening complication of antipsychotics, which typically arises in the early stages of treatment and has been attributed to the effects of dopamine blockade. The classic signs and symptoms include severe muscle rigidity and/or marked extrapyramidal signs; autonomic instability, including a high or sometimes fluctuating temperature and blood pressure; delirium; and laboratory findings of elevated creatinine kinase and leukocytosis. Atypical antipsychotics probably have a lower incidence and produce perhaps a milder form of neuroleptic malignant syndrome (Caroff et al. 2000). However, some dramatic case studies illustrate the potential for the side effect in adolescents who are only briefly exposed to even atypicals (Hanft et al. 2004). Treatment of neuroleptic malignant syndrome relies on prompt transfer to a medical setting, withdrawal of the neuroleptic, intensive supportive care, and possible treatment with dantrolene and bromocriptine. Psychotic exacerbations during this period of abrupt antipsychotic withdrawal have sometimes been treated successfully with electroconvulsive therapy.

Sedation

It is difficult to disentangle the relative contribution of the avolition of the negative syndrome in schizophrenia, possible mood disturbance, and true sedative effects of medication, particularly in the psychotic child. With this caveat in mind, high rates of fatigue and/or sedation have been consistently reported in association with nearly all antipsychotics in COS. Rates for haloperidol range from a low of 25% in an NIMH double-blind study (P. Shaw et al. 2006) to 50% and 66% in two earlier trials of the medication (Pool et al. 1976; Spencer et al. 1992). Other typical antipsychotics have been associated with even higher rates of sedation.

Unfortunately, the newer agents also seem to produce this unwanted side effect, albeit with a wide variability among the various agents. Rates of over 50% have been reported for ziprasidone and clozapine, with risperidone occupying an intermediate position (31%), and olanzapine (20%) and quetiapine (20%) having lower, but still high, rates (for a review, see Cheng-Shannon et al. 2004). Interestingly, one study linked initial sedation on olanzapine with a better clinical response at 8 weeks, suggesting the need for perseverance with fatigue and sedation occurring early in treatment (Sholevar et al. 2000). The management of sedation is empirical and requires rigorous assessment to exclude underlying psychopathology. It also relies on maintenance treatment with as low a dose as possible and attention to and encouragement of activity scheduling and constant motivation.

Weight Gain

Weight gain has been reported in association with antipsychotics since their initial use but has become a focus of more interest, given the increased general awareness of the increased morbidity and mortality accompanying obesity (Deckelbaum and Williams 2001). In their study of 50 children with psychotic symptoms, Sikich et al. (2004) found a weight gain of 7.1 kg over an 8-week period for children being treated with olanzapine—a value greater than the gain of 4.9 kg and 3.5 kg reported for risperidone and haloperidol, respectively). Such increases are well in excess of the weight gain that would be expected through normal growth during this age range. In a double-blind comparison of clozapine and olanzapine, a similar weight gain of just under 4 kg over an 8-week period was associated with both agents, corresponding to an increase of 1.5 units in the body mass index (P. Shaw et al. 2006). The most extreme weight gains occurred among those treated with clozapine: 3 children in the clozapine gained more than 10 kg, compared with only 1 child in the olanzapine group.

Among the atypical antipsychotics other than clozapine, open-label studies report greatest weight gain with olanzapine (for a recent comprehensive review of metabolic side effects of atypicals in children, see Fedorowicz and Fombonne 2005). Thus, Findling et al. (2003) reported a gain of approximately 1 kg/week over an 8-week period. A longer-term study suggested that after an initial sharp increase, weight plateaus at around 2 months and then remains more stable (Ross et al. 2003). A recent systematic review of antipsychotic use in children, regardless of diagnosis, gave estimates of increases in weight (adopting the criteria used in each individual study) occurring with the following frequencies: 4% for ziprasidone, 7% for clozapine, 17% for risperidone, and 22% for both olanzapine and quetiapine (Cheng-Shannon et al. 2004). A similar ranking emerges in adult studies. Mechanistically, the relative affinities of the novel antipsychotics for histamine H_1 receptors appear to be the most robust correlate of these clinical findings, although interactions with serotonergic and dopaminergic receptors are also likely to play a role (Wirshing et al. 1999). Elevated levels of leptin, a hormone secreted by adipocytes that partly regulates body weight, are also greater among the antipsychotics most closely linked with weight gain (Herran et al. 2001). The management of this side effect has typically relied on behavioral programs, which unfortunately have mixed evidence of success (Faulkner et al. 2003). Pharmacological interventions are also unproven; there are case reports of amantadine, topiramate, and various anorectic agents attenuating antipsychotic-induced weight gain, although none can be recommended for routine clinical use (Canitano 2005; Gracious et al. 2002).

Glycemic Control

There is an established link between impaired glycemic control and atypical antipsychotics in adult-onset schizophrenia, with several reports suggesting a similar link in children and adolescents. Sikich et al. (2004) found that olanzapine, but not risperidone or haloperidol, was associated with a trend toward an increased fasting blood glucose. In our direct comparison of clozapine and olanzapine, we found little evidence for marked hyperglycemia, although comprehensive data were available only for the 8-week double phase. The link with impaired glucose control could arise through hyperinsulinemia and the impaired sensitivity to insulin found with use of atypical antipsychotics (Sowell et al. 2002). Additionally, antipsychotics may have direct toxic effects on the pancreas. A final link between antipsychotics and type 2 diabetes mellitus could be through obesity and weight gain associated both with antipsychotic treatment and with type 2 diabetes mellitus. Despite the lack of a clear association between antipsychotics use and impaired glycemic control in COS, regular blood monitoring seems judicious, given the pediatric case report indications and findings in adult populations (Jin et al. 2004). Diabetic keto-acidosis, characterized by delirium, dehydration, and hyperventilation, has been reported in adolescents treated with olanzapine (Selva and Scott 2001).

Hyperlipidemia

Sikich et al. (2004) noted a deleterious increase in low-density lipoprotein and a decrease in high-density lipoprotein in patients randomly assigned to receive olanzapine but not risperidone or haloperidol. In the NIMH cohort, we found high levels of hypercholesterolemia and hypertriglyceridemia, with the complication occurring in 6 of 15 patients who were followed up for a 2-year period while receiving open-label clozapine. Although all cases were detected early and managed through diet and lipid-lowering agents, the high rates underscore the need for regular monitoring for this complication among children maintained on treatment with clozapine and perhaps olanzapine as well (Melkersson et al. 2004).

Hyperprolactinemia

An increase in prolactin secondary to antipsychotics reflects the D_2 receptor blockade in the tuberoinfundibular pathway that releases the tonic inhibition from dopamine upon pituitary lactotropes, leading to increased prolactin (for a review, see Pappagallo and Silva 2004). As a result, elevated prolactin levels are typically produced by the antipsychotics with greatest D_2 affinity (Saito et al. 2004). The sequelae of hyperprolactinemia range from sexual dysfunction, menstrual irregularities, and lactation to decreased bone density and possible cardiovascular disease. Wudarksy et al. (1999) found increased prolactin levels in 36 psychotic children after 6 weeks of treatment with either haloperidol or olanzapine but not clozapine. The association may be modulated by gender, because a correlation between olanzapine and prolactin levels was found among girls only in the NIMH cohort (Alfaro et al. 2002). In this study, all but one child remained asymptomatic; the girl with the highest prolactin levels developed transient galactorrhea. Although there are inconsistent findings linking elevated prolactin levels with sexual side effects, the high rate of sexual problems (22%) among adolescents taking antipsychotics suggests that routine inquiry about sexual health is required.

The most effective treatment for symptomatic hyperprolactinemia is either reduction of the dose of the antipsychotic (Masi et al. 2001) or a switch to an agent possibly less associated with the complication, such as quetiapine (J.A. Shaw et al. 2001). Dopamine agonists reinstitute the dopaminergic inhibition of prolactin release; and cabergoline has been used with success in male children with risperidone-induced hyperprolactinemia (Cohen and Biederman 2001), although bromocriptine has a more established role. Whether asymptomatic hyperprolactinemia requires intervention is more controversial, given evidence for the normalization of prolactin levels at 1-year follow-up in disruptive children being treated with risperidone (Findling et al. 2004).

Cardiovascular and Autonomic Side Effects

Several antipsychotics alter repolarization of cardiac muscle, as reflected in a prolonged cardiac-corrected (QT) interval. In turn, this may act as a risk factor for more serious arrhythmias such as torsades de pointes. Reports of sudden cardiac deaths among adults taking antipsychotics have fueled particular concern about such side effects among children. In a double-blind study comparing clozapine and olanzapine, we found higher rates of supine tachycardia among patients treated with clozapine, but no serious arrhythmias. Perhaps of greater concern, seven patients in the clozapine wing became hypertensive during the trial, compared with just one patient treated with olanzapine. Anomalies on the electrocardiogram during treatment with quetiapine have also been reported in adolescents with psychotic disorder, including transient prolongation of the QT interval and intermittent and asymptomatic atrioventricular block, which did not require intervention (McConville et al. 2003).

Side Effects Particularly Associated With Clozapine

The association between clozapine use and a precipitous fall in the body's number of granulocytes (white blood cells important in the immune response against predominately bacterial infections) is well established. In review of data on more than 1,100 patients treated with clozapine, there was an increased risk of agranulocytosis in patients under age 21 compared with those ages 21–40 (Alvir et al. 1993). A more recent synthesis reported two cases of agranulocytosis occurring among 243 children and adolescents treated with clozapine, giving a rate more in line with that seen in the adult population (Cheng-Shannon et al. 2004). Although the side effect has been reported in association with other antipsychotics, the prevalence appears to be much lower. As a result, clozapine requires intensive blood monitoring, overseen by manufacturing companies. The monitoring guidelines are complex, and the reader should refer to the relevant clozapine-monitoring service for details.

The high rates of neutropenia and agranulocytosis in children are particularly unfortunate given the severity of COS, which often means clozapine is the only effective treatment. As a result, there is considerable interest in developing strategies to maximize the opportunity for children to be reestablished on clozapine following initial withdrawal due to the development of neutropenia. We have reported on two cases of children, ages 7 and 12 years, diagnosed with very early-onset schizophrenia, who developed neutropenia when initially treated with clozapine (Sporn et al. 2003). In both cases, addition of lithium carbonate was associated with a sustained elevation of the white blood count, allowing a successful rechallenge with clozapine. It should be stressed that the rechallenge with clozapine requires intensive monitoring and is best performed in highly specialized units in close conjunction with medical colleagues and relevant clozapine-monitoring services.

Epileptiform abnormalities are commonly found in the electroencephalograms of children and adolescents taking clozapine, although frank seizures are rare. Clozapine poses the greatest risk, with seizures occurring in approximately 2% of children taking the medication. Most patients can continue taking clozapine with an adjunctive anticonvulsant, and authorities recommend using anticonvulsants prophylactically when patients are given high doses of clozapine. There is greatest experience of using valproate in this setting. We have also reported on the success of gabapentin as an anticonvulsant in clozapine-induced seizures, chosen in view of its relatively benign side-effect profile and its lack of significant drug interactions (Usiskin et al. 2000).

Hypersalivation is a distressingly common side effect of clozapine that has only rarely been reported with use of other antipsychotics. Proposed mechanisms include the action of clozapine at the muscarinic M_4 receptor, blockade of α_2-adrenoceptors, or distortion of the swallowing reflex. Treatment options include chewing gum; reduction in the dosage of clozapine; or treatment with pharmacological agents such as anticholinergics, α_2-adrenergic agonists, and, in extreme cases, botulinum toxin (Kahl et al. 2004). Other studies suggest that the addition of other antipsychotics, such as amisulpride, at low doses may be efficacious, although a double-blind study found that one of the most promising (based on results of open-label studies) agents, pirenzepine, was no more effective than placebo (Bai et al. 2001).

Early Intervention Studies

Nearly all existing research focuses on improving treatment when a patient is already involved with psychiatric services. However, there are several other potential windows for intervention. From earliest childhood, there are subtle motor and cognitive abnormalities in adults with schizophrenia, similar to the constellation of deficits found in children at high risk of developing psychosis by virtue of having a parent with schizophrenia (Cornblatt 2002). Many other studies, most notably the large epidemiological study on the course of psychosis (the Age, Beginning and Course study), have established the existence of a prodromal phase, lasting 2–5 years (Beiser et al. 1993; Hafner et al. 1998). During this time, there is a marked decline in overall functioning, and mental state is characterized by abnormalities of thought, perception, and action, which appear to be attenuated forms of the positive psychotic symptoms. Nearer the onset of established psychosis many patients have fully developed positive psychotic symptoms, but these are transient, intermittent, and self-terminating. Finally, several studies have demonstrated there is typically a long period of delay between the onset of definite psychotic symptoms and onset of treatment.

Research into interventions during the period between the development of a DSM-IV-TR psychotic disorder and receiving treatment is fueled by evidence that a longer duration of untreated psychosis is linked to poorer clinical outcome in many, but not all, studies (for a review, see Ruhrmann et al. 2005). Additionally, there are concerns that untreated psychosis is not only intensely aversive for the patient but also possibly neurotoxic (Lieberman et al. 1997; Pantelis et al. 2003). The evidence for such secondary prevention is surprisingly scant (e.g., see Kuipers et al. 2004), given that it forms the current dominant model of health service provision.

A second, more ambitious strategy attempts to identify people who are prepsychotic or prodromal and intervene during this stage to not only delay but possibly avert an eventual transition to frank psychosis. As the median age at onset of schizophrenia is 19 years, most prodromal subjects are adolescents, making the rise of preventive interventions of particular relevance to the child and adolescent psychiatrist.

The feasibility of such preventive intervention relies on the ability to accurately identify subjects who are at high risk of psychosis. The current dominant approach defines patients at ultra-high risk of developing psychosis in the near future, combining the traditional definition of genetic high risk (having a first-degree relative with a psychotic disorder) with early symptomatic and functional changes. McGorry et al. (2003) led the field in developing definitions of ultra-high risk for the development of psychosis: *state and trait factors,* which incorporate genetic high risk with a rapid, recent decline in global function and/or schizotypal personality disorder. In addition, clusters of attenuated positive symptoms (including unusual thought content/delusional ideation, suspiciousness/persecutory ideas, grandiosity) and brief, limited, intermittent psychotic symptoms are defined. Overall, approximately 40% of patients meeting these criteria will transition to psychosis (not just schizophrenia) within 12 months, with psychosis defined as the presence of positive psychotic symptoms for longer than 1 week (Yung et al. 2003). An alternative approach emphasizes so-called basic symptoms, which are subtle self-experienced neuropsychological deficits, such as thought pressure, perseverative thinking, derealization, and slight perceptual aberrations. In one study using this approach, the Cologne Early Recognition Study, investigators correctly predicted a transition to schizophrenia (not only psychosis) in 78% of cases within 4 years (Klosterkotter et al. 2001), and their work has partly formed the basis of ongoing prevention studies in Germany.

Issues of intervention are more contentious. There are several possible ethical and pragmatic objections to using psychotropics during the prodromal phase. First, it has been claimed that the evidence base for use is scant, a criticism that will be considered below. This is of particular concern, as even the best current criteria of ultra-high risk are far from perfect, carrying a high rate of false positives, which means many subjects will be potentially exposed to medications without any clear evidence that they would have developed psychosis if left untreated. Second, taking medication entails contact with psychiatric services and accepting the label of being at risk of developing psychosis, both of which are likely to carry some degree of social stigma.

One of the first studies on early intervention at the prodromal stage was conducted in the United Kingdom (Falloon 1992). In this study, all patients who were prodromal as defined by DSM-III (American Psychiatric Association 1980) criteria were given psychoeducation, and some patients additionally received low-dose antipsychotics. The study reported a 10-fold decrease in the incidence of schizophrenia in the region compared with a previous period, although the study was uncontrolled and it is unclear which components of the intervention were efficacious.

The first controlled study (McGorry et al. 2003) found that significantly fewer patients who were treated with a mix of low-dose risperidone and psychotherapy progressed to first-episode psychosis by the end of the 6-month trial period compared with a group who received nonspecific "needs-based" interventions (9.7% vs. 35.7%, respectively; $P<0.05$) (Table 9–3). However, the significant difference between the groups was not sustained at a 6-month follow-up period after the active intervention, because of an increase in the number of patients in the specific intervention group becoming psychotic. A post hoc analysis suggested that overall, subjects in the specific-intervention group who received low-dose risperidone had the lowest rates of transition to psychosis, although the numbers were small. Additionally, given the design of the study, it is difficult to determine the specific contribution of risperidone to the findings.

The Prevention Through Risk Identification, Management, and Education trial compared olanzapine with placebo and found that although olanzapine treatment reduced the transition to psychosis rate by 50% (from 35% to 17%), the reduction was not statistically significant (Woods et al. 2003). Detailed reporting on the data at 8 weeks after initial randomization suggested that there was more improvement in psychopathology in association with olanzapine treatment, given at a mean dose of 10 mg over the period (with a significant interaction of groups with scores on the PANSS and Scale of Prodromal Symptoms in a linear, mixed-model regression). However, there was also marked weight gain in the olanzapine group during this period (mean = 4 kg vs. 0.3 kg in the placebo group; $P<0.001$).

A descriptive, interim analysis of a German intervention trial comparing amisulpride with placebo indicates beneficial effects of amisulpride not only on attenuated positive symptoms but also on negative and depressive symptoms and global functioning (Ruhrmann et al. 2003). Whether these promising initial results will be sustained when the study is completed is unclear.

The potential use of nonpharmacological interventions alone in prodromal patients has also proved to be a promising avenue. Morrison et al. (2004)

Table 9–3.   Randomized trials of interventions for patients at ultra-high risk of developing psychosis

Study	Interventions	N	Outcome measures	Results	Comments
McGorry et al. 2003	NBI vs. SPI (risperidone 1.3 mg/day and CBT)	59	Development of definite psychotic symptoms	10/28 in NBI vs. 3/31 in SPI developed psychosis at 6 months Difference not sustained at 12 months	Lower rate of development of psychosis in patients who were fully adherent to risperidone (2/14 vs. 7/17)
Morrison et al. 2004	TAU vs. CT	58	Development of definite psychotic symptoms (based on PANSS)	2/35 in CT developed psychosis vs. 4/23 in TAU	96% reduction in odds of making a transition to psychosis in CT group[a]
Woods et al. 2003	Placebo vs. olanzapine	60	Development of psychosis (based on Scale of Prodromal Symptoms)	10/29 placebo vs. 5/31 olanzapine developed psychosis	Significant group difference at 8 weeks using linear mixed-models analyses.

Note.   CBT = cognitive-behavioral therapy; CT = cognitive therapy; NBI = needs-based intervention; PANSS = Positive and Negative Syndrome Scale; SNI = specific preventive intervention; TAU = treatment as usual.
[a]After adjustment for potential moderating variables.

found that 5.7% of patients receiving cognitive therapy compared with 17.4% receiving "treatment as usual" developed psychosis over a 1-year-period. In addition, the therapy appeared to reduce the intensity of the prodromal symptoms themselves.

Moreover, it is not at all clear that antipsychotics are necessarily the only, or the best, pharmacological intervention. In the Hillside Recognition and Prevention Program, adolescents were first identified as being at risk of developing psychosis on the basis of specific combination deficits of neurocognitive deficits and then were treated (Cornblatt 2002). Unlike in other studies, the adolescents did not have to display any attenuated positive symptoms. The 54 adolescents in this group were treated on an unrandomized, open-label basis with either antipsychotics or antidepressants (selective serotonin reuptake inhibitors). Interestingly, the antidepressants, often given in combination with mood stabilizers, were as effective in promoting clinical improvement as the antipsychotics. Again, large-scale, randomized trials are needed to replicate and extend these findings.

Further research into secondary and possibly even primary prevention is warranted, but no clear treatment guidelines can be given on the basis of current evidence to guide the child and adolescent psychiatrist through this controversial field.

Clinical Pearls

- Childhood-onset schizophrenia is similar to the adult form of the disorder but much rarer and usually more severe and more difficult to treat.

- Antipsychotics are the mainstay of treatment and are superior to placebo.

- Randomized controlled trials suggest a trend to superior efficacy for the atypicals olanzapine and risperidone over haloperidol in the treatment of childhood psychoses.

- For children with treatment-resistant schizophrenia, clozapine is more efficacious than haloperidol and olanzapine, especially for negative symptoms.

- All antipsychotics are associated with adverse side effects: extrapyramidal side effects with the typicals and metabolic complications with the newer atypicals.
- It is unclear whether treatment during the prodromal phase immediately preceding the onset of frank psychosis is effective.

References

Alfaro CL, Wudarsky M, Nicolson R, et al: Correlation of antipsychotic and prolactin concentrations in children and adolescents acutely treated with haloperidol, clozapine, or olanzapine. J Child Adolesc Psychopharmacol 12:83–91, 2002

Alvir JM, Lieberman JA, Safferman AZ, et al: Clozapine-induced agranulocytosis: incidence and risk factors in the United States. N Engl J Med 329:162–167, 1993

American Academy of Child and Adolescent Psychiatry: Practice parameter for the assessment and treatment of children and adolescents with schizophrenia. J Am Acad Child Adolesc Psychiatry 40(suppl):4S–23S, 2001

American Psychiatric Association: Diagnostic and Statistical Manual of Mental Disorders, 3rd Edition. Washington, DC, American Psychiatric Association, 1980

American Psychiatric Association: Diagnostic and Statistical Manual of Mental Disorders, 3rd Edition, Revised. Washington, DC, American Psychiatric Association, 1987

American Psychiatric Association: Diagnostic and Statistical Manual of Mental Disorders, 4th Edition. Washington, DC, American Psychiatric Association, 1994

American Psychiatric Association: Diagnostic and Statistical Manual of Mental Disorders, 4th Edition, Text Revision. Washington, DC, American Psychiatric Association, 2000

Armenteros JL, Whitaker AH, Welikson M, et al: Risperidone in adolescents with schizophrenia: an open pilot study. J Am Acad Child Adolesc Psychiatry 36:694–700, 1997

Bai YM, Lin CC, Chen JY, et al: Therapeutic effect of pirenzepine for clozapine-induced hypersalivation: a randomized, double-blind, placebo-controlled, cross-over study. J Clin Psychopharmacol 21:608–611, 2001

Barnes TR: A rating scale for drug-induced akathisia. Br J Psychiatry 154:672–676, 1989

Barnett M: Ziprasidone monotherapy in pediatric bipolar disorder. Poster presented at the 156th Annual Meeting of the American Psychiatric Association, San Francisco, CA, May 2003

Beiser M, Erickson D, Fleming JA, et al: Establishing the onset of psychotic illness. Am J Psychiatry 150:1349–1354, 1993

Beitchman JH: Childhood schizophrenia: a review and comparison with adult-onset schizophrenia. Psychiatr Clin North Am 8:793–814, 1985

Bitter I, Dossenbach MR, Brook S, et al: Olanzapine versus clozapine in treatment-resistant or treatment-intolerant schizophrenia. Prog Neuropsychopharmacol Biol Psychiatry 28:173–180, 2004

Canitano R: Clinical experience with topiramate to counteract neuroleptic induced weight gain in 10 individuals with autistic spectrum disorders. Brain Dev 27:228–232, 2005

Caroff SN, Mann SC, Campbell EC, et al: Atypical antipsychotics and neuroleptic malignant syndrome. Psychiatr Ann 30:314–321, 2000

Cheng-Shannon J, McGough JJ, Pataki C, et al: Second-generation antipsychotic medications in children and adolescents. J Child Adolesc Psychopharmacol 14:372–394, 2004

Chengappa KN, Shelton MD, Baker RW, et al: The prevalence of akathisia in patients receiving stable doses of clozapine. J Clin Psychiatry 55:142–145, 1994

Childs B, Scriver CR: Age at onset and causes of disease. Perspect Biol Med 29:437–460, 1986

Cohen LG, Biederman J: Treatment of risperidone-induced hyperprolactinemia with a dopamine agonist in children. J Child Adolesc Psychopharmacol 11:435–440, 2001

Cornblatt BA: The New York high risk project to the Hillside Recognition and Prevention (RAP) program. Am J Med Genet 114:956–966, 2002

Davis JM, Chen N, Glick ID: A meta-analysis of the efficacy of second-generation antipsychotics. Arch Gen Psychiatry 60:553–564, 2003

Deckelbaum RJ, Williams CL: Childhood obesity: the health issue. Obes Res 9(suppl):239S–243S, 2001

Eggers C, Bunk D: The long-term course of childhood-onset schizophrenia: a 42-year followup. Schizophr Bull 23:105–117, 1997

Engelhardt DM, Polizos P, Waizer J, et al: A double-blind comparison of fluphenazine and haloperidol in outpatient schizophrenic children. J Autism Child Schizophr 3:128–137, 1973

Falloon IR: Early intervention for first episodes of schizophrenia: a preliminary exploration. Psychiatry 55:4–15, 1992

Faulkner G, Soundy AA, Lloyd K: Schizophrenia and weight management: a systematic review of interventions to control weight. Acta Psychiatr Scand 108:324–332, 2003

Fedorowicz VJ, Fombonne E: Metabolic side effects of atypical antipsychotics in children: a literature review. Psychopharmacology 19:533–550, 2005

Findling RL, McNamara NK, Youngstrom EA, et al: A prospective, open-label trial of
olanzapine in adolescents with schizophrenia. J Am Acad Child Adolesc Psychiatry
42:170–175, 2003

Findling RL, Aman MG, Eerdekens M, et al: Long-term, open-label study of risperidone in children with severe disruptive behaviors and below-average IQ. Am J
Psychiatry 161:677–684, 2004

Frazier JA, Gordon CT, McKenna K, et al: An open trial of clozapine in 11 adolescents
with childhood-onset schizophrenia. J Am Acad Child Adolesc Psychiatry
33:658–663, 1994

Geddes J, Freemantle N, Harrison P, et al: Atypical antipsychotics in the treatment of
schizophrenia: systematic overview and meta-regression analysis. BMJ 321:1371–
1376, 2000

Glazer WM: Extrapyramidal side effects, tardive dyskinesia, and the concept of atypicality. J Clin Psychiatry 61(suppl):16–21, 2000

Gogtay N, Sporn A, Alfaro CL, et al: Clozapine-induced akathisia in children with
schizophrenia. J Child Adolesc Psychopharmacol 12:347–349, 2002

Gogtay N, Ordonez A, Herman D, et al: Dynamic mapping of cortical development before
and after the onset of pediatric bipolar illness. J Child Psychol Psychiatry (in press)

Gothelf D, Apter A, Reidman J, et al: Olanzapine, risperidone and haloperidol in the
treatment of adolescent patients with schizophrenia. J Neural Transm 110:545–
560, 2003

Gracious BL, Krysiak TE, Youngstrom EA: Amantadine treatment of psychotropic-
induced weight gain in children and adolescents: case series. J Child Adolesc
Psychopharmacol 12:249–257, 2002

Grcevich SJ, Findling RL, Rowane WA, et al: Risperidone in the treatment of children
and adolescents with schizophrenia: a retrospective study. J Child Adolesc Psychopharmacol 6:251–257, 1996

Guy W: Clinical Global Impressions, in ECDEU Assessment Manual for Psychopharmacology, Revised (NIMH Publ No 76-338). Rockville, MD, National Institute
of Mental Health, 1976, pp 218–222

Hafner H, Maurer K, Loffler W, et al: The ABC Schizophrenia Study: a preliminary
overview of the results. Soc Psychiatry Psychiatr Epidemiol 33:380–386, 1998

Hanft A, Eggleston CF, Bourgeois JA: Neuroleptic malignant syndrome in an adolescent after brief exposure to olanzapine. J Child Adolesc Psychopharmacol 14:481–
487, 2004

Herran A, Garcia-Unzueta MT, Amado JA, et al: Effects of long-term treatment with
antipsychotics on serum leptin levels. Br J Psychiatry 179:59–62, 2001

Hollis C: Adult outcomes of child- and adolescent-onset schizophrenia: diagnostic
stability and predictive validity. Am J Psychiatry 157:1652–1659, 2000

IMS Health: Retail and Provider Perspective Audit (PMATSLS2), 2002. Available at: http://www.IMSHealth.com.

Jin H, Meyer JM, Jeste DV: Atypical antipsychotics and glucose dysregulation: a systematic review. Schizophr Res 71:195–212, 2004

Kahl KG, Hagenah J, Zapf S, et al: Botulinum toxin as an effective treatment of clozapine-induced hypersalivation. Psychopharmacology 173:229–230, 2004

Kane J, Honigfeld G, Singer J, et al: Clozapine for the treatment-resistant schizophrenic: a double-blind comparison with chlorpromazine. Arch Gen Psychiatry 45:789–796, 1988

Kapur S, Remington G: Atypical antipsychotics: new directions and new challenges in the treatment of schizophrenia. Annu Rev Med 52:503–517, 2001

Klosterkotter J, Hellmich M, Steinmeyer EM, et al: Diagnosing schizophrenia in the initial prodromal phase. Arch Gen Psychiatry 58:158–164, 2001

Kolvin I: Studies in the childhood psychoses, I: diagnostic criteria and classification. Br J Psychiatry 118:381–384, 1971

Kontaxaki BJ, Roukas DK: Randomized controlled augmentation trials in clozapine resistant schizophrenia patients: a critical review. Eur Psychiatry 20:409–415, 2005

Kraepelin E: Dementia Praecox and Paraphrenia. Huntington, NY, Robert E Krieger, 1919

Kuipers E, Holloway F, Rabe-Hesketh S, et al: An RCT of early intervention in psychosis: Croydon Outreach and Assertive Support Team (COAST). Soc Psychiatry Psychiatr Epidemiol 39:358–363, 2004

Kumra S, Frazier JA, Jacobsen LK, et al: Childhood-onset schizophrenia: a double-blind clozapine-haloperidol comparison. Arch Gen Psychiatry 53:1090–1097, 1996

Kumra S, Jacobsen LK, Lenane M, et al: Childhood-onset schizophrenia: an open-label study of olanzapine in adolescents. J Am Acad Child Adolesc Psychiatry 37:377–385, 1998

Leucht S, Pitschel-Walz G, Abraham D, et al: Efficacy and extrapyramidal side-effects of the new antipsychotics olanzapine, quetiapine, risperidone, and sertindole compared to conventional antipsychotics and placebo: a meta-analysis of randomized controlled trials. Schizophr Res 35:51–68, 1999

Leucht S, Wahlbeck K, Hamann J, et al: New generation antipsychotics versus low-potency conventional antipsychotics: a systematic review and meta-analysis. Lancet 361:1581–1589, 2003

Lieberman JA, Sheitman BB, Kinon BJ: Neurochemical sensitization in the pathophysiology of schizophrenia: deficits and dysfunction in neuronal regulation and plasticity. Neuropsychopharmacology 17:205–229, 1997

Lieberman JA, Phillips M, Gu H, et al: Atypical and conventional antipsychotic drugs in treatment-naive first-episode schizophrenia: a 52-week randomized trial of clozapine vs chlorpromazine. Neuropsychopharmacology 28:995–1003, 2003

Lieberman JA, Stroup TS, McEvoy JP, et al: Effectiveness of antipsychotic drugs in patients with chronic schizophrenia. N Engl J Med 353:1209–1223, 2005

Masi G, Cosenza A, Mucci M: Prolactin levels in young children with pervasive developmental disorders during risperidone treatment. J Child Adolesc Psychopharmacol 11:389–394, 2001

McConville B, Carrero L, Sweitzer D, et al: Long-term safety, tolerability, and clinical efficacy of quetiapine in adolescents: an open-label extension trial. J Child Adolesc Psychopharmacol 13:75–82, 2003

McGorry PD, Yung AR, Phillips LJ: The "close-in" or ultra high-risk model: a safe and effective strategy for research and clinical intervention in prepsychotic mental disorder. Schizophr Bull 29:771–790, 2003

Melkersson KI, Dahl ML, Hulting AL: Guidelines for prevention and treatment of adverse effects of antipsychotic drugs on glucose-insulin homeostasis and lipid metabolism. Psychopharmacology 175:1–6, 2004

Moncrieff J: Clozapine vs. conventional antipsychotic drugs for treatment-resistant schizophrenia: a re-examination. Br J Psychiatry 183:161–166, 2003

Morrison AP, French P, Walford L, et al: Cognitive therapy for the prevention of psychosis in people at ultra-high risk: randomised controlled trial. Br J Psychiatry 185:291–297, 2004

Mozes T, Greenberg Y, Spivak B, et al: Olanzapine treatment in chronic drug-resistant childhood-onset schizophrenia: an open-label study. J Child Adolesc Psychopharmacol 13:311–317, 2003

Nicolson R, Lenane M, Brookner F, et al: Children and adolescents with psychotic disorder not otherwise specified: a 2- to 8-year follow-up study. Compr Psychiatry 42:319–325, 2001

Pantelis C, Velakoulis D, McGorry PD, et al: Neuroanatomical abnormalities before and after onset of psychosis: a cross-sectional and longitudinal MRI comparison. Lancet 361:281–288, 2003

Pappagallo M, Silva R: The effect of atypical antipsychotic agents on prolactin levels in children and adolescents. J Child Adolesc Psychopharmacol 14:359–371, 2004

Patel NC, Sanchez RJ, Johnsrud MT, et al: Trends in antipsychotic use in a Texas Medicaid population of children and adolescents: 1996 to 2000. J Child Adolesc Psychopharmacol 12:221–229, 2002

Pickar D, Litman RE, Hong WW, et al: Clinical response to clozapine in patients with schizophrenia. Arch Gen Psychiatry 51:159–160, 1994

Pool D, Bloom W, Mielke DH, et al: A controlled evaluation of loxitane in seventy-five adolescent schizophrenic patients. Curr Ther Res Clin Exp 19:99–104, 1976

Poulton R, Caspi A, Moffitt TE, et al: Children's self-reported psychotic symptoms and adult schizophreniform disorder: a 15-year longitudinal study. Arch Gen Psychiatry 57:1053–1058, 2000

Rapoport JL, Addington AM, Frangou S, et al: The neurodevelopmental model of schizophrenia: update 2005. Mol Psychiatry 10:434–449, 2005

Realmuto GM, Erickson WD, Yellin AM, et al: Clinical comparison of thiothixene and thioridazine in schizophrenic adolescents. Am J Psychiatry 141:440–442, 1984

Ross RG, Novins D, Farley GK, et al: A 1-year open-label trial of olanzapine in school-age children with schizophrenia. J Child Adolesc Psychopharmacol 13:301–309, 2003

Ruhrmann S, Schultze-Lutter F, Klosterkotter J: Early detection and intervention in the initial prodromal phase of schizophrenia. Pharmacopsychiatry 36(suppl):S162–S167, 2003

Ruhrmann S, Schultze-Lutter F, Maier W, et al: Pharmacological intervention in the initial prodromal phase of psychosis. Eur Psychiatry 20:1–6, 2005

Saito E, Correll CU, Gallelli K, et al: A prospective study of hyperprolactinemia in children and adolescents treated with atypical antipsychotic agents. J Child Adolesc Psychopharmacol 14:350–358, 2004

Selva KA, Scott SM: Diabetic ketoacidosis associated with olanzapine in an adolescent patient. J Pediatr 138:936–938, 2001

Shaw JA, Lewis JE, Pascal S, et al: A study of quetiapine: efficacy and tolerability in psychotic adolescents. J Child Adolesc Psychopharmacol 11:415–424, 2001

Shaw P, Sporn A, Gogtay N, et al: Childhood-onset schizophrenia: a double-blind, randomized clozapine-olanzapine comparison. Arch Gen Psychiatry 63:721–730, 2006

Sholevar EH, Baron DA, Hardie TL: Treatment of childhood-onset schizophrenia with olanzapine. J Child Adolesc Psychopharmacol 10:69–78, 2000

Sikich L, Hamer RM, Bashford RA, et al: A pilot study of risperidone, olanzapine, and haloperidol in psychotic youth: a double-blind, randomized, 8-week trial. Neuropsychopharmacology 29:133–145, 2004

Simpson GM, Angus JW: A rating scale for extrapyramidal side effects. Acta Psychiatr Scand Suppl 212:11–19, 1970

Sowell MO, Mukhopadhyay N, Cavazzoni P, et al: Hyperglycemic clamp assessment of insulin secretory responses in normal subjects treated with olanzapine, risperidone, or placebo. J Clin Endocrinol Metab 87:2918–2923, 2002

Spencer EK, Kafantaris V, Padron-Gayol MV, et al: Haloperidol in schizophrenic children: early findings from a study in progress. Psychopharmacol Bull 28:183–186, 1992

Sporn A, Gogtay N, Ortiz-Aguayo R, et al: Clozapine-induced neutropenia in children: management with lithium carbonate. J Child Adolesc Psychopharmacol 13:401–404, 2003

Sporn A, Gogtay N, Bobb A, et al: Clozapine treatment of childhood-onset schizophrenia: evaluation of efficacy, adverse effects, and long-term outcome. J Am Acad Child Adolesc Psychiatry (in press)

Thomsen PH: Schizophrenia with childhood and adolescent onset: a nationwide register-based study. Acta Psychiatr Scand 94:187–193, 1996

Tollefson GD, Birkett MA, Kiesler GM, et al: Double-blind comparison of olanzapine versus clozapine in schizophrenic patients clinically eligible for treatment with clozapine. Biol Psychiatry 49:52–63, 2001

Tossell JW, Greenstein DK, Davidson AL, et al: Stimulant drug treatment in childhood-onset schizophrenia with comorbid ADHD: an open-label case series. J Child Adolesc Psychopharmacol 14:448–454, 2004

Turetz M, Mozes T, Toren P, et al: An open trial of clozapine in neuroleptic-resistant childhood-onset schizophrenia. Br J Psychiatry 170:507–510, 1997

Usiskin SI, Nicolson R, Lenane M, et al: Gabapentin prophylaxis of clozapine-induced seizures. Am J Psychiatry 157:482–483, 2000

Versiani M, Bueno J, Mundim M: A double-blind comparison between loxapine and chlordiazepoxide in the treatment of anxiety. Psychopharmacol Bull 13:22–24, 1977

Volavka J, Czobor P, Sheitman B, et al: Clozapine, olanzapine, risperidone, and haloperidol in the treatment of patients with chronic schizophrenia and schizoaffective disorder. Am J Psychiatry 159:255–262, 2002

Volkmar FR: Childhood and adolescent psychosis: a review of the past 10 years. J Am Acad Child Adolesc Psychiatry 35:843–851, 1996

Weiner DM, Meltzer HY, Veinbergs I, et al: The role of M1 muscarinic receptor agonism of N-desmethylclozapine in the unique clinical effects of clozapine. Psychopharmacology 177:207–216, 2004

Wirshing DA, Wirshing WC, Kysar L, et al: Novel antipsychotics: comparison of weight gain liabilities. J Clin Psychiatry 60:358–363, 1999

Woods SW, Breier A, Zipursky RB, et al: Randomized trial of olanzapine versus placebo in the symptomatic acute treatment of the schizophrenic prodrome. Biol Psychiatry 54:453–464, 2003 [erratum: 54:497, 2003]

Woods SW, Gueorguieva RV, Baker CB, et al: Control group bias in randomized atypical antipsychotic medication trials for schizophrenia. Arch Gen Psychiatry 62:961–970, 2005

Wudarsky M, Nicolson R, Hamburger SD, et al: Elevated prolactin in pediatric patients on typical and atypical antipsychotics. J Child Adolesc Psychopharmacol 9:239–245, 1999

Yung AR, Phillips LJ, Yuen HP, et al: Psychosis prediction: 12-month follow up of a high-risk ("prodromal") group. Schizophr Res 60:21–32, 2003

Zalsman G, Carmon E, Martin A, et al: Effectiveness, safety, and tolerability of risperidone in adolescents with schizophrenia: an open-label study. J Child Adolesc Psychopharmacol 13:319–327, 2003

10

Disorders Primarily Seen in General Medical Settings

John V. Campo, M.D.

The aim of this chapter is to address the psychopharmacological management of pediatric problems and conditions that are especially likely to be introduced in general medical settings and become targets of consultation for child and adolescent psychiatrists. Psychopharmacological intervention is particularly well suited to the general medical setting, where it offers relative simplicity and cultural consistency. Challenges specific to the general medical setting include coexisting physical disease and the use of other medications, thus increasing the risk and likelihood of pharmacodynamic and pharmacokinetic drug interactions and complications (Campo and Perel 2002). Although there is a growing appreciation that health is a unitary construct that cannot and should not be parsed into *physical* and *mental* health, the reality is that our health care delivery system has been divided into sectors devoted to problems conceptualized as physical (i.e., general medical conditions) and to those viewed as primarily psychological (i.e., mental disorders). This *practical dual-*

ism presents special challenges to patients, families, and professionals in that how a particular problem or disorder is conceptualized (i.e., as *physical* or *mental*) may dictate where care will be delivered, the types of professionals involved, the reimbursement scheme, and sometimes even the content of the treatments offered. Because child and adolescent psychiatry is a medical subspecialty focused on disorders of emotion, thinking, and behavior in youth, it is critical for practitioners to be conversant in the medical differential diagnosis of psychiatric syndromes and presentations and in the delivery of psychopharmacological and somatic interventions. It is particularly crucial when treating youth with comorbid physical illness or physical presentations of disorders typically conceptualized as being *mental*.

For the sake of clarity, the chapter is divided into sections addressing current practice and existing knowledge regarding psychopharmacology for youth presenting with physical symptoms or signs that are medically unexplained or *functional* (e.g., somatoform disorders); those with other disorders conceptualized as psychiatric, yet associated with key physical functions (e.g., eating disorders, elimination disorders, and sleep disorders); those with disorders that may involve agitation or prove disruptive in traditional medical settings (e.g., delirium, anxiety, borderline personality disorder); and those being treated psychopharmacologically in the context of a coexisting general medical condition (e.g., epilepsy) or organ failure (e.g., hepatic failure).

Functional Somatic Syndromes and Somatoform Disorders

Patients with disorders conceptualized as psychiatric may present with primarily physical symptoms in general medical settings. Functional or "medically unexplained" physical symptoms are a common presentation of psychiatric disorders in primary care and specialty medical settings, where they are associated with high levels of health service use (Campo et al. 2002). Functional somatic symptoms in childhood also increase the risk of serious health consequences across the life span, including alcohol and substance abuse, early pregnancy, obesity, accidental injury, suicide, and violence (Bernstein and Shaw 1997; Birmaher et al. 1996). The biomedical model asserts that illness (i.e., the subjective sufferings and associated behaviors of our patients) is a consequence of physical disease, a biophysical process that can be demonstrated structurally or biochemically. Many pediatric patients presenting in general medical settings nevertheless suffer from somatic distress and associated impairment in the absence of explanatory physical disease in the traditional sense, with such physical symptoms commonly being described as *functional* in nature. Approximately half of preschool and school-age children report at least one somatic complaint in the previous 2 weeks, and approximately 15% endorse at least four somatic symptoms (Garber et al. 1991).

The definition of pain as an unpleasant sensory and emotional experience that is associated with tissue damage or perceived as representative of such (Basbaum and Jesell 2000) illustrates that pain is expected to be caused by demonstrable tissue pathology, yet acknowledges that pain may be subjectively experienced in the apparent absence of demonstrable pathology. Headache is the most common painful symptom of childhood and adolescence, reported at least weekly by 10%–30% of youth, and followed in frequency by functional abdominal pain (FAP), chest pain, and limb pain (Campo and Fritsch 1994). The most relevant types of headaches are migraine and tension-type headache (TTH). The diagnosis of migraine is applied in youth with the following characteristics: 1) there is a history of at least five headache attacks in which the headache lasts 1–72 hours (4–72 hours in adults); 2) the headache has at least two of the following characteristics: a) unilateral location, b) pulsating quality, c) moderate-to-severe pain intensity, d) worsened by routine physical activity; and 3) the headache is accompanied by either a) nausea or vomiting or b) photophobia and phonophobia. Migraine may or may not be accompanied by aura (i.e., focal neurological features preceding or accompanying the headache, such as visual scintillating scotoma; sensory symptoms such as numbness, tingling, or parethesias; and motor symptoms such as motor weakness or dysphasia). TTH can be episodic or chronic, and is generally bilateral, nonpulsatile, of mild-to-moderate intensity, and not especially worsened by routine physical activity (Lipton et al. 2004). Gastrointestinal symptoms such as nausea, vomiting, and bowel problems are also commonly associated with functional pain disorders and/or migraine (Abu-Arafeh and Russell 1995), with some youth developing *cyclical vomiting syndrome,* a disorder characterized by recurrent episodes of intense, unexplained vomiting that may be likely related to migraine. Fatigue is also common, especially in adolescents, but *chronic fatigue syndrome* (CFS), a functional somatic syndrome characterized by disabling fatigue for at least 6 months that is associated with concentration and short-term memory problems, sleep problems, and musculoskeletal aches and pains, is relatively uncommon (prevalence less than 1%).

Patients with medically unexplained or functional somatic symptoms may be categorized by criteria developed in general medicine for functional somatic syndromes (e.g., CFS, fibromyalgia, irritable bowel syndrome) or may be classified according to existing standards for mental disorders (e.g., somatoform disorders, panic disorder, major depressive disorder). The category of somatoform disorders was developed to classify disorders in patients with physical symptoms that suggest a physical disorder but are not fully explained by the presence of a general medical condition, the direct effects of a substance, or another mental disorder; the symptoms must cause distress or functional impairment and should not appear to be voluntarily or intentionally produced (American Psychiatric Association 2000). Seven specific somatoform disorders are described in the current nosology: somatization disorder, undifferentiated somatoform disorder, conversion disorder, pain disorder, hypochondriasis, body dysmorphic disorder, and somatoform disorder not otherwise specified. A full discussion of somatoform disorders in youth is beyond the scope of this chapter and can be found elsewhere (Campo and Fritz 2007).

The evidence base available to guide the management of youth with somatoform disorders and functional somatic symptoms is limited. There have been few randomized controlled trials (RCTs) of intervention capable of informing clinical practice. A general approach to affected youth is described elsewhere (Campo and Fritz 2001, 2007). Briefly, reassurance that the patient is not suffering from a life-threatening or otherwise serious physical disease is generally an important first step in management, because it is often important to reduce patient and family anxiety about the presenting symptoms before proceeding with intervention. The use of placebo and/or sham interventions is generally a bad idea and is discouraged for both practical and ethical reasons.

There have been no large RCTs of psychoactive medications in the treatment of pediatric somatoform disorders or functional somatic syndromes. Pharmacological management may nevertheless prove worthy of consideration for pediatric patients with functional somatic syndromes and/or somatoform disorders. It is important to remember, however, that such treatment is largely presumptive and based on experience with adults who have functional somatic syndromes and somatoform illness, and who commonly suffer from comorbid anxiety and depressive disorders. Available evidence suggests that active treatment of comorbid emotional disorder can be helpful for the associated somatic symptoms and complaints (Simon et al. 1998). Antidepressant medications have been reported to be helpful for adults with a variety of somatoform disorders and functional somatic syndromes (Fallon 2004; Stahl 2003). These include functional pain syndromes such as fibromyalgia and headache (Fishbain et al. 1998; O'Malley et al. 1999) and functional gastrointestinal disorders such as irritable bowel syndrome (Drossman et al. 2003; Jailwala et al. 2000). St. John's wort also proved superior to placebo in a study of adults with somatoform disorder (Muller et al. 2004). A few studies have also found the serotonergic tricyclic antidepressant (TCA) clomipramine (Hollander et al. 1999) and the selective serotonin reuptake inhibitor (SSRI) fluoxetine (K. Phillips et al. 2002) to be efficacious in the treatment of adults with body dysmorphic disorder. Case reports also suggest that serotonergic antidepressants may be useful in treating adolescents with body dysmorphic disorder (El-Khatib and Dickey 1995; Sondheimer 1988), but pediatric RCTs are yet to be accomplished.

Psychopharmacological interventions may be especially worthy of consideration for youth with persistent medically unexplained pain and/or gastrointestinal symptoms, particularly in the presence of psychiatric comorbidity (e.g., anxiety, depression) or when psychotherapeutic interventions have not resulted in symptomatic remission or adequate functional improvement. Pediatric functional pain syndromes are commonly associated with comorbid anxiety and depressive symptoms and disorders (Campo et al. 2004a; Egger et al. 1999; Liakopoulou-Kairis et al. 2002), suggesting that attention to comorbid psychopathology might also prove beneficial to pediatric patients with functional somatic symptoms (Campo 2005). Functional gastrointestinal disorders associated with pain have been associated with visceral *hyperalgesia* or a special sensitivity among affected individuals to gut stretch or irritation (DiLorenzo et al. 2001), and such *visceral hypersensitivity* has been linked to serotonin as a likely mediator (Camilleri 2002). In addition, medications that interfere with serotonergic neurotransmission in the gut, such as alosetron and tegaserod, have been associated with positive results in treatment trials of adults with irritable bowel syndrome. Because of the possible relationship between serotonergic neurotransmission and gut sensation, in addition to the well-observed associations among anxiety, depression, and FAP, the SSRI citalopram was evaluated as a treatment for FAP in a study of 25 affected children and adolescents; 21 (84%) of the treated youth showed evidence of a favorable treatment response based on clinician ratings of *much* or *very much* improved (Campo et al. 2004b). Improvements in child and parent ratings of abdominal pain were accompanied by improvements in ratings of anxiety, depression, and other somatic symptoms in that study. Randomized, placebo-controlled trials are needed to adequately assess whether citalopram or other SSRIs have real utility in pediatric FAP or other functional somatic disorders.

Pediatric gastroenterologists have tended to favor the use of TCAs in youth with FAP (Hyams and Hyman 1998), in keeping with adult experience (Drossman et al. 2003) and the commonly made but not fully substantiated assertion that TCAs might be more efficacious than other antidepressants in pain syndromes. Past reports of sudden death in association with the use of TCAs in children, their potential for lethality in overdose, the absence of proven efficacy in the treatment of pediatric depression (Geller et al. 1999), and the absence of published controlled trials of TCAs for youth with somatoform illness all make it difficult to recommend the use of TCAs as first-line agents for youth with functional somatic syndromes.

With regard to headache, analgesics such as acetaminophen and ibuprofen and the serotonin receptor agonist sumatriptan (in nasal spray form) have been shown to be effective in the treatment of pediatric migraine (Lewis et al. 2004). Antipsychotic medications such as prochlorperazine and chlorpromazine have been demonstrated to be efficacious in the management of acute migraine in adults, with effects at least comparable to those of sumatriptan, and perhaps better when used parenterally (Siow et al. 2005). A single open trial with 20 patients found intravenous prochlorperazine to be a promising treatment for intractable pediatric migraine (Kabbouche et al. 2001), but double-blind RCTs are yet to be conducted. Antipsychotic medications may be worthy of consideration in the management of disorders that have been associated with migraine such as cyclic vomiting syndrome, but controlled studies are lacking. With regard to headache prophylaxis, antidepressant medications have been found to prevent chronic headaches over time in adults (Tomkins et al. 2001), as have beta-blockers and the anticonvulsants divalproex sodium and topiramate (Modi and Lowder 2006). A variety of medications have been used in an effort to reduce pediatric headache frequency, severity, duration, and associated functional impairment, as well as to improve acute treatment response. Studied agents include cyproheptadine, beta-blockers such as propranolol, the antidepressants amitriptyline and trazodone (Battistella et al. 1993), and a variety of anticonvulsants, such as divalproex sodium, levetiracetam (Lewis et al. 2004), and topiramate, but the evidence-base does not permit firm conclusions to be drawn about efficacy (Hershey et al. 2002). The α_2-adrenergic agonist clonidine does not appear to be efficacious as a treatment for pediatric headache (Lewis et al. 2004).

In youth with functional somatic syndromes, including recurrent pain, who do not respond to psychotherapeutic intervention or prefer pharmacological management, our clinical approach has been to initiate treatment with an SSRI at a low dosage (e.g., citalopram or fluoxetine 10 mg/day), then increasing to a potentially therapeutic dosage over the next week (e.g., citalopram or fluoxetine 20 mg/day), and advancing to higher dosages (e.g., to 40 mg/day) at approximately week 4 in the absence of full improvement. Clinicians considering the use of antidepressant agents in youth with functional somatic syndromes and somatoform disorders should understand that this represents an off-label use. The potential risks and benefits should be reviewed with patients and families in detail, particularly the black box warning that antidepressant use can be associated with suicidal thinking and/or behavior in a small proportion of children and adolescents, especially during the early phases of treatment. The U.S. Food and Drug Administration (FDA) recommends that *ideal* follow-up and safety monitoring for SSRI use in youth take place weekly for the first month of treatment, then every other week in the second month, then at 12 weeks, with subsequent follow-up taking place as appears clinically indicated.

Although there is no published pediatric experience with the selective serotonin-norepinephrine reuptake inhibitors (SNRIs) for functional pain or other somatic symptoms, positive adult studies suggest that both venlafaxine (e.g., Kroenke et al. 2006) and duloxetine (e.g., Brannan et al. 2005) may be promising agents. Pediatric experience with duloxetine is especially limited. Mirtazapine is a novel antidepressant that may be worthy of consideration and future study in youth with functional somatic complaints, particularly FAP and/or gastrointestinal symptoms, given its ability to block the serotonin 5-HT$_3$ receptor relevant to nausea and gastrointestinal discomfort, its antihistaminic and sleep-enhancing properties, and its utility as an antidepressant and anxiolytic in adults. Table 10–1 lists several nontricyclic antidepressant medications that might prove useful in patients with functional somatic symptoms, based on theoretical considerations and/or anecdotal experience. Any use of psychoactive medication in youth with functional pain and/or somatoform disorder should be approached with caution and with the knowledge that there are limited or no empirical data to guide such off-label treatment. Patients and families require detailed explanation, and it is only reasonable to move forward within a carefully managed process of informed consent.

Given the fact that many youth with functional somatic syndromes suffer from migraine and may use anti-migraine drugs known as triptans that are serotonin receptor agonists (e.g., sumatriptan), there is reason for concern about the possibility of a serotonin syndrome in association with use of these agents along with SSRIs and other antidepressants. Although prior experience suggested that the combination of triptans with SSRIs was likely to be relatively safe (Putnam et al. 1999), a July 2006 public health advisory from the FDA warned about the risk of serotonin syndrome when triptans are used in combination with SSRIs or SNRIs. Serotonin syndrome is associated with symptoms of restlessness, tachycardia, rapid changes in blood pressure, elevated body temperature, loss of coordination, overactive reflexes, nausea, vomiting, diarrhea, and/or hallucinations. Physicians considering prescribing both a triptan and a serotonergic antidepressant are advised to weigh the potential risks and benefits of precipitating a serotonin syndrome, discuss that possibility in detail with patients being considered for such treatment, and then monitor and proceed cautiously with any patients choosing this option.

There is little available research addressing the use of psychoactive medications in pediatric CFS (Garralda and Chalder 2005). Given the common association of anxiety and depressive disorders with the symptom profile in CFS, consideration might be given to the use of antidepressant medications, including potentially more activating agents, such as bupropion, venlafaxine, and duloxetine, but these interventions would require additional study and cannot be recommended routinely.

Clinical experience also suggests that some youth suffering from physical symptoms associated with emotional arousal and anxiety may benefit from a short course of a benzodiazepine such as clonazepam or lorazepam (Campo and Fritz 2001). This can sometimes be particularly useful in somatoform patients who are beginning treatment with an SSRI or SNRI antidepressant,

Table 10–1. Antidepressant medication for functional somatic disorders

Basic Principles
"Start low and go slow"
Attempt to reach target dose in 7 days if starting dose tolerated
Reevaluate dose after 3–4 weeks at target dose

Drug class	Drug	Starting dose (mg/day)	Target dosage (mg/day)	Maximum dosage (mg/day)
SSRI	Citalopram	10	20	40
	Escitalopram	5	10	20
	Fluoxetine	10	20	40
	Fluvoxamine	25	100	300
	Paroxetine	10	20	40
	Sertraline	25	100	200
SNRI	Venlafaxine	37.5	75	375
	Duloxetine	20	40	120
Other	Mirtazapine	7.5	30	45

Note. There are no medications that have been FDA approved or tested in randomized controlled trials for youth with functional somatic disorders.
SNRI=serotonin-norepinephrine reuptake inhibitor; SSRI=selective serotonin reuptake inhibitor.

since they may be hypersensitive to bodily symptoms and sensations that sometimes accompany the initiation of such medication. Clonazepam has the advantage of being relatively long-acting, with a gradual onset of action, and can be started at a low dosage of 0.25 mg given twice a day or at bedtime, with the dosage increased to 0.5 mg given twice a day, as needed. Lorazepam has a more intermediate half-life and can be administered initially at 0.5 mg given three times a day, with the dosage increased to 1 mg three times a day, as needed. Although the available literature on the use of benzodiazepines in anxious children and adolescents is inconsistent, with few well-powered and well-controlled studies available for evaluation (Witek et al. 2005), this approach nevertheless sometimes leads to rapid symptomatic relief. It can help reassure the patient and family and demonstrate the potential contribution of emotional activation to the child's somatic distress. The azapirone buspirone is a partial agonist of the serotonin 5-HT$_{1A}$ receptor that has been demonstrated to have anxiolytic properties in adults, yet lacks substantial efficacy in panic anxiety. It has not been well studied as an anxiolytic in youth, but there have been some preliminary studies exploring its potential efficacy for FAP in adults. Buspirone can be initiated at 5 mg po bid, and the dosage can be increased by approximately 5 mg/day each week to a maximum of 60 mg/day.

For youth with persistent nausea or vomiting that is unresponsive to anxiolytics such as benzodiazepines, and/or in the presence of symptoms suggesting acute migraine, the use of an antipsychotic medication (e.g., prochlorperazine) or an antiemetic (e.g., ondansetron) may also be worthy of consideration as acute treatments. Although not as well studied as anxiolytics or antiemetics for this use, atypical antipsychotics such as aripiprazole, olanzapine, quetiapine, risperidone, and ziprasidone may prove helpful clinically in managing anxiety and associated symptoms of nausea, vomiting, and fear of eating.

Eating Disorders

Anorexia nervosa (AN) is a serious psychiatric disorder characterized by extremely low body weight and cognitive distortions of body shape and image, as well as amenorrhea in women. There are currently no FDA-approved medications for the treatment of AN. Because previous studies of amitriptyline, clomipramine, and fluoxetine have failed to show benefits for antidepressant medications in excess of placebo for acutely ill, undernourished patients with AN (Attia and Schroeder 2005), their use is not recommended as the sole or initial treatment in such circumstances. Treatment with antidepressants might nevertheless be worth considering as a means of relapse prevention and weight maintenance following nutritional support and the resolution of psychological consequences of malnutrition (Yager and Andersen 2005). Fluoxetine (20–60 mg/day) was found to be superior to placebo in decreasing core eating disorder symptoms and maintaining restored weight for at least 1 year in patients with restrictive AN who had been returned to at least 90% of expected body weight by initial nutritional and behavioral intervention (Kaye et al. 2001). Antidepressants may also be of benefit in the treatment of comorbid mood and anxiety symptoms and disorders. Available studies have primarily recruited adults and older adolescents, with few trials conducted that include children. Although it has not been especially well studied, administration of a benzodiazepine approximately 30 minutes before meals has been justified by the commonly observed anxiety experienced by patients with AN around eating (Ebeling et al. 2003). Studies of cyproheptadine for AN have yielded mixed results (Attia and Schroeder 2005), and evidence for the efficacy of lithium carbonate is lacking (American Psychiatric Association 2006).

Numerous case reports and small open-label studies suggest that atypical antipsychotic medications such as olanzapine may be useful in improving weight gain for patients with AN, including treatment-resistant patients; but randomized, placebo-controlled trials have not been completed (Barbarich et al. 2004; Powers and Santana 2004). Traditional neuroleptics such as haloperidol have also shown some promise in open trials (Cassano et al. 2003). Atypical antipsychotics may also be useful in the management of atypical eating disorders and food refusal in young children, as evidenced by the case report of a 3-year-old boy with food refusal who improved following initiation of risperidone at 0.25 mg two times a day (Schwam et al. 1998).

Psychoactive medications have also been used to reduce the frequency of disturbed eating behaviors such as binging and purging in bulimia nervosa (BN) and to manage accompanying symptoms of emotional distress. Double-blind, placebo-controlled studies of antidepressant medications for adults with BN have found efficacy for TCAs such as imipramine, SSRIs such as fluoxetine, monoamine oxidase inhibitors (MAOIs) such as phenelzine, and other novel agents such as trazodone and bupropion (American Psychiatric Association 2006). Unfortunately, no trials have been conducted in children and adolescents. Fluoxetine is the only medication approved by the FDA for the treatment of BN in adults, but it is not approved for treatment of youth with BN. Another SSRI, fluvoxamine, was shown to be superior to placebo in preventing relapse in BN (Fichter et al. 1996). Bupropion is not recommended, given its association with seizures during the treatment of purging patients with BN (Horne et al. 1988). The anticonvulsant topiramate has also been found to be efficacious in treating adults with BN (Hoopes et al. 2003) and binge-eating disorder (McElroy et al. 2003). SSRIs have also been deemed helpful in the management of adults with binge-eating disorder (Carter et al. 2003), as has sibutramine (Appolinario et al. 2003). A study of obesity in adolescents also found sibutramine plus behavior therapy to be significantly superior to placebo and behavioral treatment in effecting weight loss (Berkowitz et al. 2006).

Sleep Disorders

Pediatric sleep difficulties can negatively impact child health, mood, behavior, and learning, as well as family life (Mindell 1993). Pediatric insomnia is defined as repeated difficulty with sleep initiation, duration, consolidation, or quality that occurs despite age-appropriate time and opportunity for sleep, and results in daytime functional impairment for the child and/or the family (Mindell et al. 2006). Youth suffering from attention-deficit/hyperactivity disorder (ADHD) are particularly vulnerable to sleep difficulties, including bedtime resistance, difficulties initiating sleep, and frequent awakenings (Bullock and Schall 2005). Pediatricians involved in the treatment of youth with ADHD are especially likely to prescribe sleep medications to children (Owens et al. 2003). Insomnia is a problem for at least 1%–6% of children and adolescents in the general population (up to 30%, if problems with bedtime refusal and night wakings are included), affects as many as 75% of youth with neurodevelopmental disabilities, and is the cited reason for approximately 3% of pediatric visits (Mindell et al. 2006; Owens et al. 2003). More than half the pediatricians in a recent survey acknowledged prescribing sleep medications to children and approximately 75% recommended the use of over-the-counter (OTC) sleep aids (Owens et al. 2003). Insomnia is also a common problem among medically hospitalized children and adolescents, and requests for help in its management are common for pediatric psychiatrists working in medical settings.

A recent conference of experts concluded that the treatment of pediatric insomnia is an unmet medical need, but that sound safety and efficacy data are lacking, despite the widespread use of OTC, hypnotic, and other psychoactive medications for pediatric sleep problems (Mindell et al. 2006). The highest-priority groups regarding insomnia appear to be youth with pervasive developmental disorders (PDDs), ADHD, mood disorders, and anxiety disorders. Other relevant sleep disorders for which pharmacological management might prove useful include delayed sleep phase syndrome and insomnia associated with specific medical conditions and their treatment. Despite the lack of approved medications or controlled studies of hypnotics in children and adolescents, a variety of agents are commonly recommended or prescribed by pediatricians (Owens et al. 2003). Antihistamines are probably the most commonly recommended OTC medication, followed by melatonin and a variety of herbal remedies such as chamomile tea or valerian root. Despite the lack of efficacy data and concern expressed about their safety (Klein-Schwartz 2002), α_2-adrenergic agonists such as clonidine appear to be the most commonly prescribed pediatric sleep medications, followed by antihistamines, antidepressants, benzodiazepines, and other prescription hypnotics; a few practitioners acknowledge prescribing barbiturates, chloral hydrate, and antipsychotics as pediatric sleep agents.

There is consensus that the use of sound sleep practices such as the avoidance of caffeine, the maintenance of an age-appropriate sleep-wake schedule, and elimination of access to late-night television viewing in the bedroom should serve as the foundation for any subsequent interventions. In general, the use of behavioral interventions should be the next consideration, as suggested by an evidence base that supports the techniques of extinction and graduated extinction, and the value of parental psychoeducation. Clinical judgment is required in this context, however, given that some children with conditions such as ADHD or PDD might not prove to be good candidates for beginning with a behavioral approach alone. It is also important to identify the underlying cause of sleep disturbance, when possible, prior to initiating treatment. Although there is little supportive data, behavioral and pharmacological approaches might be productively combined.

There are currently no systematically studied agents approved for use as hypnotics in children and adolescents. Considerable interest has developed in the use of melatonin for pediatric insomnia. Melatonin is a naturally occurring indole neurotransmitter derived from serotonin and its precursor, tryptophan. It is synthesized in the pineal gland, with darkness stimulating and bright light suppressing its secretion. Melatonin acts on the suprachiasmatic nucleus in the anterior hypothalamus, where it influences circadian rhythms and is capable of shifting sleep phase, apparently with little influence on sleep architecture. Not surprisingly, melatonin has been reported to be effective in the management of sleep-wake cycle problems related to jet lag, shift work, and delayed sleep phase syndrome (Herxheimer and Petrie 2002; Stores 2003), though a recent review did not support its efficacy for secondary sleep disorders (i.e., those associated with medical, neurological, or substance-related problems) and sleep disorders accompanying sleep restriction (Buscemi et al. 2006). Exogenous, synthetic melatonin has a half-life of 30–60 minutes and

388 Clinical Manual of Child and Adolescent Psychopharmacology

apparently promotes sleep onset within 30–40 minutes of administration. Its use has been advocated for sleep problems in youth with neurodevelopmental disorders on the basis of several published reports showing a significant decrease in time-to-sleep onset for melatonin-treated youth (Jan et al. 1999), but sample sizes have been small and well-designed RCTs are few (L. Phillips and Appleton 2004).

In studies of melatonin at a dose of 5 mg for the treatment of school-aged children with chronic, idiopathic insomnia, melatonin significantly advanced the sleep-wake rhythm and improved parental global ratings of child health compared with placebo, with a trend toward an increase in total sleep time (Smits et al. 2003). Dose-response studies have not been performed, and a maximal dosage has not been well defined, but the dose in published studies has ranged from 0.3 mg to 10 mg, with most reports suggesting a dose of 2–3 mg, with subsequent increases if ineffective (Ivanenko et al. 2003; Jan et al. 1999). Melatonin has been considered safe for short-term use based on available evidence, and adverse effects are said to be unusual (Herxheimer and Petrie 2002). However, safety assessment of melatonin has been limited, and there is no information about the safety of long-term use (Stores 2003). Sedation and headache have been the most commonly reported side effects (Jan et al. 1999; Smits et al. 2003; Stores 2003). Although there have been reports of an increase in seizures with melatonin use in the neurodevelopmentally disabled (Sheldon 1998), there is also evidence that melatonin may be helpful in managing sleep problems in epileptic children (Gupta et al. 2005). Adding to the uncertainty is the fact that melatonin is an unlicensed drug and is sold as a food supplement, raising concerns about variability in preparations and possible impurities. The development of melatonin receptor agonists such as ramelteon, a recently approved agent for insomnia in adults, has thus generated considerable interest, presumably due to concerns about quality-control issues and the pharmacokinetic profile of melatonin.

Sedating antihistamines such as diphenhydramine (25–50 mg orally) and cyproheptadine (2–4 mg orally) continue to be used as sleep aids in school-aged children, though paradoxical excitation and sleeplessness in some patients, as well as reports of daytime drowsiness, irritability, and cognitive blunting, have resulted in some dissatisfaction with their use, particularly in youth with developmental disabilities (Turk 2003). Tolerance may also develop (Younus and Labellarte 2002). Cyproheptadine may be of use as a sleep aid for youth being treated with stimulants for ADHD, given its potential to improve sleep and increase appetite and weight (Daviss and Scott 2004).

Benzodiazepines are the most widely prescribed sedative-hypnotics in adults, and lorazepam and midazolam are approved agents for sedation in children but have not been studied or approved as treatments for pediatric insomnia (Younus and Labellarte 2002). Ideally, a hypnotic medication will help induce sleep rapidly and maintain sleep quality without producing sedation or other adverse cognitive effects the following day, making it difficult to recommend the use of benzodiazepines with particularly long half-lives. If a decision is made to use a benzodiazepine, it is generally wise to begin with relatively low doses of an intermediate-acting agent such as lorazepam (0.25–0.5 mg at bedtime) for children and adolescents. Benzodiazepines may suppress Stage IV, or slow-wave, sleep, making them potentially useful in sleep disorders associated with slow-wave sleep such as sleepwalking or night terrors (Witek et al. 2005). One small study suggested the short-acting benzodiazepine midazolam may be a promising treatment for pediatric night terrors (Popoviciu and Corfariu 1983). Potential adverse effects include disinhibition, withdrawal phenomena (including rebound insomnia), cognitive impairment, and psychomotor impairment (Younus and Labellarte 2002).

The anticonvulsant gabapentin (100–300 mg initially), developed as a gamma-aminobutyric acid analog, may also deserve consideration as a hypnotic, given a wide therapeutic index, low potential for drug-drug interactions, and a relatively favorable side-effect profile, but pediatric studies of the drug in this capacity are not available.

Newer nonbenzodiazepine hypnotics such as zolpidem, zaleplon, zopiclone, and eszopiclone have not been studied in children and adolescents but are becoming more popular than benzodiazepines in adult clinical practice because of what appears to be a more favorable risk-benefit profile, their lack of active metabolites, and less rebound insomnia upon withdrawal. These drugs are type 1 benzodiazepine receptor agonists and generally lack the muscle relaxant and anticonvulsant properties of benzodiazepines. There is little in the way of literature to guide pediatric use. Zaleplon appears to be the most rapidly eliminated of these medications, with less reported cognitive impairment or sedation compared with zolpidem (Younus and Labellarte 2002).

Numerous antidepressant medications have been used to manage pediatric insomnia, though again with little empirical support. Trazodone (25–50 mg initially) has been used to improve sleep in depressed patients and in patients with sleep difficulties who are taking SSRIs, but the potential for priapism has limited its use in males. The related drug nefazodone also has sedative properties but has been associated with liver toxicity, making its use as a hypnotic ill-advised, especially in children. Mirtazapine (7.5–15 mg initially) is another novel antidepressant with antihistaminic and sedating properties that is not approved as a hypnotic but may prove useful as a pediatric sleep aid (Younus and Labellarte 2002). A small open-label study of mirtazapine suggested it may be of some help with sleep in youth with PDDs (Posey et al. 2001), but randomized, placebo-controlled trials in pediatric patients with sleep disorders have not been accomplished. TCAs such as amitriptyline or imipramine have also been used in clinical settings to manage pediatric sleep problems, but concerns related to toxicity in overdose, cardiovascular complications, and sudden death make their use less appealing, given alternatives. Of the TCAs, doxepin and trimipramine are particularly antihistaminic and sedating.

The α_2-adrenergic receptor agonist clonidine is commonly used as a sleep aid by general pediatricians (Schnoes et al. 2006) and has also been reported to be useful for sleep difficulties in developmentally disabled children (Ingrassia and Turk 2005). The drug has gained popularity for sleep problems in stimulant-treated youth with ADHD, but caution is warranted because of the need for cardiovascular monitoring, the potential for adverse cardiovascular effects, and reports of sudden death for youth treated with clonidine and a stimulant (Cantwell et al. 1997). Clonidine at dosages ranging from 0.05 to 0.15 mg/day was also examined in a small open trial in preschool children with posttraumatic stress disorder (PTSD) and appeared to be associated with improvements in nightmares and insomnia (Harmon and Riggs 1996). Guanfacine, another sedating α_2-adrenergic receptor agonist that may have less potential for adverse effects, has been reported to suppress nightmares in a child with PTSD (Horrigan 1996).

The use of traditional or atypical antipsychotics for isolated insomnia is generally frowned upon, but these drugs may prove especially helpful as sleep aids for patients with PDD, psychosis, or bipolar mood disorders. The phenothiazine promethazine has been used as a sedative in children, but it is neither approved nor studied as a hypnotic in children (Younus and Labellarte 2002).

Because of an unfavorable safety profile, a narrow therapeutic index, and the potential for "hangover," the use of barbiturates or nonbarbiturate hypnotics such as chloral hydrate cannot be recommended.

Elimination Disorders

Enuresis

Enuresis is defined as the repeated voiding of urine during the day or at night into the bed or clothes in the absence of a medical cause, with current diagnostic criteria requiring that the child be at least 5 years of age, that the frequency be at least twice per week for 3 months, and that the disorder cause significant distress or functional impairment (Mikkelsen 2001). Although approximately 5%–7% of children older than 5 years wet the bed, the spontaneous remission rate is approximately 15% per year, an especially important point to communicate to parents in discussing the risks and benefits associated with treatment, particularly with regard to the use of medication. It is also critical to realize that the best-studied and most effective treatment for nocturnal enuresis is not pharmacological, but rather the bell-and-pad method of behavioral treatment. The use of an enuresis alarm has been demonstrated to be significantly superior to no treatment or placebo, reducing bedwetting by an average of 4 nights per week, with a number needed to treat (NNT) of 2 to achieve 14 consecutive dry nights and a relapse rate of approximately 50% after stopping treatment, which indicates it offers significantly better results than control interventions (Glazener et al. 2003). Education about the disorder is helpful in all cases, and parents should be counseled to withhold punishment (Fritz et al. 2004).

Numerous studies have documented the efficacy of desmopressin given intranasally (10–60 µg) or orally (100–600 µg) (Glazener et al. 2003; Mikkelsen 2001). Desmopressin reduces wet nights per week by an average of at least 1 or 2, with a NNT of 7 to achieve 14 consecutive dry nights (Glazener et al. 2003). Unfortunately, there is a high relapse rate once the medication is stopped, suggesting that treatment must be ongoing until spontaneous remission occurs. Long-term administration is generally considered safe, though there have been rare reports of hyponatremia and hyponatremia-induced seizures and mental status changes. Because these adverse events seem to have occurred in the context of excessive fluid intake, some caution desmopressin-treated youth to avoid consuming more than 8 ounces of fluid before bedtime.

The TCA imipramine has been used for many years as a treatment for enuresis, with a recent systematic review suggesting that it reduces wet-nights-per-week by at least one, with a NNT of 6 to achieve 14 consecutive dry nights. As with desmopressin, the relapse rate for imipramine is quite high upon drug discontinuation. Because of the risk of cardiac conduction abnormalities and the dangers associated with TCAs in overdose, desmopressin has largely replaced imipramine as the most commonly prescribed medication for enuresis. The availability of an oral preparation of desmopressin has also made administration considerably easier. Reports have also explored the use of medications such as carbamazepine, oxybutynin (Mikkelsen 2001), and atomoxetine (Shatkin 2004), though desmopressin and imipramine are clearly the best studied of the drugs used to treat this condition.

In sum, behavioral intervention should be identified as a first-line treatment for enuretic children, with ongoing pharmacological treatment considered only in refractory cases, when environmental factors make such treatment difficult or impossible, or when dictated by patient and family preference in the context of a risk-benefit ratio judged as acceptable by the clinician and family. Desmopressin may be a reasonable choice as a short-term choice for sleepovers or camping trips.

Encopresis

Encopresis refers to the repeated passage of feces into inappropriate places such as clothing or the floor, whether involuntary or intentional, with at least one event occurring per month for at least 3 months in a child of a chronological age or equivalent developmental level of at least 4 years. Medical treatment of encopresis has typically involved evacuation of the distal colon (i.e., bowel cleanout) followed by the ongoing use of laxatives, and is most productively combined with behavioral treatments and toileting programs. Psychoactive medications have not played a direct role in the management of encopresis, but clinical experience suggests that youth with refractory encopresis deserve careful assessment for comorbid psychopathology, particularly chronic depression. Aggressive treatment of comorbid psychopathology with antidepressant or antipsychotic medication may prove necessary, if not sufficient, to remedying the encopresis.

Agitation and Delirium

Agitation

Agitation refers to a relatively nonspecific constellation of behaviors that can impair patient functioning, interfere with caregiving, and/or pose a risk to the safety of the patient or others, and can be seen in a variety of different clinical situations (Yildiz et al. 2003). The agitated patient most often appears emotionally distressed, restless, inattentive, and tense, with characteristics that include loud speech; an angry, irritable, or threatening demeanor; increased muscle tension, motor activity, or pacing; and physiological signs of autonomic arousal such as elevated heart rate. The differential diagnosis is broad (see Table 10–2) and includes delirium, dementia, substance intoxication or withdrawal, other medical conditions (e.g., hyperthyroidism, hypoglycemia), psychotic states and mood disorders, anxiety disorders, disruptive behavior disorders (e.g., conduct disorder), personality disorders, and neurodevelopmental disorders. Despite the importance of the problem, there is surprisingly little in the way of systematic research on the assessment or management of agitation in pediatric settings.

A comprehensive discussion of the assessment and management of pediatric agitation is beyond the scope of this chapter, but there is no substitute for careful assessment. After establishing the nature and severity of the patient's agitation, the clinician should make a presumptive descriptive or phenomenological diagnosis (e.g., delirium, anxiety, mania), followed by a careful medical assessment investigating possible physical etiologies for the presentation (e.g., alcohol withdrawal as an etiology for delirium, hyperthyroidism as the cause of marked anxiety). Even though a clear physical etiology cannot always be identified, it is essential that the clinician consider the hypothesis that the patient's symptomatic or syndromic presentation may be the consequence of an unrecognized general medical condition or substance (Campo 1993). Understanding the specific etiology of the presentation may prove critical to appropriate intervention (e.g., substance intoxication or withdrawal). Beyond specific interventions tailored to the etiology of the patient's

Table 10–2.   Differential diagnosis of agitation

Delirium

Dementia

Substance intoxication/withdrawal

Other physical disorder

Psychosis

Mood disorder

Anxiety disorder

Neurodevelopmental disorder

Disruptive behavior disorders (e.g., conduct disorder)

Personality disorders

presentation, nonspecific symptomatic management is most often necessary (see Table 10–3).

Delirium

Delirium is a powerful clue to the presence of an unrecognized general medical condition that is responsible for the child's agitation and thus deserves special comment. The term refers to a disturbance or impairment in arousal or consciousness that most often develops acutely and that may be associated with a reduced ability to focus or shift attention, disorientation, disorganized thinking, fluctuations in level of consciousness, memory problems, marked changes in activity level, sleep-wake cycle disturbances, emotional distress, and problems with reality testing, such as hallucinations. Traditional teaching maintains that young children and the elderly are especially vulnerable to delirium, but there is little evidence to support the claim that youth are especially vulnerable. Delirium has been associated with increased lengths of stay and increased morbidity and mortality for hospitalized adults, with mechanistic explanations including increased central noradrenergic activity, an imbalance between dopaminergic and cholinergic systems in the brain with a resultant excess of dopaminergic activity, and direct impairment of neuronal function (Eisendrath and Shim 2006).

In many respects, the biggest single challenge in dealing with pediatric delirium is its recognition (Martini 2005). Children and adolescents suffering from a delirium may be dismissed as "naughty," "difficult," or simply misbehaving in the face of the stress associated with medical care or hospitalization.

Table 10–3.   Management of agitation

Identify and treat underlying etiology

Nonspecific intervention

    Honest interaction to establish and maintain credibility

    Empathic, nonjudgmental listening, and information gathering

    Avoidance of intense eye contact or deliberate provocation

    Support and reassurance

    Frequent orientation for confused or disoriented patients

    Establishment of a familiar, nonthreatening environment

    Minimizing of extraneous noise and stimulation

    Control of physical pain

    Kind but firm limits that emphasize the safety of all

Adequate staffing

    Appropriate use of safety officers

    Show of force when necessary to encourage self-control

Judicious pharmacotherapy

    Antipsychotic medications

        Haloperidol and traditional antipsychotics

        Atypical antipsychotics

    Benzodiazepines

        Lorazepam

    Combination treatment

        Antipsychotic + benzodiazepine

Even though it is inadequately studied and often overlooked clinically, delirium is common in hospitalized and physically ill youth. It represents a true emergency in that it can indicate the presence of a rapidly deteriorating and potentially fatal physical condition (Prugh et al. 1980; Turkel and Tavare 2003). Consequently, delirium should always engender a careful medical workup and evaluation, since identifying and treating the physical cause of the delirium is the foundation of successful treatment. Risk factors for delirium in adult patients include the presence of prior brain injury or damage, the use of multiple medications (particularly anticholinergics), substance intoxication or withdrawal, burns, hypoalbuminemia (i.e., protein-bound drugs may be more bioavailable), multiple serious medical problems, and organ failure (e.g., hepatic or renal failure) (Trzepacz 1996; Tune et al. 1992). Reversible causes of delirium such as hypoxia, hypoglycemia, narcotic overdose, alcohol withdrawal, or infection are especially important to identify and treat promptly. Thiamine should be administered when there is concern about alcohol withdrawal.

In addition to attempting to identify and rectify the cause of the patient's delirium, the clinician should undertake efforts to manipulate the patient's surroundings in conjunction with any psychopharmacological management (see Table 10–3). Ensuring constant and adequate supervision to maintain the patient's safety and making arrangements to have a parent, family member, or other trusted individual present to help comfort and orient the child are likely to be the most important interventions in pediatric delirium. Staff and family members should provide ongoing support and reassurance and make every effort to create a familiar, less-threatening environment. This can involve limiting noise and overstimulation, maintaining adequate, soft lighting in the patient's room, and controlling any physical pain (Ryan 1998). Medically hospitalized delirious youth should be constantly supervised, given the potential dangerousness of the condition. Intravenous access is generally wise, providing appropriate supervision of the patient is maintained.

Aside from addressing the medical etiology of the patient's delirium and the supportive measures outlined above, pharmacological treatment with antipsychotic medication has been considered the mainstay of active intervention ("Practice Guideline for the Treatment of Patients With Delirium" 1999), though there is little in the way of empirical study to guide active management in the pediatric population. In addition to the more commonly used traditional antipsychotics, atypical antipsychotics have been increasingly used. Benzodiazepines—most notably lorazepam—are also widely used, either alone or in combination with antipsychotic medication. Practicalities of medication management for the agitated patient are addressed below.

Practical Management

Despite the lack of high-quality empirical support for specific medications in the management of pediatric agitation, situations in which pharmacotherapy appears to be prudent are common, even when a specific etiology for the agitation has not been identified. Medication should not be used simply as a means of restraint per se, as a substitute for adequate supervision, as a convenience for caring professionals, or as a misguided punishment for disturbing behaviors. Sedation alone should not be the focus of intervention; instead, the aim should be behavioral control. Realistic goals of pharmacotherapy include the following: minimize disruptive behaviors and prevent escalation to violence; treat patient anxiety and emotional distress; and specifically target any identified, underlying psychiatric or physical condition. Given the lack of systematic research in this area, the reader is cautioned to review the medication package insert and all medication-related decisions on a case-by-case basis. Although the judicious use of medication to control agitation in the medical setting often appears reasonable and relatively safe, the fact remains that pediatric experience is somewhat limited and there is little guidance regarding the real risk of relatively rare, yet potentially catastrophic adverse reactions such as multifocal ventricular tachycardia. Given the relative safety of oral administration and the very real risks of the physical restraint sometimes necessary to administer medication intramuscularly, it is exceptionally important to remember that, although parenteral administration is sometimes necessary, most agitated patients can be persuaded to accept and take an oral medication (Yildiz et al. 2003).

Under ideal circumstances, it is generally wise to begin with a low dose of the medication chosen to help manage the patient's agitation. Gradually titrate the medication upward, approximately every 30 minutes until the desired effect is reached, thus minimizing the risk of excessive sedation or other adverse effects. A systematic approach should emphasize the competing priorities of *doing no harm* alongside the very real need for behavioral control and the *risk of doing nothing*. Marked agitation may thus call for more aggressive dosing, given the need to take decisive action in the face of potentially threatening and dangerous agitated behaviors, balancing these concerns against a realistic appraisal of drug safety for a given patient.

Traditional Antipsychotics

The traditional antipsychotic haloperidol has been the most commonly used agent for delirium across the life span, and is often used for nonspecific agitation as well. There is a long history of experience with the drug in the physically ill, given its availability in oral, intramuscular, and intravenous formulations. Haloperidol also has few active metabolites and limited anticholinergic effects, and produces relatively less sedation than other antipsychotics. Some evidence indicates that, when used judiciously, haloperidol can decrease the duration of delirium and reduce the length of hospital stay for adults (Eisendrath and Shim 2006).

The recommended pediatric dose of haloperidol is 0.025–0.075 mg/kg, generally not to exceed 2.5 mg in younger children and 5 mg in adolescents (Sorrentino 2004). In general, a dose of 0.5 mg may be sufficient for the delirious school-age child or adolescent with mild agitation, with higher doses of 1–2 mg indicated for moderate agitation, and up to 5 mg for more severe agitation in adolescents (Ryan 1998). Intravenous administration is not FDA-approved, but there is some indication that this route of administration is less likely to be associated with extrapyramidal side effects (EPS) (Menza et al. 1988). When given intravenously, the drug should not be administered at a rate greater than 1 mg/minute (Eisendrath and Shim 2006). Total daily doses of 1–2 mg for oral administration or divided every 4–6 hours intravenously are generally sufficient for maintenance until delirium has cleared, though higher doses may occasionally be needed. Using a relatively low, scheduled maintenance dose is preferable to relying entirely on "as needed" dosing that waits for a patient to become acutely agitated or distressed prior to administration. The medication can then be gradually tapered once the patient's condition has been stabilized. A recent report documents the use of low-dose intravenous haloperidol (0.15–0.25 mg) as a successful treatment of delirium in two critically ill preschool children (Schieveld and Leentjens 2005), and earlier reports suggest a dose of 0.25 mg administered slowly intravenously in very young children, with a subsequent maintenance dosage of 0.05–0.5 mg/kg/day (Brown et al. 1996). In a retrospective review of haloperidol use in 26 pediatric burn patients, the mean single dose reported was 0.057 mg/kg (range=0.013–0.278 mg/kg), with the most commonly reported adverse effects being dystonic reactions, which were most likely to occur with extended use of the medication (Ratcliff et al. 2004).

The safety record of haloperidol under controlled conditions in the medical setting appears to be reassuring, given the scope of its use. The most significant concerns are potential lengthening of the QT interval (QTc) and the risk of multifocal ventricular tachycardia or torsades de pointes, which has been reported when using both high and low doses and when administering both intravenous and oral formulations (Jackson et al. 1997; Sharma et al. 1998). Abnormal serum levels of magnesium and potassium may increase risk. Ideally, a baseline electrocardiogram (ECG) should be obtained when administering antipsychotic medications to the delirious pediatric patient, particularly when using intravenous haloperidol. Consideration should also be given to checking and monitoring serum magnesium and potassium. The ECG and length of the QTc should be monitored across the course of treatment. Other adverse effects associated with haloperidol include EPS and akathisia. Although the antihistamine diphenhydramine has fallen out of favor in the management of agitation because of concern that it produces significant anticholinergic effects that may negatively affect cognition and exacerbate delirium, its sedative properties and relative safety make it a good choice in the management of EPS in the agitated patient.

The butyrophenone droperidol has also been used in the management of delirium and acute agitation in the past, based on a more rapid onset of action and greater sedative properties. But its pediatric use has declined because the FDA mandated a black box warning in 2001 on the basis of associated lengthening of the QTc, torsades de pointes, and sudden death. Droperidol is not offered in an oral preparation—it requires intramuscular or intravenous administration—and is also more likely to be associated with hypotension than haloperidol ("Practice Guideline for the Treatment of Patients With Delirium" 1999). Droperidol has a somewhat shorter half-life than haloperidol. The initial pediatric dosage recommendation for droperidol has been similar to that of haloperidol, at 0.03–0.07 mg/kg/dose, with a maximum initial dose for children of 2.5 mg.

Low-potency phenothiazines such as chlorpromazine have also been used to manage agitation and delirium in pediatric settings, but they have more anticholinergic effects, are more sedating, and are more likely to produce hypotension than haloperidol, particularly when administered parenterally. The low-potency neuroleptics are also more likely to lower the seizure threshold than haloperidol, which may be an important consideration in medically compromised patients and/or in situations where the etiology of the agitation is unknown.

Atypical Antipsychotics

The atypical antipsychotic medications (e.g., aripiprazole, olanzapine, paliperidone, quetiapine, risperidone, ziprasidone) are being more commonly prescribed for the management of agitation and delirium in adults. They appear to have a superior short-term safety record and possibly offer greater efficacy compared with traditional neuroleptics (Battaglia 2005; Yildiz et al. 2003). Expert opinion increasingly considers atypical antipsychotic medications as first-line agents in the management of agitation for patients with a primary psychiatric disorder such as bipolar disorder or schizophrenia (Allen et al. 2005). A few small, open studies and case reports suggest that the use of antipsychotic medications, particularly risperidone and olanzapine, may offer potential benefits for adults with delirium, but large well-designed studies are yet to be conducted (Boettger and Breitbart 2005). Few case reports document the successful use of risperidone in pediatric delirium (Sipahimalani and Masand 1997), and one case report of delirium in an HIV-infected adolescent found initial treatment with risperidone to be ineffective prior to successful management with haloperidol (Scharko et al. 2006).

Atypical antipsychotics appear to be better tolerated than traditional neuroleptics, at least with regard to short-term use, with lower risks of EPS and tardive dyskinesia in adults. However, their use has been associated with orthostasis, as well as weight gain and prominent metabolic adverse effects when administered chronically. Aripiprazole comes in both liquid and tablets, including a rapidly dissolving preparation, with initial single oral dose being 2.5–10 mg. Olanzapine may be administered orally as a tablet or as a rapidly dissolving tablet, and may also be administered intramuscularly (see below); initial oral dose is generally 2.5–5 mg. Risperidone may be initiated at initial oral doses of 0.25–1 mg and is available in tablets, rapidly dissolving tablets, and liquid form. Ziprasidone is available only as a capsule, with an initial oral dose of 20 mg recommended; an injectable form is also available (see below). Quetiapine is available only in tablet form, with beginning doses ranging from 25 to 100 mg.

The availability of injectable atypical antipsychotics such as olanzapine, ziprasidone, and aripiprazole has raised questions about their role in the acute management of agitation, but there is woefully little research to guide management. It should also be remembered that the necessity of using parenteral medications in agitated and delirious patients has probably been overemphasized. Most agitated patients can be persuaded to take oral medication if the basic principles of crisis management and patient stabilization are properly followed and treated as the foundation of any intervention (Yildiz et al. 2003). A retrospective chart review of intramuscular ziprasidone administered to 49 pediatric psychiatric inpatients for agitation suggested that the drug was effective and well tolerated at a dose of 10–20 mg (all youth under age 14 received 10 mg) without reported adverse events (Staller 2004). Another small case series focusing on three children, ages 12–13 years, who were administered 10 mg of intramuscular ziprasidone for agitation suggested that the drug may be effective, although syncope was reported in one of the cases (Hazaray et al. 2004). Ziprasidone has antihistaminic properties that contribute to its sedative effects. The drug has been associated with orthostatic hypotension, tachycardia, dizziness, and less commonly syncope in adults. Other reported adverse effects include nausea, headache, and dizziness. The biggest apprehension about its use involves prolongation of the QTc, raising at least theoretical concerns about its use in physically ill patients who may be taking a variety of other medications. Intramuscular olanzapine has been associated with hypotension but appears unlikely to prolong the QTc. Olanzapine has some anticholinergic effects that could prove problematic in the management of anticholinergic delirium. Aripiprazole injection, unlike olanzapine, has a low risk for anticholinergic effects; therefore, this drug may prove more suitable in the management of anticholinergic delirium.

As noted, prolongation of the QTc can occur with the traditional antipsychotics (e.g., droperidol, haloperidol, mesoridazine, pimozide, thioridazine), as well as with the atypical agents. It is recommended that electrocardiographic monitoring of the QTc take place, particularly during the treatment of physically ill youth. Although clinical judgment may dictate otherwise in an emergent situation, obtaining an ECG prior to initiating treatment is the ideal in order to identify congenital or preexisting drug-related QTc prolongation. This is particularly critical when antipsychotics are being prescribed in combination with other medications that can increase drug levels (e.g., olanzapine or pimozide with a cytochrome P450 (CYP) 1A2 inhibitor; haloperidol, pimozide, or ziprasidone with a CYP3A4 inhibitor). Standards for QTc monitoring are available elsewhere (Blair et al. 2004; Labellarte et al. 2003).

Benzodiazepines

Benzodiazepines are perhaps the most frequently used agents to provide sedation and management for acutely agitated patients, and they may also be quite useful in the management of delirium, but this practice is lacking a firm evidence base in youth (Witek et al. 2005). Adverse effects include sedation, ataxia, and confusion. The adverse effects of greatest concern in medical settings are respiratory depression and paradoxical disinhibition. Caution should be exercised when there is greater potential for respiratory depression, as with a patient with pulmonary disease or when dealing with alcohol or opiate intoxication. Although concerns that the use of benzodiazepines may result in paradoxical behavioral disinhibition cannot be dismissed on the basis of anecdotal evidence and limited empirical support (Petti et al. 1982), the practical likelihood of disinhibition is probably overstated (Hughes and Kleespies 2003), particularly if one considers the risk of akathisia when administering antipsychotic medications.

Lorazepam appears to be the most commonly used agent in pediatric emergency room settings, probably because of its relatively short half-life, rapid onset of sedative action, lack of active metabolites, and availability of multiple routes of administration (i.e., oral, sublingual, intramuscular, intravenous, and rectal) (Sorrentino 2004). The impact of benzodiazepine administration can sometimes be dramatic, particularly in circumstances such as alcohol withdrawal or catatonia. A recent update of the Expert Consensus Guidelines on the Treatment of Behavioral Emergencies recommends benzodiazepines as the preferred intervention for agitation when there is no provisional diagnosis, when no data are available, or when benzodiazepines may have specific benefits, as in alcohol withdrawal (Allen et al. 2005). Typical initial doses range from 0.5 mg for smaller children and not particularly urgent circumstances to 2 mg for markedly agitated adolescents, with a dosage guideline of 0.05–0.1 mg/kg/dose and an initial maximum of 2 mg per dose (Sorrentino 2004).

Diazepam has also been used in the management of agitation and can be administered orally, parenterally, and rectally, though intramuscular administration is not recommended because of difficulties with absorption. With regard to dose equivalence, 1 mg of lorazepam is generally considered equivalent to 5 mg of diazepam and 0.25 mg of clonazepam (Cummings and Miller 2004). Midazolam is a short-acting benzodiazepine that can be administered orally or parenterally, although its especially short half-life makes it a somewhat less appealing agent for use in the agitated patient.

Benzodiazepines are especially useful in treating the markedly anxious patient in a medical setting, given their apparent efficacy and relative safety.

Even though the use of benzodiazepines in such circumstances is not particularly well established scientifically and their use may prolong recovery time from general anesthesia, the drugs have a solid track record as a means of decreasing anxiety preoperatively and in hospitalized patients, with a side-effect profile that appears to be more favorable than that of agents such as opiates and barbiturates (Witek et al. 2005). In managing the anxious patient, the use of a fixed-dose regimen is generally recommended in order to avoid rebound effects and better manage patients who may be unable to express the need for an anxiolytic (Eisendrath and Shim 2006). Some concern about respiratory depression associated with the use of benzodiazepines is certainly justified, but this risk must be balanced against the potential negative impact of excessive anxiety on the work of breathing in patients with pulmonary disease and who are being weaned from mechanical ventilation. Although traditional antipsychotics are not necessarily free of effects on respiration, atypical agents may be beneficial in the short-term management of anxiety in hospitalized patients. When there is sufficient time to allow for use of medication with a less rapid onset of action, the use of SSRIs or even buspirone may be worth considering, given that they are not associated with the adverse effect of respiratory depression.

In the unusual circumstance of catatonia in children or adolescents—a confusing presentation characterized by motoric immobility and/or excessive, seemingly purposeless motor activity, mutism and/or extreme negativism, echolalia and/or echopraxia, and other peculiarities of voluntary movement—administration of a benzodiazepine may prove both enlightening and potentially lifesaving, with one case report documenting improvements following oral doses of lorazepam as low as 0.5 mg (Pruett and Rizvi 2005). Data about the use of benzodiazepines to manage aggression are limited, with one small study finding some benefits associated with benzodiazepines in managing angry outbursts in youth with conduct disorder (Gleser et al. 1965), but another noting an increase in aggressive behaviors with benzodiazepine use (Petti et al. 1982).

Combination Treatment

Treatment with a combination of a traditional neuroleptic (e.g., haloperidol) and a benzodiazepine (e.g., lorazepam) appears to be superior to use of either agent alone in the management of agitation in adults, and may reduce the likelihood of EPS or akathisia in comparison with antipsychotic medication alone (Yildiz et al. 2003). In a recent survey, experts recommended that haloperidol should almost always be administered along with a benzodiazepine in the agitated patient, except in the most medically compromised patient, but they were less likely to recommend combining benzodiazepines with atypical antipsychotics (Allen et al. 2005). For example, the dangerously combative adolescent with no presumptive diagnosis combined with inadequate information about his or her condition might be aggressively managed acutely with 5 mg of haloperidol and 2 mg of lorazepam. Should intramuscular administration prove necessary, haloperidol and lorazepam are reportedly compatible when drawn up in the same syringe and can be administered together (Sorrentino 2004). However, consultation with the hospital pharmacy is recommended if consideration is given to mixing medications.

Borderline Personality Disorder

Although personality disorders are ubiquitous and not limited to the medical setting, the presence of significant character pathology can be especially disruptive in acute-care medical settings and in the context of a chronic physical condition such as diabetes mellitus. The *Cluster B* personality disorders are characterized by affective instability and impulsivity, with the prototype being borderline personality disorder (BPD). *Borderline personality disorder* refers to a pervasive pattern of instability in interpersonal relationships, affect, and self-image that is associated with potentially self-damaging impulsivity (American Psychiatric Association 2000). Common characteristics include marked affective instability; unstable interpersonal relationships; attachment issues resulting in frantic efforts to avoid a subjective sense of abandonment; identity disturbance; reckless behaviors; recurrent suicidal thinking or behavior; self-mutilation; chronic feelings of emptiness; periods of intense, inappropriate anger; and a tendency to develop paranoid ideation or dissociative symptoms during stressful life circumstances. Patients with BPD are particularly vulnerable in medical settings, not only with regard to the various threats and stressors presented by physical illness and its demands, but also with regard to the opportunity to use physical illness in a care-eliciting fashion, much as direct threats of self-harm or self-injurious behavior may mobilize those in proximity to the patient.

A comprehensive discussion of the management of BPD in hospitalized youth is beyond our scope, but it is worth noting that although the evidence base is limited, experience with adults suggests that affected youth may benefit from the use of a variety of psychopharmacological agents that target affective instability, impulsivity, and impulsive aggression (McClellan and Hamilton 2006). Medications such as the antidepressants, particularly SSRIs and non-TCAs such as the MAOIs, have been found to reduce patient ratings of anger and hostility (Binks et al. 2006). However, the use of MAOIs poses special challenges in this population, given that the need for dietary compliance may prove difficult for a patient with BPD. Because affective instability appears to be core to the disorder, interventions useful in bipolar disorder have been proposed and studied, with a review of available studies in adults suggesting that anticonvulsants such as divalproex and lamotrigine may have a stabilizing effect. (MacKinnon and Pies 2006). A reduction in impulsive aggression has also been reported with divalproex (Hollander et al. 2005) and topiramate (Nickel et al. 2004), and a recent review suggests that both anticonvulsants and antidepressants show weak evidence of efficacy in the ongoing management of aggressive behavior in adults (Goedhard et al. 2006).

In addition to the modest and less-than-conclusive results reported with antidepressants and anticonvulsants in BPD, perhaps the greatest limitation of these agents is their relatively slow onset of action. When a relatively rapid and enduring response is required in treating the youthful patient with a Cluster B personality disorder or traits, the most credible option appears to be the use of antipsychotic medication, primarily the atypical antipsychotics. Randomized, placebo-controlled trials in adults with BPD have demonstrated efficacy for olanzapine (Soler et al. 2005) and aripiprazole (Nickel et al. 2006), and the results of an open trial suggest that quetiapine may be a promising treatment for associated impulsivity as well (Villeneuve and Lemelin 2005). Atypical antipsychotics are currently the most commonly prescribed medications for the management of maladaptive aggression in children and adolescents, with risperidone being the best-studied drug for the ongoing management of aggressive youth (Findling et al. 2005). Studies conducted with adult subjects suggest efficacy for antipsychotics in the management of aggressive behavior, with atypical agents generally performing better than the traditional antipsychotics (Goedhard et al. 2006). Longer-term adverse effects associated with atypical antipsychotics include weight gain, hyperlipidemia, hyperglycemia, and hyperprolactinemia, and many of these adverse effects may create special challenges for patients with specific physical disorders such as preexisting diabetes mellitus or obesity.

General Medical Conditions and Organ Failure

Chronic physical disease is increasingly common in childhood, with approximately 1%–3% of youth experiencing significant functional impairment associated with a chronic physical health condition (Gortmaker et al. 1990). Not only does the presence of physical disease increase the risk of associated psychiatric problems and disorders (Dew 1998; Gortmaker et al. 1990; Rutter et al. 1970), but comorbid psychiatric disorders can also negatively impact the course of physical disease. For example, youth with diabetes mellitus are at elevated risk of developing psychiatric disorders (Kovacs et al. 1997), and comorbid depression increases the risk of treatment nonadherence, repeat hospitalization (Garrison et al. 2005), and development of specific disease-related complications such as diabetic retinopathy (Kovacs et al. 1995).

Psychiatric disorder may impact physical health in a variety of ways. First, it can negatively impact patient adherence to the prescribed treatment regimen and interfere with living a healthy lifestyle. Depression in adults with physical disease apparently increases medical nonadherence by a factor of three, and is associated with poor health outcomes (DiMatteo et al. 2000). Second, psychiatric disorders may have a negative impact on the disease process itself, as with diabetes, in which psychiatric disorder may negatively impact metabolic control (Dantzer et al. 2003), or with asthma, in which anxiety, with associated hyperventilation and emotional arousal, may facilitate bronchoconstriction in vulnerable individuals (Smoller et al. 1999). If so, it follows that aggressive management of comorbid psychiatric disorder in the physically ill could potentially improve physical health status.

The approach outlined here is addressed in greater detail elsewhere (Campo and Perel 2002) and should not be mistaken to be comprehensive, since the potential for specific drug-disease and drug-drug interactions is enormous. The risks associated with the use of psychoactive drugs in the physically ill child are poorly understood, and the thoughtful clinician is reminded that the *absence of evidence* should not be misconstrued as *evidence of absence*. Individual clinicians are cautioned about the need to individualize treatment, to carefully consult prescribing information for each agent considered for use, and to search the medical literature accordingly. A working diagnostic formulation and the delineation of clear target symptoms are critical prior to initiating treatment. Education of patients and families is no less important when dealing with the physically ill, and is likely more so. The psychiatric diagnostic workup should be reviewed in the context of the child's overall health status, with the goal being the truly shared decision-making that can only follow meaningful informed consent.

Details of the medication under consideration should be reviewed, including potential adverse effects, drug interactions, dosing, time to effect, need for monitoring, and uncertainties. Relevant considerations in selecting a psychoactive medication have been sensibly outlined by Preskorn (1999) and include safety, efficacy, tolerability, cost, and simplicity of administration. Because the pharmacodynamic effects of a given medication may be multiple, physically ill youth may be at special risk for adverse effects due to potential impact on the existing disease process. Moreover, they are at greater risk for drug-drug interactions, which can be pharmacodynamic (e.g., serotonin syndrome) and/or pharmacokinetic in nature, with the potential impact of such interactions increasing if at least one of the drugs in question has a low or narrow therapeutic index. Although pharmacokinetic interactions between drugs can impact all aspects of drug handling, including absorption, distribution, biotransformation, and excretion, the most common drug-drug interactions relevant to pediatric psychopharmacology are related to the biotransformation of highly lipid soluble compounds by the CYP enzyme system. Adverse drug interactions have been associated with considerable morbidity, increased lengths of hospital stay, higher costs, and mortality (Classen et al. 1997), making it critical to determine and document all the prescription and nonprescription medications, contraceptive agents, and herbal or natural remedies being taken.

Physical disease and organ failure can interfere with drug absorption, distribution, metabolism, and elimination and are important considerations in choosing and managing psychoactive medications. A physical condition can also influence a variety of different aspects of drug handling. Although organ failure need not be a contraindication for the use of most psychoactive medications, their use in the seriously ill patient requires careful monitoring and a willingness to modify drug dose or administration schedule.

Cardiovascular Disease

Cardiovascular disease can create significant challenges for the psychopharmacologist, and it is critical to attend to possible cardiovascular effects of psychoactive medications in patients with preexisting disease. Congestive heart failure can reduce drug clearance by reducing renal or hepatic perfusion, and volume of distribution may increase in association with retained fluid (Rubey and Lydiard 1999). Cardiac conduction abnormalities may be especially problematic, as in congenital prolongation of the QTc, which could increase the risk of sudden death when using drugs that can prolong the QTc. This is an important consideration with the use of both traditional and atypical antipsychotics, which have been associated with lengthening of the QTc and the development of multifocal ventricular tachycardia (i.e., torsades de pointes), with the potential to progress to ventricular fibrillation and sudden death. Because the antipsychotic pimozide may inhibit cardiac conduction via calcium channel blockade, it should not be used in combination with other calcium channel blockers such as nifedipine (Alpert et al. 1997). Antipsychotics with anticholinergic, antihistaminic, and α-adrenergic blocking effects, such as chlorpromazine, thioridazine, and clozapine, have also been associated with hypotension and tachycardia. TCAs in therapeutic doses can have significant cardiac effects, including on conduction (e.g., class I antiarrhythmic effects), and can increase heart rate and blood pressure, as well as add to the risk of conduction abnormalities and sudden death; these drugs can also prove especially deadly in overdose (Geller et al. 1999). Despite being generally considered benign from a cardiovascular perspective, the SSRIs have been associated with a modest slowing of heart rate, with rare reports of sinus bradycardia in adults (Settle 1998). Other antidepressants such as venlafaxine and bupropion may be associated with increases in blood pressure, but these effects have not been especially well studied in youth (Glassman 1998). Alpha-adrenergic agonists such as clonidine can decrease systolic blood pressure, heart rate, and cardiac output, and arrhythmias and sudden death have been reported in association with its use (Cantwell et al. 1997). Conduction abnormalities have also been associated with the use of lithium (Dunner 2000). Psychopharmacological agents with cardiovascular effects should thus be used cautiously in the physically ill and monitored closely, both clinically and electrocardiographically.

Pulmonary Disease

Pulmonary disease and respiratory disorders can also affect the way that psychoactive drugs are handled by the body. Hypoxia and hypercarbia can have an impact on the pharmacokinetics of psychoactive medications, primarily via changes in serum pH (Rubey and Lydiard 1999). Anxiety is common in the face of pulmonary disease and respiratory failure. Benzodiazepines can be a rapid and effective treatment for acute anxiety, but their potential for respiratory depression and associated hypercarbia in the patient with pulmonary disease creates a dilemma for the clinician dealing with an anxious patient who has pulmonary disease. The consequent reduction in anxiety may decrease symptoms, calm the patient, and prove beneficial in helping the mechanically ventilated patient wean from the ventilator; yet balancing the potential risks and benefits can be difficult. The drugs appear to be most dangerous at higher doses, when administered parenterally, or when given in combination with drugs such as opiates that can also depress respiratory drive, but safe use of the benzodiazepines does appear to be possible in patients with pulmonary disease (Smoller et al. 1999). It is nevertheless important to be aware that epidemiological studies report an increased risk of death for asthmatic patients prescribed antipsychotics and other sedatives, which raises concerns about the potential for negative effects on respiration and pulmonary function (Joseph 1997). Lorazepam may be preferable to diazepam, because it possibly has a lower tendency to induce respiratory depression (Denault et al. 1975). For chronic management of anxiety in patients with pulmonary disease, the SSRIs and the anxiolytic nonbenzodiazepine buspirone may be worth careful consideration, given that respiratory depression has not been associated with their use (Craven and Sutherland 1991; Rubey and Lydiard 1999). Cystic fibrosis is a systemic disease with prominent pulmonary manifestations. Affected youth have a genetic defect that may be associated with abnormalities of the ion channels involved in electrolyte transport, suggesting that patience and some degree of caution are warranted in dosing lithium in youth with cystic fibrosis (Brager et al. 1996). It should also be noted that psychotropic drugs with anticholinergic effects can reduce bronchial secretions and may potentially exacerbate underlying pulmonary disease.

Gastrointestinal Disease

Gastrointestinal disease that affects mucosal integrity or gut motility can alter drug absorption (Leipzig 1990). Particularly, delays in gastric emptying can impact drug absorption, given that most psychoactive drugs are weak bases, and absorption may be limited until the acidic stomach contents are emptied into the more alkaline small intestine. On the other hand, increases in intestinal motility as seen in diarrheal illnesses can effectively limit the absorption of other drugs such as lithium. The volume of distribution for a drug can be affected by changes in nutritional status and protein binding, as well as by the patient's fluid balance. For example, dehydration can reduce a drug's volume of distribution (e.g., lithium), whereas edematous states (e.g., congestive heart failure, ascites) can increase the volume of distribution for water-soluble or protein-bound drugs (Rubey and Lydiard 1999).

Liver Disease

Liver disease and hepatic failure present special challenges because most psychoactive drugs, with the notable exceptions of lithium and gabapentin, are lipophilic and thus require biotransformation in the liver to convert to more water-soluble compounds capable of excretion. Drug metabolism in the liver can be affected by parenchymal loss, changes in enzyme induction or inhibition, and changes in blood flow. Hepatic failure and portal hypertension can lead to reduced first-pass extraction and biotransformation of psychoactive drugs, resulting in potentially higher drug plasma levels after oral administration and increasing the risk of adverse drug effects and toxicity, particularly for drugs with a low or narrow therapeutic index. Because of reduced protein synthetic capabilities, liver disease can decrease the volume of distribution for highly protein-bound drugs, such as most of the antidepressants, some benzodiazepines, and haloperidol, thus increasing the risk for toxicity despite otherwise normal-appearing plasma levels. Medications with the potential for hepatoxicity such as carbamazepine, chlorpromazine, divalproex/valproate, nefazodone, and pemoline should be avoided if the patient has existing liver disease. Despite a scarcity of systematic research in this area, dose reductions are usually in order when prescribing psychoactive medications to patients with hepatic failure, beginning with a 25%–50% reduction from the typical dose and then titrating clinically (Campo and Perel 2002; Rubey and Lydiard 1999).

Kidney Disease

Kidney disease and renal failure present fewer problems for the psychophar-macologist than hepatic disease in general, most notably because renal elimi-nation is critical for only a handful of psychoactive drugs (e.g., lithium). However, because most psychoactive drugs and their metabolites have not been adequately evaluated in renal failure, a thoughtful, individualized ap-proach to each patient is recommended. In general, mild-to-moderate renal impairment does not require dosage or schedule adjustments. Lithium is the most notable exception because it is excreted essentially unchanged in the urine; it is readily dialyzable due to its small molecular size. Consequently, it can be administered as a single dose immediately after dialysis in patients with renal failure, though careful monitoring of blood level is required. Because most psychoactive drugs are primarily dependent on hepatic metabolism, dosage adjustments are usually unnecessary in the presence of mild-to-mod-erate impairments in renal function, but it must be remembered that clini-cally significant metabolites of specific psychoactive agents may accumulate in end-stage renal disease. In such circumstances, increases in administration interval and possible dose reduction should be contemplated. Drugs that can be affected by changes in renal function include clonidine, many of the TCAs and benzodiazepines and their metabolites, paroxetine, and venlafaxine, so care must be exercised in the face of renal failure and dosage adjustments may be necessary (Campo and Perel 2002; Rubey and Lydiard 1999). Drug vol-ume of distribution can also be affected by associated edema and hypoalbu-minemia in renal failure.

Neurological Disorders

Neurological disorders such as epilepsy are common conditions associated with exceptionally high rates of comorbid psychiatric disorder, particularly mood disorders. This comorbidity is likely a consequence of both the disease and its treatment, considering that several anticonvulsants, particularly the barbiturates, have been associated with depression, suicidal ideation, overac-tivity, and disruptive behaviors (Brent et al. 1987; Campo and Perel 2002). Given the high rates of psychiatric disorders in patients with epilepsy, it is im-portant to realize that many psychoactive drugs can lower seizure threshold, especially the antidepressants bupropion and clomipramine, the antipsychotic clozapine, and the mood stabilizer lithium (Alldredge 1999). The use of stimulants in epileptic children with ADHD has generated concerns about lowering seizure threshold, particularly when these drugs are prescribed at higher doses. However, clinical experience suggests that treatment with methylphenidate at typical doses is generally both safe and effective, especially if the child is seizure-free at the time the stimulant is initiated (Gross-Tsur et al. 1997). Clonidine has also been associated with seizures in overdose and can lower seizure threshold as well, but it has been used at therapeutic doses without prominent difficulties (Thiele et al. 1999). Using the lowest possible dose of psychoactive medication is recommended in pediatric epilepsy, given that drug-induced seizures are generally dose-related. A few reports suggest that active treatment of comorbid psychiatric disorders in patients with epilepsy may improve seizure control (Dailey and Naritoku 1996). Results of animal experiments suggest that antipsychotic medications may delay neuronal recovery after traumatic brain injury, whereas stimulant treatment might facilitate recovery (Feeney et al. 1982).

Diabetes Mellitus

Diabetes mellitus has been associated with high rates of psychiatric disorders, particularly emotional disorders (Kovacs et al. 1997), which can negatively impact treatment adherence and the pathophysiology of the disease process (Garrison et al. 2005). These findings suggest that active treatment could potentially improve physical health outcomes. Treatment of depressed diabetic adults with SSRIs (Carney 1998) and alprazolam (Lustman et al. 1995) has been associated with improved glycemic control. SSRIs may reduce glucose levels in diabetic persons independent of insulin level, and may be associated with some risk of hypoglycemia initially. Of special note is the fact that atypical antipsychotics such as clozapine and olanzapine have been associated with increased appetite, weight gain, and the deterioration of glycemic control in diabetic patients, which suggests that clinicians should exercise caution in their use (Wirshing et al. 1998). Because youth with diabetes may be at increased risk for tardive dyskinesia when treated with traditional neuroleptics, treatment decisions may be somewhat constrained and require considerable clinical judgment (Ganzini et al. 1991).

Clinical Pearls

- Clinicians should entertain the hypothesis that any given patient's psychiatric presentation could be due to an unrecognized general medical condition.

- Because pediatric psychopharmacology trials have not included youth with physical disorders, practice must be guided by accumulated clinical experience.

- Antidepressant medications are worthy of additional study as treatments for pediatric somatoform and functional somatic disorders.

- Antidepressant medications are generally not helpful in anorexia nervosa until nutritional stabilization has been accomplished.

- The prescription of medication for the management of pediatric insomnia is widespread, but sound safety and efficacy data are lacking.

- The single most effective, safe, and durable treatment for enuresis is behavioral intervention using the enuresis alarm, not medication.

- Though research is lacking, benzodiazepines and antipsychotics, alone or in combination, are commonly used to manage pediatric agitation.

- Physically ill youth are at heightened risk for both pharmacodynamic and pharmacokinetic adverse effects from psychoactive medications.

References

Abu-Arafeh I, Russell G: Prevalence and clinical features of abdominal migraine compared with those of migraine headache. Arch Dis Child 72:413–417, 1995

Alldredge BK: Seizure risk associated with psychotropic drugs: clinical and pharmacokinetic considerations. Neurology 53(5, suppl 2):S68–S75, 1999

Allen MH, Currier GW, Carpenter D, et al: The expert consensus guideline series. Treatment of behavioral emergencies 2005. J Psychiatr Pract 11(suppl):5–108, 2005

Alpert JE, Bernstein JG, Rosenbaum JF: Psychopharmacologic issues in medical settings, in Massachusetts General Hospital Handbook of General Hospital Psychiatry. St. Louis, Mosby, 1997, pp 249–303

American Psychiatric Association: Diagnostic and Statistical Manual of Mental Disorders, 4th Edition, Text Revision. Washington, DC, American Psychiatric Association, 2000

American Psychiatric Association: Treatment of patients with eating disorders, third edition. Am J Psychiatry 163(suppl):4–54, 2006

Appolinario JC, Bacaltchuk J, Sichieri R, et al: A randomized, double-blind, placebo-controlled study of sibutramine in the treatment of binge-eating disorder. Arch Gen Psychiatry 60:1109–1116, 2003

Attia E, Schroeder L: Pharmacologic treatment of anorexia nervosa: where do we go from here? Int J Eat Disord 37(suppl):S60–S63, 2005

Barbarich NC, McConaha CW, Gaskill J, et al: An open trial of olanzapine in anorexia nervosa. J Clin Psychiatry 65:1480–1482, 2004

Basbaum AI, Jesell TM: The perception of pain, in Principles of Neural Science, 4th Edition. Edited by Kandel ER, Schwartz JH, Jesell TM. New York, McGraw-Hill, 2000, pp 472–491

Battaglia J: Pharmacological management of acute agitation. Drugs 65:1207–1222, 2005

Battistella P, Ruffilli R, Cernetti R, et al: A placebo controlled crossover trial using trazodone in pediatric migraine. Headache 33:36–39, 1993

Berkowitz RI, Fujioka K, Daniels SR, et al: Effects of sibutramine treatment in obese adolescents: a randomized trial. Ann Intern Med 145:81–90, 2006

Bernstein G, Shaw K: Practice parameters for the assessment and treatment of children and adolescents with anxiety disorders. J Am Acad Child Adolesc Psychiatry 36(suppl):69S–84S, 1997

Binks CA, Fenton M, McCarthy L, et al: Pharmacological interventions for people with borderline personality disorder. Cochrane Database Syst Rev (1):CD005653, 2006

Birmaher B, Ryan N, Williamson D, et al: Childhood and adolescent depression: a review of the past 10 years, part I. J Am Acad Child Adolesc Psychiatry 35:1427–1439, 1996

Blair J, Taggart B, Martin A: Electrocardiographic safety profile and monitoring guidelines in pediatric psychopharmacology. J Neural Transm 111:791–815, 2004

Boettger S, Breitbart W: Atypical antipsychotics in the management of delirium: a review of the empirical literature. Palliat Support Care 3:227–237, 2005

Brager NP, Campbell NR, Reisch H, et al: Reduced renal fractional excretion of lithium in cystic fibrosis. Br J Clin Pharmacol 41:157–159, 1996

Brannan SK, Mallinckrodt CH, Brown EB, et al: Duloxetine 60 mg once-daily in the treatment of painful physical symptoms in patients with major depressive disorder. J Psychiatr Res 39:43–53, 2005

Brent DA, Crumrine PK, Varma RR, et al: Phenobarbital treatment and major depressive disorder in children with epilepsy. Pediatrics 80:909–917, 1987

Brown RL, Henke A, Greenhalgh DG, et al: The use of haloperidol in the agitated, critically ill pediatric patient with burns. J Burn Care Rehabil 17:34–38, 1996

Bullock GL, Schall U: Dyssomnia in children diagnosed with attention deficit hyperactivity disorder: a critical review. Aust N Z J Psychiatry 39:373–377, 2005

Buscemi N, Vandermeer B, Hooton N, et al: Efficacy and safety of exogenous melatonin for secondary sleep disorders and sleep disorders accompanying sleep restriction: meta-analysis. BMJ 332:385–393, 2006

Camilleri M: Serotonergic modulation of visceral sensation: lower gut. Gut 51(suppl):i81–i86, 2002

Campo JV: Medical issues in the care of child and adolescent inpatients, in Handbook of Behavior Therapy in the Psychiatric Setting. Edited by Bellack AS, Hersen M. New York, Plenum, 1993, pp 373–406

Campo JV: Coping with ignorance: exploring pharmacologic management of pediatric functional abdominal pain. J Pediatr Gastroenterol Nutr 41:569–574, 2005

Campo J, Fritsch S: Somatization in children and adolescents. J Am Acad Child Adolesc Psychiatry 33:1223–1235, 1994

Campo J, Fritz G: A management model for pediatric somatization. Psychosomatics 42:467–476, 2001

Campo JV, Fritz GK: Somatoform disorders, in Lewis's Child and Adolescent Psychiatry: A Comprehensive Textbook, 4th Edition. Edited by Martin A, Volkmar FR, Lewis M. Baltimore, MD, Lippincott Williams & Wilkins, 2007, 633–647

Campo JV, Perel JM: Pediatric psychopharmacology in the consultation-liaison setting, in Pharmacotherapy for Child and Adolescent Psychiatric Disorders, 2nd Edition, Revised and Expanded. Edited by Rosenberg D, Davanzo PA, Gershon S. New York, Marcel Dekker, 2002, pp 635–678

Campo JV, Comer D, Jansen-McWilliams L, et al: Recurrent pain, emotional distress, and health service use in childhood. J Pediatr 141:76–83, 2002

Campo JV, Bridge J, Ehmann M, et al: Recurrent abdominal pain, anxiety, and depression in primary care. Pediatrics 113:817–824, 2004a

Campo JV, Perel J, Lucas A, et al: Citalopram treatment of pediatric recurrent abdominal pain and comorbid internalizing disorders: an exploratory study. J Am Acad Child Adolesc Psychiatry 43:1234–1242, 2004b

Cantwell DP, Swanson J, Connor DF: Case study: adverse response to clonidine. J Am Acad Child Adolesc Psychiatry 36:539–544, 1997

Carney C: Diabetes mellitus and major depressive disorder: an overview of prevalence, complication, and treatment. Depress Anxiety 7:149–157, 1998

Carter WP, Hudson JI, Lalonde JK, et al: Pharmacologic treatment of binge eating disorder. Int J Eat Disord 34(suppl):S74–S88, 2003

Cassano GB, Miniati M, Pini S, et al: Six-month open trial of haloperidol as an adjunctive treatment for anorexia nervosa: a preliminary report. Int J Eat Disord 33:172–177, 2003

Classen DC, Pestotnik SL, Evans RS, et al: Adverse drug events in hospitalized patients. JAMA 277:301–306, 1997

Craven J, Sutherland A: Buspirone for anxiety disorders in patients with severe lung disease. Lancet 338:249, 1991

Cummings MR, Miller BD: Pharmacologic management of behavioral instability in medically ill pediatric patients. Curr Opin Pediatr 16:516–522, 2004

Dailey JW, Naritoku DK: Antidepressants and seizures: clinical anecdotes overshadow neuroscience. Biochem Pharmacol 1323–1329, 1996

Dantzer C, Swendsen J, Maurice-Tison S, et al: Anxiety and depression in juvenile diabetes: a critical review. Clin Psychol Rev 23:787–800, 2003

Daviss WB, Scott J: A chart review of cyproheptadine for stimulant induced weight loss. J Child Adolesc Psychopharmacol 14:65–73, 2004

Denault M, Yernault JC, Coster AD: Double blind comparison of the respiratory effects of parenteral lorazepam and diazepam in patients with chronic obstructive lung disease. Curr Med Res Opin 2:611–615, 1975

Dew MA: Psychiatric disorder in the context of physical illness, in Adversity, Stress, and Psychopathology. Edited by Dohrenwend BP. New York, Oxford University Press, 1998, pp 177–218

DiLorenzo C, Youssef N, Sigurdsson L, et al: Visceral hyperalgesia in children with functional abdominal pain. J Pediatr 139:838–843, 2001

DiMatteo MR, Lepper HS, Croghan TW: Depression is a risk factor for noncompliance with medical treatment: meta-analysis of the effects of anxiety and depression on patient adherence. Arch Intern Med 160:2101–2107, 2000

Drossman DA, Toner BB, Whitehead WE, et al: Cognitive-behavioral therapy versus education and desipramine versus placebo for moderate to severe functional bowel disorders. Gastroenterology 125:19–31, 2003

Dunner DL: Optimizing lithium treatment. J Clin Psychiatry 61(suppl):S76–S81, 2000

Ebeling H, Tapanainen P, Joutsenoja A, et al: A practice guideline for treatment of eating disorders in children and adolescents. Ann Med 35:488–501, 2003

Egger H, Costello E, Erkanli A, et al: Somatic complaints and psychopathology in children and adolescents: stomach aches, musculoskeletal pains and headaches. J Am Acad Child Adolesc Psychiatry 38:852–860, 1999

Eisendrath SJ, Shim JJ: Management of psychiatric problems in critically ill patients. Am J Med 119:22–29, 2006

El-Khatib H, Dickey T: Sertraline for body dysmorphic disorder. J Am Acad Child Adolesc Psychiatry 27:251–260, 1995

Fallon B: Pharmacotherapy of somatoform disorders. J Psychosom Res 56:455–460, 2004

Feeney DM, Gonzalez A, Law WA: Amphetamine, haloperidol, and experience interact to affect rate of recovery after motor cortex injury. Science 217:855–857, 1982

Fichter M, Kruger R, Rief W, et al: Fluvoxamine in prevention of relapse in bulimia nervosa: effects on eating-specific psychopathology. J Clin Psychopharmacol 16:9–18, 1996

Findling RL, Steiner H, Weller EB: Use of antipsychotics in children and adolescents. J Clin Psychiatry 66(suppl):29–40, 2005

Fishbain DA, Cutler RB, Rosomoff HL, et al: Do antidepressants have an analgesic effect in psychogenic pain and somatoform pain disorder? A meta-analysis. Psychosom Med 60:503–509, 1998

Fritz G, Rockney R, Work Group on Quality Issues: Practice parameter for the assessment and treatment of children and adolescent with enuresis. J Am Acad Child Adolesc Psychiatry 43:1540–1550, 2004

Ganzini L, Heintz RT, Hoffman WF, et al: The prevalence of tardive dyskinesia in neuroleptic treated diabetics: a controlled study. Arch Gen Psychiatry 48:259–263, 1991

Garber J, Walker L, Zeman J: Somatization symptoms in a community sample of children and adolescents: further validation of the Children's Somatization Inventory. Psychol Assess 3:588–595, 1991

Garralda ME, Chalder T: Practitioner review: chronic fatigue syndrome in childhood. J Child Psychol Psychiatry 46:1143–1151, 2005

Garrison MM, Katon WJ, Richardson LP: The impact of psychiatric comorbidities on readmissions for diabetes in youth. Diabetes Care 28:2150–2154, 2005

Geller B, Reising D, Leonard HL, et al: Critical review of tricyclic antidepressant use in children and adolescents. J Am Acad Child Adolesc Psychiatry 38:513–516, 1999

Glassman AH: Adverse cardiovascular effects of antidepressants. J Clin Psychiatry 59(suppl):13–18, 1998

Glazener CM, Evans RE, Peto JH: Effects of interventions for the treatment of nocturnal enuresis in children. Qual Saf Health Care 12:390–394, 2003

Gleser GC, Gottschalk LA, Fox R, et al: Immediate changes in affect with chlordiazepoxide: chlordiazepoxide administration in juvenile delinquent boys. Arch Gen Psychiatry 13:291–295, 1965

Goedhard LE, Stolker JJ, Heerdink ER, et al: Pharmacotherapy for the treatment of aggressive behavior in general adult psychiatry: a systematic review. J Clin Psychiatry 67:1013–1024, 2006

Gortmaker SL, Walker DK, Weitzman M, et al: Chronic conditions, socioeconomic risks, and behavioral problems in children and adolescents. Pediatrics 85:267–276, 1990

Gross-Tsur V, Manor O, van der Meere J, et al: Epilepsy and attention deficit hyperactivity disorder: is methylphenidate safe and effective? J Pediatr 130:40–44, 1997

Gupta M, Aneja S, Kohli K: Add-on melatonin improves sleep behavior in children with epilepsy: randomized, double-blind, placebo-controlled trial. J Child Neurol 20:112–115, 2005

Harmon RJ, Riggs PD: Clonidine for posttraumatic stress disorder in preschool children. J Am Acad Child Adolesc Psychiatry 35:1247–1249, 1996

Hazaray E, Ehret J, Posey DJ, et al: Intramuscular ziprasidone for acute agitation in adolescents. J Child Adolesc Psychopharmacol 14(3):464–470, 2004

Hershey A, Powers S, Vockell A, et al: Effectiveness of topiramate in the prevention of childhood headaches. Headache 42:810–818, 2002

Herxheimer A, Petrie KJ: Melatonin for the prevention and treatment of jet lag. Cochrane Database Syst Rev (2):CD001520, 2002

Hollander E, Allen A, Kwon J, et al: Clomipramine vs. desipramine crossover trial in body dysmorphic disorder: selective efficacy of a serotonin reuptake inhibitor in imagined ugliness. Arch Gen Psychiatry 56:1033–1039, 1999

Hollander E, Swann AC, Coccaro EF, et al: Impact of trait impulsivity and state aggression on divalproex versus placebo response in borderline personality disorder. Am J Psychiatry 162:621–624, 2005

Hoopes SP, Reimherr FW, Hedges DW, et al: Treatment of bulimia nervosa with topiramate in a randomized, double-blind, placebo-controlled trial, part 1: improvement in binge and purge measures. J Clin Psychiatry 64:1335–1341, 2003

Horne RL, Ferguson JM, Pope HG Jr, et al: Treatment of bulimia with bupropion: a multicenter controlled trial. J Clin Psychiatry 49:262–266, 1988

Horrigan JP: Guanfacine for PTSD nightmares. J Am Acad Child Adolesc Psychiatry 35:975–976, 1996

Hughes DF, Kleespies PM: Treating aggression in the psychiatric emergency service. J Clin Psychiatry 64(suppl):10–15, 2003

Hyams JS, Hyman PE: Recurrent abdominal pain and the biopsychosocial model of medical practice. J Pediatr 133:473–478, 1998

Ingrassia A, Turk J: The use of clonidine for severe and intractable sleep problems in children with neurodevelopmental disorders: a case series. Eur Child Adolesc Psychiatry 14:34–40, 2005

Ivanenko A, Crabtree VM, Tauman R, et al: Melatonin in children and adolescents with insomnia: a retrospective study. Clin Pediatr 42:51–58, 2003

Jackson T, Ditmanson L, Phibbs B: Torsades de pointes and low dose oral haloperidol. Arch Intern Med 157:2013–2015, 1997

Jailwala J, Imperiale T, Kroenke K: Pharmacologic treatment of the irritable bowel syndrome: a systematic review of randomized, controlled trials. Ann Intern Med 133:136–147, 2000

Jan JE, Freeman RD, Fast DK: Melatonin treatment of sleep-wake cycle disorders in children and adolescents. Dev Med Child Neurol 41:491–500, 1999

Joseph KS: Asthma mortality and antipsychotic or sedative use: What is the link? Drug Saf 16:351–354, 1997

Kabbouche M, Vockell A, LeCates S, et al: Tolerability and effectiveness of prochlorperazine for intractable migraine in children. Pediatrics 107:E62, 2001

Kaye WH, Nagata N, Weltzin TE, et al: Double-blind placebo-controlled administration of fluoxetine in restricting- and restricting-purging-type anorexia nervosa. Biol Psychiatry 49:644–652, 2001

Klein-Schwartz W: Trends and toxic effects from pediatric clonidine exposures. Arch Pediatr Adolesc Med 156:392–396, 2002

Kovacs M, Mukerji P, Drash A, et al: Biomedical and psychiatric risk factors for retinopathy among children with IDDM. Diabetes Care 18:1592–1599, 1995

Kovacs M, Goldston D, Obrosky DS, et al: Psychiatric disorders in youths with IDDM: rates and risk factors. Diabetes Care 20:36–44, 1997

Kroenke K, Messina N III, Benattia I, et al: Venlafaxine extended release in the short-term treatment of depressed and anxious primary care patients with multisomatoform disorder. J Clin Psychiatry 67:72–80, 2006

Labellarte MJ, Crosson JE, Riddle MA : Relevance of prolonged QTc measurement to pediatric psychopharmacology. J Am Acad Child Adolesc Psychiatry 42:642–650, 2003

Leipzig RM: Psychopharmacology in patients with hepatic and gastrointestinal disease. Int J Psychiatry Med 20:109–139, 1990

Lewis D, Ashwal S, Hershey A, et al: Practice parameter: pharmacological treatment of migraine headache in children and adolescents. Report of the American Academy of Neurology Quality Standards Subcommittee and the Practice Committee of the Child Neurology Society. Neurology 63:2215–2224, 2004

Liakopoulou-Kairis M, Alifieraki T, Protagora D, et al: Recurrent abdominal pain and headache: psychopathology, life event and family functioning. Eur Child Adolesc Psychiatry 11:115–122, 2002

Lipton R, Bigal M, Steiner T, et al: Classification of primary headaches. Neurology 63:427–435, 2004

Lustman PJ, Griffith LS, Clouse RE: Effects of alprazolam on glucose regulation in diabetes: results of a double blind placebo controlled trial. Diabetes Care 18:1133–1139, 1995

MacKinnon DF, Pies R: Affective instability as rapid cycling: theoretical and clinical implications for borderline personality and bipolar spectrum disorders. Bipolar Disord 8:1–16, 2006

Martini DR: Commentary: the diagnosis of delirium in pediatric patients. J Am Acad Child Adolesc Psychiatry 395–398, 2005

McClellan JM, Hamilton JD: An evidence-based approach to an adolescent with emotional and behavioral dysregulation. J Am Acad Child Adolesc Psychiatry 45:489–493, 2006

McElroy SL, Arnold LM, Shapira NA, et al: Topiramate in the treatment of binge eating disorder associated with obesity: a randomized, placebo-controlled trial. Am J Psychiatry 160:255–261, 2003

Menza MA, Murray GB, Holmes VF: Controlled study of extrapyramidal reaction in the management of delirious medically ill patients: intravenous haloperidol versus intravenous haloperidol plus benzodiazepines. Heart Lung 17:238–241, 1988

Mikkelsen EJ: Enuresis and encopresis: ten years of progress. J Am Acad Child Adolesc Psychiatry 40:1146–1158, 2001

Mindell JA: Sleep disorders in children. Health Psychol 12:151–162, 1993

Mindell JA, Emslie G, Blumer J, et al: Pharmacologic management of insomnia in children and adolescents: consensus statement. Pediatrics 117:e1223–e1232, 2006

Modi S, Lowder DM: Medications for migraine prophylaxis. Am Fam Physician 73:72–78, 2006

Muller T, Mannel M, Murck H, et al: Treatment of somatoform disorders with St John's wort: a randomized, double-blind and placebo-controlled trial. Psychosom Med 66:538–547, 2004

Nickel MK, Nickel C, Mitterlehner FO, et al: Topiramate treatment of aggression in female borderline personality disorder patients: a double-blind, placebo-controlled study. J Clin Psychiatry 65:1515–1519, 2004

Nickel MK, Muehlbacher M, Nickel C, et al: Aripiprazole in the treatment of patients with borderline personality disorder: a double-blind, placebo-controlled study. Am J Psychiatry 163:833–838, 2006

O'Malley PG, Jackson JL, Santoro J, et al: Antidepressant therapy for unexplained symptoms and symptom syndromes. J Fam Pract 48:980–990, 1999

Owens JA, Rosen CL, Mindell JA: Medication use in the treatment of pediatric insomnia: results of a survey of community based pediatricians. Pediatrics 111:e628–e635, 2003

Petti TA, Fish B, Shapiro T, et al: Effects of chlordiazepoxide in disturbed children: a pilot study. J Clin Psychopharmacol 2:270–273, 1982

Phillips K, Albertini R, Rasmussen S: A randomized placebo-controlled trial of fluoxetine in body dysmorphic disorder. Arch Gen Psychiatry 59:381–388, 2002

Phillips L, Appleton L: Systematic review of melatonin treatment in children with neurodevelopmental disabilities and sleep impairment. Dev Med Child Neurol 46:771–775, 2004

Popoviciu L, Corfariu O: Efficacy and safety of midazolam in the treatment of night terrors in children. Br J Clin Pharmacol 16(suppl):97S–102S, 1983

Posey DJ, Guenin KD, Kohn AE, et al: A naturalistic open-label study of mirtazapine in autistic and other pervasive developmental disorders. J Child Adolesc Psychopharmacol 11:267–277, 2001

Powers PS, Santana C: Available pharmacological treatments for anorexia nervosa. Expert Opin Pharmacother 5:2287–2292, 2004

Practice guidelines for the treatment of patients with delirium. American Psychiatric Association. Am J Psychiatry 156 (5, suppl):1–21, 1999

Preskorn SH: Outpatient Management of Depression: A Guide for the Practitioner, 2nd Edition. Caddo, OK, Professional Communications, 1999

Pruett JR, Rizvi ST: A 16-year-old girl with excited catatonia treated with low-dose lorazepam. J Child Adolesc Psychopharmacol 15:1005–1010, 2005

Prugh D, Wagonfeld S, Metcalf D, et al: A clinical study of delirium in children and adolescents. Psychosom Med 42:177–195, 1980

Putnam GP, O'Quinn S, Bolden-Watson CP, et al: Migraine polypharmacy and the tolerability of sumatriptan: a large scale, prospective study. Cephalalgia 19:668–675, 1999

Ratcliff SL, Meyer WJ, Cuervo LJ, et al: The use of haloperidol and associated complications in the agitated, acutely ill pediatric burn patient. J Burn Care Rehabil 24:472–478, 2004

Rubey RN, Lydiard RB: Pharmacological treatment of anxiety in the medically ill patient. Semin Clin Neuropsychiatry 4:133–147, 1999

Rutter M, Tizard J, Whitmore K: Education, Health, and Behavior. London, Longman Group, 1970

Ryan EP: Psychiatric emergencies in the pediatric setting, in Handbook of Pediatric Psychology and Psychiatry, Vol I. Edited by Ammerman RT, Campo JV. Boston, MA, Allyn & Bacon, 1998, pp 91–124

Scharko AM, Baker EH, Kothari P, et al: Case study: delirium in a girl with human immunodeficiency virus-associated dementia. J Am Acad Child Adolesc Psychiatry 45:104–108, 2006

Schieveld JNM, Leentjens AFG: Delirium in severely ill young children in the pediatric intensive care unit (PICU). J Am Acad Child Adolesc Psychiatry 44:392–394, 2005

Schnoes CJ, Kuhn BR, Workman EF, et al: Pediatric prescribing practices for clonidine and other pharmacologic agents for children with sleep disturbance. Clin Pediatr 45:229–238, 2006

Schwam JS, Klass E, Alonso C, et al: Risperidone and refusal to eat. J Am Acad Child Adolesc Psychiatry 37:572–573, 1998

Settle EC: Antidepressant drugs: disturbing and potentially dangerous adverse effects. J Clin Psychiatry 59(suppl):25–30, 1998

Sharma ND, Rosman HS, Padhi D, et al: Torsades de pointes associated with intravenous haloperidol in critically ill patients. Am J Cardiol 81:238–240, 1998

Shatkin JP: Atomoxetine for the treatment of pediatric nocturnal enuresis. J Child Adolesc Psychopharmacol 14:443–447, 2004

Sheldon SH: Pro-convulsant effects of oral melatonin in neurologically disabled children. Lancet 351:1254, 1998

Simon GE, Katon W, Rutter C, et al: The impact of improved depression treatment in primary care on daily functioning and disability. Psychol Med 28:693–701, 1998

Siow H, Young W, Silberstein S: Neuroleptics in headache. Headache 45:358–371, 2005

Sipahimalani A, Masand PS: Use of risperidone in delirium: case reports. Ann Clin Psychiatry 9:105–107, 1997

Smits MG, van Stel HF, van der Heijden K, et al: Melatonin improves health status and sleep in children with idiopathic chronic sleep-onset insomnia: a randomized placebo-controlled trial. J Am Acad Child Adolesc Psychiatry 42:1286–1293, 2003

Smoller JW, Simon NM, Pollack M, et al: Anxiety in patients with pulmonary disease: comorbidity and treatment. Semin Clin Neuropsychiatry 4:84–97, 1999

Soler J, Pascual JC, Campins J, et al: Double-blind, placebo-controlled study of dialectical behavior therapy plus olanzapine for borderline personality disorder. Am J Psychiatry 162:1221–1224, 2005

Sondheimer A: Clomipramine treatment of delusional disorder, somatic type. J Am Acad Child Adolesc Psychiatry 27:188–192, 1988

Sorrentino A: Chemical restraints for the agitated, violent, or psychotic pediatric patient in the emergency department: controversies and recommendations. Curr Opin Pediatr 16:201–205, 2004

Stahl S: Antidepressants and somatic symptoms: therapeutic actions are expanding beyond affective spectrum disorders to functional somatic syndromes. J Clin Psychiatry 64:745–746, 2003

Staller JA: Intramuscular ziprasidone in youth: a retrospective chart review. J Child Adolesc Psychopharmacol 14:590–592, 2004

Stores G: Medication for sleep-wake disorders. Arch Dis Child 88:899–903, 2003

Thiele EA, Gonzalez-Heydrich J, Riviello JJ: Epilepsy in children and adolescents. Child Adolesc Psychiatr Clin N Am 8:671–694, 1999

Tomkins G, Jackson J, O'Malley P, et al: Treatment of chronic headache with antidepressants: a meta-analysis. Am J Med 111:54–63, 2001

Trzepacz PT: Delirium: advances in diagnosis, pathophysiology, and treatment. Psychiatr Clin North Am 19:429–448, 1996

Tune L, Carr S, Hoag E, et al: Anticholinergic effects of drugs commonly prescribed for the elderly: potential means for assessing risk of delirium. Am J Psychiatry 149:1393–1394, 1992

Turk J: Melatonin supplementation for severe and intractable sleep disturbance in young people with genetically determined developmental disabilities: short review and commentary. J Med Genet 40:793–796, 2003

Turkel SB, Tavare CJ: Delirium in children and adolescents. J Neuropsychiatry Clin Neurosci 15:431–435, 2003

Villeneuve E, Lemelin S: Open-label study of atypical neuroleptic quetiapine for treatment of borderline personality disorder: impulsivity as main target. J Clin Psychiatry 66:1298–1303, 2005

Wirshing DA, Spellberg BJ, Erhart SM, et al: Novel antipsychotics and new onset diabetes. Biol Psychiatry 44:778–783, 1998

Witek MW, Rojas V, Alonso C, et al: Review of benzodiazepine use in children and adolescents. Psychiatr Q 76:283–296, 2005

Yager J, Andersen AE: Anorexia nervosa. N Engl J Med 353:1481–1488, 2005

Yildiz A, Sachs GS, Turgay A: Pharmacologic management of agitation in emergency settings. Emerg Med J 20:339–346, 2003

Younus M, Labellarte MJ: Insomnia in children: when are hypnotics indicated? Paediatr Drugs 4:391–403, 2002

Index

*Page numbers printed in **boldface** type refer to tables or figures.*

Dexmethylphenidate *(continued)*
  for attention-deficit/hyperactivity
    disorder, 40, 59–60
  dosage of, **42**, 59
  efficacy of, **49**, **53**, 59–60
  pharmacokinetics of, 59
  plasma levels of, 59
Dextroamphetamine, 20, 61–62, 82
  adverse effects of, growth slowdown,
    65
  for attention-deficit/hyperactivity
    disorder, 40, 61–62, 67
    efficacy of, 45, **46**, **47**, **50**, 67
  for disruptive behavior disorders
    and aggression, **109**, **115**, 120
  dosage of, **43**, **109**
Dextrostat. *See* Dextroamphetamine
Diabetes mellitus, 406, 412
  atypical antipsychotic–induced,
    113, **116**, 126, 247, **249**,
    357–358, 412
  beta-adrenergic antagonist–induced
    hypoglycemia in, **117**, 125, 127
  psychopharmacotherapy in, 412
Diabetic ketoacidosis, 358
*Diagnostic and Statistical Manual of
  Mental Disorders* (DSM-IV-TR),
  99
  anxiety disorders in, 144
  attention-deficit/hyperactivity
    disorder in, 37, **38–39**
  conduct disorder in, **103–104**
  disruptive behavior disorder not
    otherwise specified in, **105**
  oppositional defiant disorder in,
    102
  pervasive developmental disorders
    in, 266
  somatoform disorders in, 378

Diagnostic Interview Schedule for
  Children, 170
Diarrhea, drug-induced
  atypical antipsychotics, **116**
  divalproex, 241, **242**
  lithium, 233, 282
  selective serotonin reuptake
    inhibitors, 158
  in serotonin syndrome, 382
Diazepam, 402
Diet–drug interactions
  with amphetamines, 62
  cytochrome P450–related, 6
  with lithium, 235
  with monoamine oxidase inhibitors,
    200
Diphenhydramine, for sleep
  disturbances, 388
Disinhibition, drug-induced
  benzodiazepines, **149**, 170, 183,
    402
  buspirone, 181
Disruptive behavior disorders (DBDs),
  99–134
  aggression in, 99–100, 105 (*See also*
    Aggression)
  antisocial personality disorder and,
    104–105
  conduct disorder, 101–102,
    103–104
  course and outcome of, 104–105
  differential diagnosis of, 102–104
  epidemiology of, 101–102
  family interventions for, 133
  nonmedication interventions for,
    130–131, 134
  not otherwise specified, 99, 102, **105**
  oppositional defiant disorder, 101,
    102

Vitamin E, for extrapyramidal
symptoms, 352
VNS (vagal nerve stimulation), for
depression, 213
Volume of distribution of drug, 2, **3**
Vyvanse. *See* Amphetamines

Warfarin, drug interactions with
antidepressants, 206
methylphenidate, 57
Weakness, lithium-induced, 282
Weight changes
in anorexia nervosa, 384
drug-induced
antipsychotics, 17, 113, 114,
116, 126, 245, 287, 309,
356–357, 400, 405
aripiprazole, 246, **247**, 273,
287
clozapine, 251, 309, 356, 357
olanzapine, 247, 248, 249,
249, 272, 287, 309,
356–357
quetiapine, 251, **251**, 287,
309, 357
risperidone, **253**, 271, 272,
287, 309, 313, 356–357
ziprasidone, 287, 309, 357
atomoxetine, 322
carbamazepine, 238
clomipramine, 274
lithium, 234
mirtazapine, 203
mood stabilizers, **117**, 123,
127
selective serotonin reuptake
inhibitors, **148**, 159,
318
stimulants, 57, 64–65, **116**

valproic acid, 240, 241, 282
venlafaxine, **149**, 165
Withdrawal from drug, 6

Yale-Brown Obsessive Compulsive Scale
(Y-BOCS), 161, 179, 276, 316
Yale Global Tic Severity Scale
(YGTSS), 306, 310, 311

Zaleplon, for sleep disturbances, 389
Ziprasidone, 244
adverse effects of, 253–254, 255,
255, 273, 309, 356, 357, 401
for agitation and delirium, 399–401
approved indications and off-label
use of, **23**
for bipolar disorder, 253–255
studies supporting use in youths,
254
for disruptive behavior disorders
and aggression, **109**, 112, **115**
dosage of, **109**, 400
formulations of, 254, 400
injectable, 400–401
for maladaptive behaviors in
pervasive developmental
disorders, 273
mechanism of action of, 273
for nausea/vomiting, 384
patient evaluation before initiation
of, 254
for schizophrenia, 345
for tics, 307–308, **308**, 313
Zoloft. *See* Sertraline
Zolpidem, for sleep disturbances, 389
Zonisamide, for bipolar disorder, 235, 243
Zopiclone, for sleep disturbances, 389
Zydis. *See* Olanzapine
Zyprexa. *See* Olanzapine